THE
GENESIS OF
NEUROSCIENCE
BY
A. EARL WALKER, MD

Edward R. Laws, Jr., MD, and
George B. Udvarhelyi, MD,
Editors

Cover: A manuscript leaf from the translation by James Breasted of the *Edwin Smith Papyrus. Published in Facsimile and Hieroglyphic Transliteration with Translation and Commentary.* Chicago, Ill: University of Chicago Press, 1930

Library of Congress Catalog
ISBN: 1-879284-62-6

Printed in U.S.A.

The American Association of Neurological Surgeons
22 South Washington Street
Park Ridge, Illinois 60068-4287

Warren R. Selman, MD, Chairman
AANS Publications Committee

Gay L. Palazzo, AANS Staff Editor

AANS3.5M398

CONTENTS

However, the distinction between the anatomy and physiology of any system or organ is a recent and artificial one, and they cannot be separated in the writings of the earlier authors.

Clarke and O'Malley, p 756

AANS Publications Committee

Warren R. Selman, MD, Chairman

Michael L.J. Apuzzo, MD

Julian E. Bailes, Jr., MD

Daniel L. Barrow, MD

Joshua B. Bederson, MD

Edward C. Benzel, MD

T. Forcht Dagi, MD

John G. Golfinos, MD

Howard H. Kaufman, MD

Christopher M. Loftus, MD

Robert J. Maciunas, MD

Ian McCutcheon, MD

Setti S. Rengachary, MD

Acknowledgments

It should become readily apparent to anyone reading this book that its production has been a true labor of love. We would like to take this opportunity to thank the many people involved in having this project come to fruition.

First of all, Agnes Marshall Walker, Dr. Walker's widow, worked hand in hand with him in the development of the manuscript, many portions of which she typed herself. She is responsible for the original idea of having the book published and for providing the manuscript, the illustrations, and the material that appears in the appendix and many of the references. She has fostered the development of virtually every phase of this project and all of us should be grateful that this work has resulted in a fitting tribute to an outstanding neuroscientist.

The publication of the book has been facilitated by the American Association of Neurological Surgeons (AANS). The AANS Publications Committee, chaired first by Dr. Dan Barrow and then by Dr. Warren Selman, approved the concept of developing and publishing the book, and once again the project could not have been completed without the support of the organization and the many skilled people who work in the area of publications and publications development. In Baltimore, Dr. George Udvarhelyi worked on the manuscript and on the references and was assisted by the professionals at the Welch Memorial Library at the Johns Hopkins University School of Medicine. In Charlottesville, Dr. Laws was assisted by Margaret Laws, who did the initial copyediting, by Pamela Leake, who prepared many of the original parts of the manuscript and the bibliography, and by the National Library of Medicine and its personnel who helped with some of the illustrations. The AANS Publications Office in New Hampshire created the final product and we are grateful to Ms. Gay Palazzo and the staff in the New Hampshire office for their efforts and their skill. Everyone who has been involved in the creation of this book feels a sense of pride, and we hope that the book will be as enjoyable for its readers as it was for those of us who played a role in having it published.

Edward R. Laws, Jr., MD, FACS
Professor of Neurosurgery
Professor of Medicine
University of Virginia
Charlottesville, Virginia

George B. Udvarhelyi, MD, FACS
Professor Emeritus of Neurosurgery
The Johns Hopkins University
School of Medicine
Baltimore, Maryland

Foreword

Over the last ten years of my late husband's life, Dr. A. Earl Walker was invited to give a series of lectures on the retrospective history of neurology and neurosurgery to the University of New Mexico medical students. These presentations were very popular and well received with an ever-increasing audience. Even the staff physicians were attending with keen interest and enthusiasm. With numerous requests for copies of his notes, Dr. Walker realized that he had the makings of a manuscript or publication. With this in mind, our travels around the world soon included various medical libraries. Not a few of these had medical books and journals so antiquated and hidden on the shelves far below the library basement level that it was often hard to discern them from other foreign objects. Books had to be handled with extreme care as they were so fragile and brittle. Some of the parchment books were in better condition, although stiff and difficult to open. One needed a solid background in old English and foreign languages to translate many of these. The usage of medical terms, instruments, and pharmacopeia, for instance, not infrequently was puzzling as the probe continued through the dust-laden publications. The spelling of ancient words or names of authors and scientists often changed with the language spoken at the time. Mistakes were made and, in some cases, continue to this day! Even the published dates of these early manuscripts were totally at the discretion of the translator or interpreter. It could be very frustrating, yet every effort was made to search all these priceless antiquities to reveal their rightful claims.

To me this was a very special experience, like no other in our years together. As I typed and re-typed edited copies of my husband's work, I would sneeze and fondly recall our time exploring the "bowels" of neuroscience history.

Agnes Marshall Walker
Albuquerque, New Mexico

Introduction

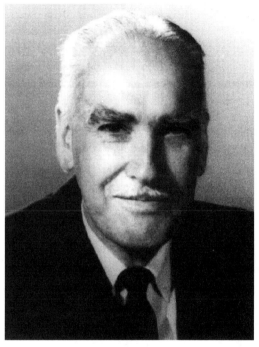

A. Earl Walker, MD
(1907-1995)
Professor of Neurosurgery, The Johns Hopkins
University School of Medicine, 1947-1972

A. Earl Walker was one of the giants of an era of modern neuroscience that bridged developments in clinical and basic aspects of disease of the nervous system. It is appropriate in this introduction to reflect upon Dr. Walker's life and his contributions. He came to this country from Canada for further training in neurosurgery, mostly at the University of Chicago, although he spent time with a Rockefeller Fellowship at Yale University, in Amsterdam and Brussels. He returned to join the faculty of the University of Chicago and rose to full professorship in the early 1940s. At the time that Dr. Walker began his training in neurosurgery, neuroscience was just coming of age as a discipline. From the beginning of his career, Earl Walker recognized the importance of integrated and collaborative research within the neurosciences. He had the good fortune to begin work in a scientific era when the specialties of neuropathology, electroencephalography, and clinical neurophysiology emerged as independent disciplines. Under the guidance of such outstanding individuals as Percival Bailey, Roy Grinker, and Stephen Polyak, he assimilated exciting discoveries in new fields of knowledge and became one of the young leaders in the generation of neurosurgeons who applied experimental findings of the neurological sciences to clinical neurosurgery. *The Primate Thalamus*, a monograph published in 1938, is considered one of the seminal contributions related to this structure of the brain. Dr. Walker applied the scientifically controlled findings of his laboratory work to clinical neurosurgery, contributing to our understanding of the organization of the spinothalamic tract and of the role of mesencephalic tractotomy and pedunculotomy in controlling painful conditions and movement disorders; he also described in scholarly fashion clinical entities including congenital dermal sinuses, congenital aplasia of the foramen of Magendie, cerebellar hemangiomas, tumors of the temporal bone, tentorial herniation, and the physiology of concussion. His monograph on *Penicillin in Neurology* in 1946 was the first comprehensive study of the effects of the drug on the central nervous system, and served as the basis for experimental models of epilepsy in animals. His attention subsequently turned to the study of post-traumatic epilepsy, conducting long-term studies on patients with this particular condition. He described the natural history of head injury and post-traumatic epilepsy extending over 40 years. He became interested in cerebral metabolism associated with head injury, described the common association of cervical spine fracture with head injury, and documented measures necessary to determine brain death.

Dr. Walker was appointed Professor of Neurosurgery at the Medical School of the Johns Hopkins University and Chief of Neurosurgery at the Johns Hopkins Hospital, following Dr. Walter Dandy's death in 1947. During his tenure he established an outstanding resident training program in neurosurgery with strong emphasis on research and medical scholarship. He established a laboratory for the study of experimental epilepsy, and contributed many important publications related to the fascinating study of neural connections of the brain. He also established a neurometric laboratory studying modern techniques such as the cerebral scintiscan, electromyography, clinical neurophysiology, the use of diagnostic ultrasound, and the possibilities of telethermalcoagulation with induction-heat in stereotactic surgery. He maintained an active neurosurgical pathological laboratory which was expanded in the early 1960s to include electron microscopy, histochemistry, and enzyme chemistry of the central nervous system. He has to his credit the original observations related to the hypophysectomy for cancer and hemispherectomies. The *Stereotaxy of the Human Brain* edited by Dr. G. Schaltenbrand and Dr. Walker represents one of the most scholarly approaches to this special area of neurosurgery.

Dr. Walker left Hopkins in 1972 and accepted a Visiting Professorship at the University of New Mexico in Albuquerque. It was during the last 20 years of his life that he returned to his original love, namely the history of neurosciences. This contribution is the result of a painstaking disciplined life of a man who did not submerge himself in the trivial pleasures of retirement, but concentrated on further elucidations of the evolution of neurosciences. Another reason prompting the publication of this book is that, in our opinion, it represents a rapidly disappearing scholarly effort, namely a work written by one individual. There is no confusing and uneven perspective related to the opinions of multiple contributors; there is instead, the continuity of a steady flow of ideas as seen through the eyes of a man of great knowledge and integrity; *The Genesis of Neuroscience* has been studied and put into a narrative form after careful evaluation of the historical literature. Dr. Walker amassed hundreds of references, of which all were read by him; summaries have been recorded on small index cards. We know that during the years that this work was in production, he spent innumerable hours in libraries working on old books and manuscripts, using parts of his vacation time to spend long hours in the library of the British Museum, of the Royal College of Surgeons, hospital libraries in Paris, and many other places. During a slow process of careful digestion of all of the amassed data and publications of the past, he traced the development of ideas which were finally applied to clinical neuroscience. We know that the impact of a book written by a single individual, representing his experience, mistakes, and some inevitable biases, has a special impact on its readers. There are several examples of such books. Mr. Northfield's *Neurosurgery* represents his lifetime experience at the London Hospital; at Johns Hopkins, the book of Dr. Frank Ford, *Neurology of Infancy and Childhood*, is one man's experience and was once the "bible" of pediatric neurology; Dr. Frank Walsh's monumental contribution to neuro-ophthalmology was typed by Dr. Walsh himself and was a testimony to individual productivity, representing his rich clinical experience, his insight, and his diagnostic and therapeutic conclusions. Under the magnifying glass of our modern times, these efforts may have included occasional errors, but the impact of the unique experience of these pioneers and the individual flavor of their contributions makes them landmarks in the medical literature.

We feel that we should give some justification for the publication of this posthumous work of Dr. A. Earl Walker. In our present time, scientific publications are mushrooming in all corners of the civilized world and are filling cyberspace. The discipline of neurosurgery is no exception, even though it represents a relatively small component of the vast empire of neurosciences. The last two decades have been characterized by innumerable textbooks consisting of large volumes with as many as 100 contributors whose opinions and experiences are rarely well coordinated. We feel that Dr. Walker's posthumous contribution is an exception.

There are several reasons we believed that this book should be published and be made available to the future generations of neuroscientists. The first justification of our efforts is to pay tribute to Dr. Walker, with whom we had the privilege to work and whom we admired as a role model for his vision, integrity, and dedication to a scholarly professional life. He produced more than 400 scientific publications and was known in every corner of the world for his dedication to improving the quality of our discipline. In 1952, he and his collaborators published *A History of Neurological Surgery*, one of the original contributions to the history of our discipline. During the next 45 years, we witnessed an extraordinary expansion of technical innovations and new discoveries in basic neurosciences which permitted the exploration of every corner of the human brain with ever increasing safety. Dr. Walker always emphasized the importance of the historical perspective; new generations were able to explore unknown territories only by standing on the shoulders of the great giants of the past. Dr. Walker decided to spend the last few years of his life exploring the contributions of individuals whose powers of observation, insight, and persistence created the foundation of the neurosciences.

The final reason for the publication of this book, especially under the aegis of the American Association of Neurological Surgeons, is to provide the young neuroscientist with a different approach and philosophy. It is hoped that the entrance into the digital age with all its promises and pitfalls will not eliminate the stimulating, fascinating account of past contributions put into the right perspective. It may help to balance the pervasive aspects of technology, in emphasizing the proper assessment of intellectual evolution of our discipline.

Dr. Walker died suddenly. The manuscript he left behind needed some reorganization and editing. In addition, the references had to be rearranged in proper order. We have also added a number of illustrations which Dr. Walker's file did not contain. We are sure that he planned to write a short epilogue, but we do not think that he wanted to speculate about the future. He always preferred to present the facts, hoping that they would speak for themselves. We sincerely hope that this scholarly work will help young clinical and basic neuroscientists to respect the power of observation and the conceptual thinking of contributors from the past. They may enjoy the product of one man's personal experience, intellectual honesty, and dedicated scholarship.

We have greatly enjoyed our involvement with this posthumous work of Dr. Walker. We hope that it will contribute to the legacy of his professional excellence contained in his many publications and of his organizational talent remembered in many parts of Asia, South America, Europe, and Africa. The impact of his integrity and intellectual honesty will remain with all who had the privilege to work with him.

George B. Udvarhelyi, MD, FACS
Edward R. Laws, Jr., MD, FACS
January 1998

1

Origins of Neuroscience

Because the newer methods of treatment are good, it does not follow that the old ones were bad; for if our honorable and worshipful ancestors had not recovered from their ailments, you and I would not be here today.

—Confucius

The Beginning of Neurological History

Information regarding the health practices of an ancient people who left no written records of their activities must be sought in their paintings, sculptures, artifacts, and paleopathology. Consequently, the medical historian's interpretation of these mute evidences of disease is open to error, both of observation and interpretation. Graphic evidence of ancient disease may well be biased by the beliefs of the populace. These graphic arts were often preserved in caves; although they gave some indication of the lifestyle of the people, they rarely depicted their diseases. As a result, any evidence of disease in the bones of these people requires critical analysis and interpretation. Moreover, the disorders of people smaller in stature and more susceptible to endemic and epidemic diseases may have been more deadly than the same ailments at the present time. Certainly, the bones of the workers of primitive times suggest that they died at an early age from infections, trauma, or warfare. The bones of the sturdier upper classes interred in ornate graves are indicative of a longer life.

When graphic methods of communication were developed, ancient medical practices were recorded on bark or wood by a tribal chief, medicine man, priest, or their scribes. The notations, probably consulted and modified from time to time, soon became so dog-eared or marked up that new and annotated copies had to be written. After some years, the text, handed down from father to son or master to pupil, might have little resemblance to the original version. Yet, the recorded successful medical therapy for certain diseases became accepted as tribal practice. The remedies would relate to the agent suspected as responsible for the illness; if a malicious sprite, it would be appeased or driven away by incantations, terrifying masks, nauseating herbals, or foul-smelling or ill-tasting substances. That these measures were often successful was more likely due to the benign nature of the disorder in a young person than to any specific effect of the therapy. Nevertheless, a favorable result would be attributed to the prescriptions of the medicine man.

Because primitive people often ascribed illness to evil spirits, the tribal priest administered to the sick. Moreover, as the common people believed that disease was divine punishment for some transgression, it was logical to appease the gods with supplications and gifts for the priests. Thus, the roots of medicine became firmly entangled in the religious practices of the populace. In Biblical times, it was the priest who made the medical diagnoses. "And the priest shall look on the plague in the skin . . . and when the hair . . . is turned white . . . it is the plague of leprosy, and the priest shall look on him and pronounce him unclean."

As the tribe organized, its various functions became more specialized and a certain member, by birth or appointment, assumed the role of medicine-man, shaman, sorcerer, exorcist, witch-doctor, or whatever name was applied to the healer. Thus, priestly activities became separated from medical practices. The shaman, looked upon as a high officer, was consulted before any tribal decision was made. As the result of wise counseling, the medicine-man occasionally acquired a great reputation and attracted a large following. He might be venerated long after his lifetime and to a degree unwarranted by his achievements. Temples erected in his name attracted the sick from afar, who, if relieved, would leave a plaque bearing his or her symptoms, the cure, and extolling the virtues of the treatment. By such written testimony, the therapy would be passed to others.

In addition to the mediations of the priests and medicine men, especially if their therapies were failing, a more dramatic means of eradicating evil spirits developed. This stemmed from the observation that a wounded body bled, presumably letting out the sprites, noble or malicious, of the injured individual. In the case of an ailing person, the blood was considered to contain sprites responsible for the illness. Their elimination seems to have been the basis for bleeding, done by scarification, cupping, or venesection. The results of scarification may be seen even today in the faces of some primitive peoples—the Melanesians, Polynesians, Eskimos, and Brazilian Indians. Cupping, by cutting the skin and sucking or applying a gourd or horn, was a widespread practice. Venesection, carried out with a knife, obsidian stone, glass, or flint, was common in Africa and Indonesia, with usually a vein in an arm or leg being incised. In some form, the practice of letting blood was used by many primitive and modern people to treat a poorly understood ailment.

Prehistoric Operations on the Skull

The art of surgery, besides being practiced in homes and at times in the temple, was being developed on the battlefields. Although written records are not available, marks on the skull are evidence of the arms used in ancient warfare. Before the introduction of gunpowder, the warrior's arms consisted of clubs, slings, spears, swords, and missiles. As most battles were fought hand-to-hand, the weapons were often aimed at the head. As a result, the cranial vault was commonly fractured. It should be recognized however, that a blunt blow to the head that produced coma but did not break the bone would be construed as impounding evil spirits which might be released by opening the skull. The many per-

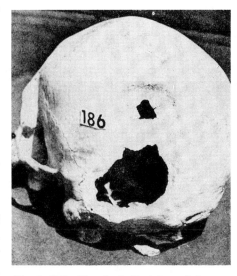

Fig. 1-1. Prehistoric skull with cranial defects and evidence of healing. (From the collection of A. Earl Walker)

forated but not fractured crania found in the crypts of Western Europe and South America probably attest to the deadly wars and the art of the wound-surgeons. Other explanations for the defects (e.g., ceremonial stigmata and prophylactic measures) are less likely.

Man-made defects in the skulls of people who lived thousands of years ago in Czechoslovakia, Denmark, England, France, Germany, Hungary, the Iberian peninsula, Italy, Poland, Russia, and Switzerland are evidence of the widespread practice. Although some skulls of these neolithic people were too fragmented to be reconstructed, others were well preserved, with thickening about the margins of the holes—undoubted evidence of the premortem origin. The first fenestrated skulls found in France in the 19th century were assumed to have resulted from combat; that they might have been purposely manmade was suggested by Prunières who, in a prehistoric burial cave near Lozère, found a skull with a large defect, the smooth margins of which suggested healing (Fig. 1-1). Other skulls with man-made holes were found soon after in various parts of Europe. The defects were most frequently in the left parietal region, occasionally in the occipital or frontal bones, but rarely in the temporal bone. The holes were commonly oval, with the long axis in the anteroposterior plane; less frequently, the defect was round or irregular in shape. Most of the perforations were singular, but in some skulls as many as five holes were present. The size of the cranial

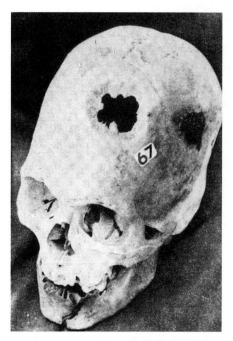

Fig. 1-2. Prehistoric skull with multiple irregular cranial defects made with crude instruments. (From the collection of A. Earl Walker)

defect varied from a few centimeters to almost half of the skull; one cranium had a hole measuring 13 × 10 cm. Not all of the defects in the prehistoric skulls were made before death; some borings may have caused the fatality, and some holes for various reasons were probably bored after the demise of the individual (Fig. 1-2).

The instruments used for perforating the skull are not known—sharp stones were available to the earliest skull-borers; metal scrapers were probably used later. Pointed stones tied to a shaft and rapidly rotated between the hands may have served as the primitive perforators or drills (Fig. 1-3). Most of the holes seem to have been made by scraping with a rough or serrated stone. With such a raspatory, the outer table of the skull could be removed to the diploic channels within a few minutes. The inner table could be similarly grated or left to slough later. Rarely, the defect was made by drilling a series of small holes in a circle and breaking the intervening bone; even less commonly, rectangular defects were made by cutting or sawing. Occasionally, the skull had an inverted "T" scraped in the sincipital region, probably representing some type of tribal mark.

How the patient was controlled during these procedures is unknown. Perhaps the victim was unconscious as a result of the head injury, drugged with wine, or choked into insensibility. Whatever the method, it must not have been extremely painful or associated with prolonged suffering, for in some neolithic sites about one fourth of the population had been subjected to the procedure.

The prehistoric perforated skulls found in the burial grounds of Europe were of a people who lived several thousand years before the Christian era. At about the same time in the New World, somewhat similar procedures were being carried out on the sandy coast of Peru, where centuries ago people of high culture had tilled the fertile soil. Although no written records of this early civilization exist, the materials found in their burial caverns on this peninsula bear evidence of their culture. In the early 20th century, Tello excavated some of the tombs in Paracas, unearthing archeological findings indicative of a highly developed race.

The fardels, or cloth coffins, of these people contained fine wool and cotton material made into luxurious clothes of many colors. Pottery, baskets, bone, and stone articles evidenced a certain degree of artistry.

Two findings of medical interest in the Paracan skulls were noted. First, almost all of the skulls were perforated and deformed. Practically 90%

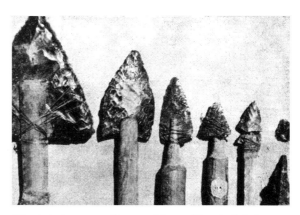

Fig. 1-3. Stone trephines used for making skull defects. (From the collection of A. Earl Walker)

of the skulls had cranial defects. The holes were probably made by scraping with a tumi (Fig. 1-4). Whether the person was anesthetized by some means or drugged is uncertain. A number of plants with anesthetizing properties have been found in Peru. The natives of that region used the flowers of Datura fecos, which contains scopolamine, to produce a numbness of the skin. The cocoa bean, "the divine plant of the Incas," was an ingredient of poultices applied to the head to deaden the scalp. It is not known whether the ancient Peruvians knew of these numbing agents. Although it has been suggested that the Peruvians induced general anesthesia with alcoholic drinks or narcotic drugs, the evidence is lacking. The technique used to perforate the skull is better known, since a number of instruments were found in the burial caverns. Later ceramic art depicts the use of an instrument termed a "tumi" that was used to perforate the calvarium.

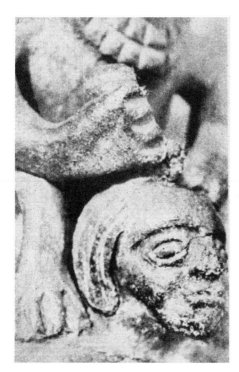

Fig. 1-4. Sculpture (pre-Colombian) showing a tumi in use performing a craniectomy. (From the collection of A. Earl Walker)

That infection was unusual might be related to the circumstances of the operation—a healthy individual, a clean surgical field, and instruments that had never been used on an infected wound. In the tombs of Paracas, antiseptic salts of mercury were found which could have been applied to the dressings. Arsenic and copper sulfate also appear to have been known, as well as a number of herbs used for ointments and cocoa-leaf tablets for chewing. Certainly, when embalming, the ancient Indians of Peru used substances rich in cinnamic acid which have antiseptic properties. Thus, the shaman had drugs to cleanse the site of operation, herbs to anesthetize the scalp, and dressings with agents having antibiotic properties to prevent putrefaction.

Within the tombs of Paracas were found a number of tools used in cranial operations. The tumi-chisel of hardened copper gouged out the calvarium in more than 90% of the skulls examined. With this instrument, in a few minutes, a hole of any size could be made in both layers of the skull. In rare instances, the defect in the skull was made by drilling a circle of perforations and breaking or cutting the intervening bone (Table 1).

Bleeding may have been controlled by a cord tied around the head just above the ears or by digital compression. Astringent vegetable products were also available; a common shrub, pumacucu, which contains tannic acid, has been used by native surgeons to stop bleeding from wounds.

TABLE 1
PARACAN PERFORATED SKULLS*
(based on a sample of Graña et al's cases)

Sex	
Male	28
Female	1
Side of Defect	
Right	6
Left	15
Right and Left	6
Other	2
Size of Defect	
Large	16
Medium	8
Small	4
Uncertain	1
Survival	
Yes	14
No	11
Uncertain	4

* Includes six thought to be postmortem defects.

6

Needles made from bone were found in Paracas, as well as one specimen with cotton sutures in place. In another person, who apparently died soon after an operation, the scalp margins were approximated by tying together groups of hairs from opposing sides of the wound. The incision was covered with rolls of cotton cloth. In the cranial defect, a gold or silver plate was sometimes found.

The type of cranial defect varied . In a series reported by Graña et al in 1954, studying the trepanation of skulls in Peru, 194 openings in the skull were circular, 26 were oval, 40 triangular, three quadrangular, six rectangular, four polygonal, and 20 irregular in shape. The cranial defect was commonly located in the central or parietal region, although some were present in other parts of the convexity (Fig. 1-5). In the series of Graña et al, the left side

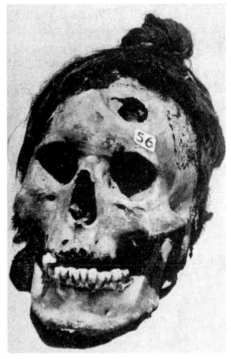

Fig. 1-5. Paracan skull with cranial defect made with a tumi chisel. (From the collection of A. Earl Walker)

was perforated in 161 instances, the right in 71, and both sides in 83. Multiple defects were common, some apparently being made simultaneously and some seriatim as many as five times. In about a quarter of the cases, the outer table of the skull only was removed, with the inner table remaining intact. It is noteworthy that males predominated over females 4:1. The mortality rate from this surgical procedure in Paracas was not excessive, probably less than 10% to 15%; precise figures based on evidence of bony regeneration are not available because the authors include in their series skulls from other regions operated upon hundreds of years later.

The second finding of medical note in the Paracan skulls is the extremely high incidence (90%) of artificial cranial deformation (Fig. 1-6). The molding was either a frontal or occipital flattening, both of which tended to elongate the skull. The mechanics of the deformation are known from the finding in the caverns of Paracas of a number of babies' skulls still in the deforming appliance. It would seem that occipital or occipital-and-frontal splints were applied to the head in early infancy until the desired cephalic contour had been obtained. The relationship of artificial cranial deformation to trepanation is conjectural.

The Rationale of Cranial Perforation

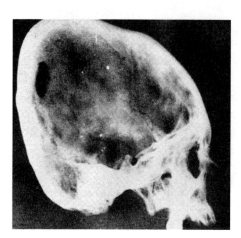

Fig. 1-6. Radiograph showing artificial deformation of the skull, a custom also practiced in Paracas. (From the collection of A. Earl Walker)

The skull has fascinated people for ages. In dwellings at Jericho in Palestine, intact or fragmented skulls of people of the 7th century BC have been found. These trophies of "skull cults" may have been used to ward off evil, to prevent injury and disease, for ancestor worship, as family heirlooms, religious tenets, martial trophies, or even as relics of cannibalism. Whatever the reason, the custom persisted well into the Christian era, as evidenced by the ossariums of central Europe.

As the ritualistic storage of skulls became an established custom, another form of cranial fetish developed, namely, the substitution of parts of the skull for the whole as objects of veneration. Thus, "skull caps" or amulets of various sizes and shapes were thought to bestow the powers of the original owners upon their new possessors. These relics were probably excised shortly after the demise of the individual and were worn as a souvenir or for decoration. Obviously, after such excisions, the cut margins of the hole in the calvarium show no evidence of healing.

Skull defects have been produced by rodents who gnawed away the margins of cranial foramina, particularly the foramen magnum, sufficiently to enter and use the intracranial cavity as a nest. In such circumstances, teeth marks along the margins of the defect may identify the intruder.

Prehistoric people, being warlike and engaging in hand-to-hand combat, must have seen the scalp torn or avulsed and pieces of bone knocked out of or loosened from the skull. Probably most of these victims died on the battlefield, but some, even with a hole in the head, survived, for such perforated skulls with thickened margins about a defect have been found in the burial grounds in many parts of the world. Radiating fracture lines attest to their traumatic origin. Some perforated crania, however, had no evidence of trauma.

At first, the discovery of such prehistoric cracked or defective skulls attracted little attention, as they were thought to be the result of combat. Prunières in 1874 attested to the man-made nature of the holes in the skulls found in France. Broca was less certain of their origin except for the obviously traumatized skull with fracture lines. Interest was revived in South America and Europe, as more prehistoric skulls were found and led to a re-examination of the problem. Zaragosa Rubiria and Vara Lopez concluded that, in Spain, primitive man operated upon traumatized heads, since many of the cranial defects were at the site of fractures. Whether the operation was done to hasten healing by removing necrotic or infected tissue, relieve pain, or let out devils was unknown. In the case of perforations in an otherwise intact skull, they suggested that the defect was made for medical reasons, such as the relief from cranial tumor, infection, headache, epilepsy, or insanity. Other causes— empiric, magic, therapeutic, and religious—may have occasioned the skull boring. Zaragosa Rubiria and Vara Lopez both noted that in cases in which the perforated skull showed no evidence of healing, the operation might have been fatal or the trephination may have been done postmortem to obtain amulets or, for more fanciful reasons, to get a piece of brain or bone for its curative or protective properties.

A number of other cranial or cerebral disorders may produce a hole in the skull. Diseased states, such as infection, neoplasm, and congenital anomalies, may cause cranial defects, the nature of which may be difficult to identify in ancient skulls. Although infectious complications such as osteomyelitis have been suspect, Graña et al reported that Soto made radiological studies of the skulls which showed the pockmarked appearance of osteomyelitis in a few cases and concluded that infection was not a serious or frequent problem.

In primitive tribes, scalp and cranial mutilations were often performed as a social, tribal, or religious rite. Perhaps the most common of these was the sincipital "T" which was carved in the midline occipital region even in modern times. It has been considered a religious ritual or a mark of the individual's rank in the tribe.

In their detailed and well-illustrated 1954 monograph on prehispanic trephining, Graña et al gave the results of a study of 250 perforated skulls from more than 2,000 skulls available in Peru. They concluded that some, if not all, of the trephinations were made for medical therapeusis. Of 250 skulls, 25.6% had cranial trauma as evidenced by fracture lines or depressed bone and 18.2% had evidence of a brain tumor manifested by thinning of the cranial vault, ballooning of the posterior fossa, and decalcification and destruction of the sella turcica. In 1926, Moodie had reported fewer cases, but he used more rigid criteria. Graña et al stated that cranial osteomyelitis was evident in 6.8% and that 20% of the skulls were deformed. They stated that eight crania had been used for surgical practice after death, but the evidence might equally be interpreted as indicating operative mortalities. Based on the finding of impacted teeth, they deduced that the craniotomy was performed in such cases for the relief of toothache. Because in approximately one half of the skulls there was no obvious cause for the defect, Graña et al argued forcefully that these individuals must have had serious disturbances such as headache, vomiting, dizziness, unsteady gait, convulsions, and other neurological complaints; otherwise, if conscious, they would not have consented to having a hole bored in their head. Yet, at a time when clubs, stones, and balls of metal were weapons of warfare, it was probable that many blows to the head produced a loss of consciousness with severe brain damage with or without fracturing the skull. Based upon current experience with such injuries, not more than half of traumatized and comatose victims would have sustained skull fractures. Accordingly, it is possible that trephination at the site of scalp contusion or laceration was performed for the relief of closed head injuries. However, Graña et al believed that if the head was perforated to release devils, the defect would have been made in the same place in all cases. As it was not, they concluded that the operators were not intent upon releasing evil spirits but rather were seeking a hematoma, sequestrum, abscess, or tumor in various parts of the head.

Unless the result in the majority of cases was successful and, at times, spectacular, Graña et al argued that the procedure would have been abandoned. But they point out that trepanation was practiced by a cultured population for 3000 years. One might surmise that skull boring in the New World was as therapeutic as blood letting in the Old World!

However, further analysis of the data presented by Graña et al discloses some interesting observations. First, with a sex ratio so predominately male and only one-fourth of the cases (mainly males) having head injuries, one wonders why there were not more females in the remaining three-quarters who presumably died of somatic or neurological causes. The marked predominance of defects in the left central region, if made to relieve localized cerebral disease (which at the present time is not more common in the left hemisphere) is difficult to explain unless it simply indicates that most of the operators were right-handed. Certainly, the fact that seven of nine individuals thought to have brain tumors lived long enough after a craniotomy to have bone proliferate around the margins of the cranial defect is a tribute to the skill of the surgeons. That nine of 29 persons in a cemetery had brain tumors is difficult to explain unless the burial grounds served as a center for neurological disease. Some other explanation, perhaps that the cemetery was used by a cult that venerated artificial cranial defects, may explain the skull changes which Graña et al interpreted as indicating a brain tumor.

Obviously, as Sigerist pointed out, the situation with regard to skull boring in prehistoric and primitive races is complex. Certainly the operators were quite skillful, whether they were performing a tribal or religious rite or were attempting to relieve a pathological state within the head.

Early Asiatic and Mediterranean Medical Practices

Assyrian and Babylonian Medicine

The earliest information regarding the nervous system comes from the practices of the ancient civilizations along the Euphrates and Tigris rivers. The Assyrians who codified medical care were aware of the effects of a blow to the head and the fatal nature of injury to the upper cervical spine. Moreover, they compressed the neck, thereby occluding the carotid arteries, to produce unconsciousness while performing circumcision.

Although it is said that the ancient Babylonian practitioner usually confined attention to just one disorder, there is no evidence that brain afflictions received special treatment. Heroditus wrote that in early Babylonian and Egyptian times, the sick were exposed in the marketplace so that passersby might tell of cures which they had attained for that affliction. Later, the priests recorded these testimonials in a "sacred book" which eventually became the accepted medical code. Perhaps these texts formed the basis of Greek medical practice and were eventually incorporated into the Hippocratic writings. In addition to Babylonian temple clinics, physicians, trained in state schools and licensed by examination, gave medical advice and performed surgery and midwifery in their homes or offices because the letting of blood in the temple was taboo. The therapy for cranial and spinal injuries, which must have been common, was not recorded, perhaps because the outlook was so bleak.

Persian Medicine

In ancient Persia, priests cared for both the spiritual and somatic ills of the people. By the late 5th century BC, Persian physicians had access to Greek medicine, for Darius had conquered many Grecian islands. In the social and political organization, the practice of medicine was regulated. The apprentice physician was required to gain experience by treating infidels and foreigners. If their care was judged to be satisfactory, after a year or two, the physician was considered qualified to treat the citizens of Persia. If the candidate failed to cure the worthless people, he was denied a license and had to seek some other means of gaining a livelihood.

It is of interest that Heroditus observed on the battlefield that the skulls of the Persians, who wore a skull cap to protect their heads from the sun, were so thin that a pebble would pierce them, whereas the skulls of their Egyptian enemies whose heads were shaven from childhood were too tough to break even with a rock. He concluded that exposure to the sun was responsible for the hard Egyptian skulls.

Little is known of Persian medicine in the next centuries, until the fall of the Roman Empire. After that time, the medical practices of Greece and

Rome were kept alive in the deserts of Asia Minor. Because of his presumed heretic concepts, Nestorius, the Patriarch of Constantinople (the eastern capital of the Roman Empire), was forced to flee to Edessa. With Greek manuscripts, Nestorius established a school that flourished until closed in 489 AD. Most of Nestorius' followers settled in Gunde-Shapur, a small city in Asia Minor under the control of Persia. With the approval in 530 AD of the Persian monarch Kavadhi I, these followers established a medical center which, with Syrian translations of Hippocrates, Galen, and Aristotle, attracted medical students from afar. As the Roman schools closed in the next century, the Persian monarchs, quite interested in medicine and literature, extended asylum to their sages. Thus, by the end of the 6th century, Gunde-Shapur, with Greek, Jewish, Persian, and Hindu teachers expounding Syriac and Aramaic translations of ancient Greek and Roman manuscripts, became the intellectual and medical center of the East. A hospital, the Bisamaristan, was built and served as a model for later hospitals at Baghdad and Damascus. When the Moslems conquered the Persian Empire, however, interest in medicine shifted to Baghdad in the East and Cordoba in the West.

Biblical Times

That the Bible has many references to illness is to be expected, but few diseases now recognized can be identified. Even epilepsy, the manifestations of which are so striking that it has been described in practically all civilizations and by all historians, cannot be diagnosed with certainty. Many Biblical characters have been assumed to have had epileptic attacks. The best known reference in the Gospels is the story of the father who brought his son afflicted with an unclean spirit to Jesus, saying: "He is possessed by a spirit which makes him speechless. Whenever it attacks him, it dashed him to the ground, and he foams at the mouth, grinds his teeth, and goes rigid." Although many writers consider Raphael's "Transfiguration" to represent this scene, some maintain that the picture does not depict a "real" convulsion but rather a hysterical attack.*

The Hebrew word "napbal," meaning to fall, is considered by some authorities to refer to an epileptic attack. If we accept this interpretation, Rabbi Schlomo Izchaki "Rashi" points out that the patriarch Abraham suffered an attack of epilepsy. The passage to which he refers is found in Genesis 17:3 "And Abram fell on his face: and God talked with him, saying. . . ." In this pronouncement Abraham, who was 99 years old, was told that he would be made exceedingly fruitful and that the Land of Canaan would be his everlasting possession. But upon a condition—a covenant which was to be kept by Abraham and all of his generation, namely that "every man child among you shall be cir-

*It should be kept in mind that Rafael's art represents the painter's concept of a vaguely described event that had occurred 1,500 years earlier.

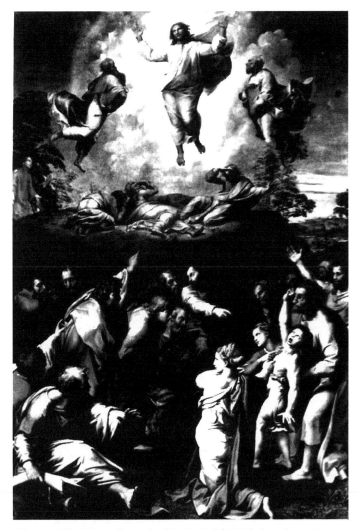

Fig. 1-7. The "Transfiguration" by Rafael (1517) thought to show an epileptic attack in an individual who is "possessed." (Vatican Museums, Rome)

cumcised." If this was a psychomotor seizure as has been suggested, consider its impact throughout the centuries (Fig. 1-7).

Apoplexy, another common ailment, is stated by Rashi to be the fatal kiss of God. In the Old Testament, Sarah, Moses, Aaron, and Miriam all "died through the mouth of God." Other neurological disorders, such as hydrophobia, are mentioned in vague terms.

Oriental Medicine

The head is the storage chamber for the essence of all knowledge.

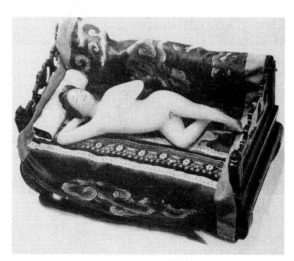

Fig. 1-8. Ancient Chinese physicians did not perform physical examination, but rather had patients describe symptoms and their location using figurines like this one. (From the collection of A. Earl Walker)

About 2700 BC, in early China, when priests and sorcerers looked after the ailments of the populace, an emperor, recognizing that knowledge of the body was lacking, authorized human dissection. No mention was made, however, of examining the head or the brain. At that time, medical therapy was based on herbal practices; somewhat later, acupuncture was introduced as a healing art. That procedure consisted of the insertion of various types of needles into specific points of the trunk, limbs, or head, depending upon the complaints of the patient. These needles were left in place for some time, twirled about or adjusted in order to obtain the desired relief. Often a ball of dried leaves (moxa) was burnt at specific points on the skin to produce a small blister. Later, acupuncture and moxa were applied at appropriate places to induce topical anesthesia of sufficient degree to allow surgical procedures to be performed. Until the Christian era, the Chinese used only herbals to complement these practices. In desperate cases, certain poisons (e.g., nux vomica and arsenic) might be administered.

The Chinese healer examined the human body, paying particular attention to the body temperature as determined by palpation and the character of the pulse (Fig. 1-8). In the 2nd century BC, a text on fevers became the standard reference for hundreds of years. About 300 AD, Wang Shu analyzed the variability of the pulse in order to prescribe and prepare the appropriate ingredients from the plants of China. A number of these medications, such as rhubarb, iron, castor oil, koalin, aconite, camphor, cannabis indica, chaulmoogra oil, and ephedra vulgaris were introduced later to Western medical practice.

The importance of medicine in the life of the Chinese may be gauged by the attitude of the emperors toward the healing arts. Wu Ti, in the 2nd century BC, is said to have had 850 volumes on medicine in his imperial library. At that time, the practice of medicine was strictly regulated; an examination assessed the candidate's knowledge and determined the salary that the physician should receive. During the golden age of China, in the T'ang dynasty of the 7th century AD, printing was introduced, signature stamps and, somewhat later, folded sheets to replace the scroll were used—the forerunners of books. Movable type was invented before the Gutenberg Bible was printed in Europe. Gunpowder, previously used for fireworks in the Sung dynasty (1161 AD), was shown to have great destructive power. The "south-pointing needle" was invented to guide mariners in the 12th century.

Because Confucian philosophy decreed that the human body was sacred and to be returned whole and sound, anatomy was poorly understood and surgery generally neglected. In an ancient text, the head was described as consisting of "skin, bones, and brain," indicating the meager knowledge of the nervous system.

However, a few references to "brain surgery," bizarre as they may seem, are to be found in the literature of the early part of the Christian era. Needham states that "they [the people of Da-Chew] have clever physicians who by opening the brain and extracting worms, can cure Mew-Sand." However, it is not clear what this affliction was.

Fanciful accounts of other craniotomies in China are found in the tales translated by Brewitt-Taylor. The famous Hua T'o is said to have operated upon a man who had a lump between his eyes which itched intolerably. Upon incising the tumor, a canary flew out, whereupon the man was cured. In spite of Hua T'o's discovery of anesthesia induced by cannabis fully 1700 years ago, Chinese surgery never advanced, presumably because of the firmly established belief in herbal medicine, manipulative techniques, and the prevalent Confucian dogma that if a Chinese body was not whole, the person could not enter the western sky. This belief often caused the Chinese to leave this earthly vale prematurely, albeit anatomically intact.

Although Osler concluded that "Chinese medicine leaves the impression of the appalling stagnation and sterility that may affect a really intelligent people for a thousand years," the ancient Chinese did make some significant advances. Besides acupuncture, the Chinese practiced inoculation for smallpox in the 11th century and used anesthesia for surgical procedures.

Hindu Practices

The scientific world owes a great debt to India. Consider that our system of calculating is based upon "Arabic" numerals engraved in the Rock Edicts of Ashoka a thousand years before the Arabs plagiarized them. Aryabhata and other Hindu mathematicians introduced the decimal system in the early Christian era Although used by the Arabs and Mayas earlier, the concept of "zero"—probably the most valuable of mathematical constructs—was the brainchild of the Hindus in the 9th century AD. Algebra, developed in India about the same time as in Greece, was popularized in Europe by the Arabs who derived their knowledge from the Hindus. And the statement that "The sphere of the stars is stationary and the earth by its rotation produces the daily rising and setting of planets and stars"was written by a Hindu a thousand years before Copernicus in 1543 published his treatise on the revolution of the planets about the sun.

The interchange of science and art between the Western civilizations (e.g., Greece, Iran, and Mesopotania) and the Eastern cultures (e.g., China, India, and adjacent lands) in the pre-Christian era was probably greater than indicated in Western textbooks. Throughout the ages, there seem to have been episodes when Asian and European civilizations mixed: the pre-Christian wandering of the Scythians, the conquests of Alexander the Great, the invasion of Huns, Goths, and Visigoths, and the western invasion by the Moors and the subsequent Crusades.

The intermingling of these different peoples was evident in their culture, architecture, religion, art, military strategy, and burial customs. The Hindus made a lasting contribution to the welfare of the early civilizations that came in contact with them. Long before the European peoples established public health systems, the Hindus had instituted sanitation and medical care for their people. As early as 600 BC, Hindu physicians recognized muscles, ligaments, nerve plexuses, fascias, fatty and vascular tissue, various membranes, and lymphatic tissues, and had fabricated sutures. Although they had some knowledge of digestive functions and considerable insight into the reproductive system, the cephalic parts were dismissed in one sentence, "the head is threefold—skin, bones and brain." Disorders now considered to originate in the nervous system were attributed to the heart, which the early Hindus thought to be the seat of emotions. Consequently, the brain and its casings were of peripheral interest. Illness was attributed to a disorder of the humors—air, phlegm, water, and blood—which could be remedied by charms or herbs.

In the golden days of India, the Hindus considered the practice of medicine, which had its origin in the earlier Vedic herbal and incantational therapies, as one of the more exalted professions. The candidate for a medical education could come from any of the first three upper castes—priestly, martial or agricultural, and business—and even from the shudras or serving class, provided that he met certain strict physical, intellectual, and personal requirements. The initiate had to take a vow of good intent, much like the Hippocratic Oath. After a probationary period of 6 months, the pupil began a five-to six-year apprenticeship to a master physician and studied the texts (samhitas), editions, or rewritings of Caraka, Susruta, and later the glossary of the two Vaghattas (physicians of the late pre- or early Christian eras). At the conclusion of this course, the candidate was required to take a difficult examination. If he passed, the student was given final instructions regarding his personal and professional conduct at a graduation ceremony.

After the death of Buddha in 480 BC, anatomical dissection was prohibited and the lot of the surgeon, and even the physician, declined both professionally and socially, so they were no longer regarded as deities in the community.

Surgical procedures in India, as in most other lands, were performed mainly by trained attendants to repair the ravages of war wounds inflicted by arrows and, less commonly, by spears or swords. Later, that branch of the healing art was incorporated into the physician's practice.

A number of historians have concluded that India was the birthplace of medicine as well as other sciences. Long before medicine flourished on the Mediterranean shores, the Hindus were practicing humane care of the sick. In a fragmented manuscript, *Ayurveda* (the science of life), disease is considered to be a humoral disturbance. The earliest complete medical work is generally conceded to be the *Charaka Samhita*. This compendium, consisting largely of questions and answers, presumably given by Caraka (or Charaka, Scirak, Scarab, or Zarach—names he was variously called by the Arabs) has been attributed to writers of the first millennium BC, or even as late as the 1st century AD. The original works were lost but revisions are extant. Translations from Sanskrit into Persian and Arabic script were made in the early Christian era.

Caraka discussed many medical subjects, but concerning surgery, only the cauterization and suturing of wounds. At that time, medicine in India, as in Greece, was intimately intertwined with philosophy. Therefore, Caraka discussed mind and matter, which he thought were composed of six elements—earth, water, fire, air, ether, and spirits. These were the basic humoral elements through which fluids activated the body. The diagnosis of disease was made by inspection, palpation, and auscultation of the heart; appropriate herbal preparations and intoxicating beverages made from various substances (e.g., honey, sugar, rice, barley, and grapes) were prescribed. Of neurological interest are the references to the skull, spine, cranial bones, and cranial matter (brain), although there is no evidence that their functions were appreciated. Many neurological disorders are said to have been known, including epilepsy, apasmara (five types), facial paralysis, headache, deafness, monoplegia, migraine, general paresis of the insane, aphonia, atrophy of muscles, convulsions, and tremor.

In the great compendium of Susruta, probably written at the time of Buddha, several centuries before Hippocrates, a physical examination is described, the variations of the pulse enumerated, and urine tests outlined. Treatment consisted of fasting, diet, baths, enemas, inhalations of many kinds, and the application of leeches.

Susruta advised medical students to dissect and become acquainted with the internal organs, for he stated that surgery should be a part of the physician's knowledge and not relegated to lesser trained artisans. Susruta is perhaps best known for his description of the repair of nasal and aural wounds, which were common in those days of hand-to-hand saber conflict, although there is no account of intracranial operations. Susruta did operate on many other parts of the body. He had a vague concept of the bacterial origin of leprosy and of the transmission of disease from man to man. Perhaps these thoughts may have been the reason why, before operating, he cut his nails, cropped his hair and beard, and put on a clean gown.

Many neurological disorders are referred to in Susruta's Samhita—convulsions, tetanus, paralysis, hemiplegia, facial palsy, sciatica, chorea, and syncope—as well as other disorders not clearly identified (Keswani). Even Parkinson's syndrome, "vepathu," is said to have been mentioned, although this disorder was not recognized in Europe until a century ago. Surgical operations were performed upon patients rendered insensitive by certain drugs. The Hindus were acquainted with cannabis and datura, which may have been ingredients in their soporific agents. Numerous and varied surgical instruments, including needles used to close wounds, were at hand.

Although in India, some surgery (especially plastic surgical repairs) was admirably carried out, the few recorded operations on the head are rather mystical. An ancient Persian manuscript refers to an Indian physician named Sarbat or Sarnab, who had spent some time with Aristotle. During his stay, a patient was seen who had an earwig which had "attached itself to the brain." Aristotle administered a drug which rendered the person unconscious, and Sarbat opened the skull and removed the offending earwig. Ballala related how a powerful king of Dhara suffered from a cerebral affliction (in some versions of the story said to be a saphara, or catfish) inside his skull. The king was stupefied with a powder, his skull was opened, and the offending object was removed. In another treatise written at the end of the first millennium AD, Hindu surgeons are said to have successfully trephined the skull of a king after administering a drug which rendered him insensitive to the procedure. Fanciful as these accounts are, such tales are sufficiently numerous to suggest that Hindu surgeons did successfully open the skull.

Even if India was not the birthplace of medicine and surgery, as a number of historians have concluded, the ancient Hindus made significant contributions to the health sciences. Many Greek physicians recognized and admired the knowledge of the Hindus. Hippocrates is said to have borrowed much of his Materia medica from India. It is noteworthy that Alexander the Great kept a number of Hindu physicians in his camp to treat conditions unknown to his Greek doctors. Certainly, the medical knowledge of the Hindus and Greeks became intermingled when the works of Charaka and Susruta were translated from Sanskrit to Arabic and Persian. Thus the Arabians—Avicenna, Rhazes, and Serapion—were well acquainted with the Eastern care of the sick. It is difficult to say how much Hindu medicine was influenced by Greek and Persian practices and how much the wisdom of India advanced Western medicine. Probably, there were mutual contributions.

Egyptian Practices

Each year, the Egyptians used mathematical and geometric principles to survey the land inundated by the Nile flood. Possibly, as some historians have suggested, they got their knowledge of arithmetic from Ur of the Chaldees. Their system of calculations using strokes for units and a symbol for 10, with a new symbol for each additional decimal increment, was cumbersome; 999 required 27 symbols. However, the Egyptians multiplied and divided even with fractions. They calculated the area of squares, cubes, and circles as well as estimating the value of pi as 3.16.

After centuries of observing the heavens and the time of appearance of the planets and stars, the Egyptians devised a calendar based upon agricultural cycles: four months, each of 30 days, for the rise, fall, and recession of the Nile, four months for cultivating crops, and four months for harvesting with an additional five days at the end of that season. This calendar was off six hours every year, an error which was not corrected until the introduction of the "Julian calendar" at the beginning of the Christian era.

The early healing practices were entrusted to the magic of the priests and, later, to specialists who confined their activities to surgery, gastrointestinal upsets, obstetrics, or ocular disorders, leaving the general health and hygienic problems (including cosmetology of poor people) to uneducated practitioners.

The first specific Egyptian references to the brain are found in a manuscript dating from about 4200 BC. This scroll, written in hieroglyphics, presumably by priests of the Nile Valley, described the preparation of the dead. Of neurological interest is the set of instructions for the care of the head. A hook was passed through the nares into the skull so that the brain could be removed piecemeal and the intracranial cavity was then filled with spices. The embalmers' assessments of the function of the fragmented brain are not given.

About 3000 BC, in the court of King Zoser, a vizier by the name of Imhotep, said to have been a skillful black sage and priest physician, developed a successful health cult. His accomplishments became so renowned that in the course of time he was venerated as a god. Within a few centuries of his death, it is said that his followers erected temples in which to heal the sick as well as to perform priestly duties. Perhaps, as some suggest, Imhotep or one of his disciples wrote the original treatise upon which the manuscript discovered later by Edwin Smith was based. In that manuscript, some 48 wounded persons were described, 17 of whom had injuries of the nervous system.

The treatment of wounds of the spinal cord and brain may be illustrated by a few histories taken from Breasted's translation of this papyrus.

> If thou examinest a man having a wound in his head, penetrating to the bone of his skull but not having a gash, thou shouldst palpate his wound; shouldst thou find his skull uninjured, not having a perforation, a split or a smash in it, thou shouldst say regarding him: "One having a wound in his head while his wound does not have two lips . . . nor a gash, although it penetrates to the bone of his head. An ailment which I will treat." Thou shouldst bind it with fresh meat the first day and treat afterwards with grease (honey) and lint every day until he recovers . . .

It is interesting to note that the early Egyptians knew of the hemostatic properties of muscle and advised a dressing impregnated with honey, which may have some antiseptic properties, after bleeding had stopped.

Fractured skulls, even if associated with meningeal irritation, were also acceptable for treatment.

> If thou examinest a man having a gaping wound in his head, penetrating to the bone and perforating his skull, thou shouldst palpate his wound; shouldst thou find him unable to look at his two shoulders and his breast, and suffering with stiffness in his neck . . . Thou shouldst say regarding him: "One having a gaping wound in his head, penetrating to the bone, and perforating his skull, while he suffers with stiffness in the neck. An ailment which I will treat." Now after thou hast stitched* it, thou shouldst lay fresh meat upon his wound the first day. Thou shouldst not bind it. Moor him to his mooring stakes until the period of his injury passes by. Thou shouldst treat it afterward with grease, honey and lint every day, until he recovers.

If the dural membranes were penetrated, however, the case was considered more serious.

> If thou examinest a man having a gaping wound in his head, penetrating to the bone, smashing his skull, and rending open the brain of the skull, thou shouldst palpate his wound. Shouldst thou find that smash which is in his skull like these corruptions which form in molten copper, and something therein throbbing and fluttering under thy fingers, like the weak place of an infant's crown before it becomes whole—when it has happened there is no throbbing and fluttering under thy fingers until the brain of his [the patient's] skull is rent open—and he discharges blood from both his nostrils, and he suffers with stiffness in his neck . . . Thou shouldst say concerning him: "An ailment not to be treated."

The surgical procedures were simple—merely an approximation of the

---

*This translation has been questioned, as sutures were a later development. Fresh meat (muscle) has served as a styptic until modern times.

wound edges. For some unknown reason, trephining was not practiced; only one perforated skull has been found in Egypt.

The writers of the *Edwin Smith papyrus* had a superficial knowledge of the nervous system. They described the membranes covering the convoluted cerebral hemispheres. When one side of the brain was damaged, the opposite limbs were paralyzed. That spinal injuries produced a different type of paralysis was known because the papyrus described paraplegia, urinary incontinence, and emissio seminis as the result of a fractured neck. Presumably, the condition was considered hopeless since only the external application of meat, honey and other substances was advised.

Subsequent medical treatises—the *Ebers* and *Neb-Sext papyri*—discussed only general issues with passing reference to epilepsy. From these few manuscripts, the ancient Egyptian knowledge of anatomy and function of the brain is difficult to gauge. Their art of embalming must have given them some insight into the general appearance of the brain and organs of the thorax and abdomen. They seemed to have some idea of control of movement by the brain but no specific understanding of the function of the nervous system. In spite of their limited knowledge of the structure of the body, they were well advanced in preventative medicine. Their attention to personal hygiene and to the cleansing of the alimentary tract with emetics and enemas may have been the reason that they were considered one of the healthiest nations of their time.

Although Egypt remained a major power for centuries, few medical advances were made after the golden age of around 1200 BC. As the power of the Pharaohs waned, the clergy maintained their favored position. With this decline, a succession of conquerors overran the country until in 30 BC, it became a province of Rome. From the blue Nile, health practices, so prominent in early times, passed to the islands of the Aegean Sea and adjacent lands, not to return to Africa for almost two thousand years.

Greek Practice of Medicine

Some 3000-4000 years before the Christian era, the people of the Mediterranean were developing civilizations that spread throughout the Western world. Of their healing arts little is known. The influence on Greek medicine of the earlier developed healing arts in the East and Egypt has been recognized in the medical practice described by Homer (c. 700 BC). The poems of Homer indicate that the warriors dressed the superficial wounds of their comrades. That Homer does not discuss injuries of the brain and spinal cord is probably an indication that such wounds were considered to be fatal. More of the Greek concepts of anatomy and functioning of the nervous system is to be gained from the philosophers who at that time engaged in discussion of many aspects of the human existence. One of the more remarkable was Praxagorus, who lived in the 6th century BC and who conceived of the essence of things in numbers and various natural elements. He conceived of life as composed of earth, air, fire, and water—elements which might be dry, cold, hot, or moist. These attributes might be combined with humors—blood, bile, phlegm, and black bile, the proportions of which determined the state of the health.

Alcmaeon, who dissected both living and dead animals, believed that the sensory receptors (e.g., eye and ears) had a canal to the seat of sensation in the brain to transmit external impressions. A constriction of this canal system caused sensory, motor, and/or intellectual disturbances. Alcmaeon implied that each sense was individually represented in the brain, but connected to a common pool, the *sensorium commune,* or a kind of soul. Later pre-Hippocratic physicians propounded various theories regarding the heart and brain without clarifying the role of the soul.

The early Greeks, according to the tales of Pindar, had a spa at Epidaurus to which the sick were brought. There, a physician-priest, Asclepiades, became so well known for his medical achievements that it was said that he "cured so many people—even raising a man from the dead—that Pluto, God of Hades, complained to Zeus that hardly anyone was dying any more." His followers built a temple at Epidaurus to which the sick came from all the Greek Isles for medical care. In the Golden Age of Greece, such an out-

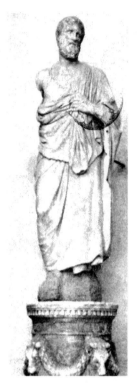

Fig. 1-9. Sculpture depicting Hippocrates. (From the collection of A. Earl Walker)

standing and famous man, as his following increased, might be venerated as a god. Thus it is not surprising that after a century or so, the renowned Asclepiades was deified as the son of Apollo. Members of his cult were called Asklepians or Asclepiades. These disciples built temples at spas along the sunny coast of the blue Aegean Sea where hydrotherapists under the direction of an Asclepiad massaged tired business men from the cities of Greece and gave encouraging psychotherapy. All manner of ills were treated by diet, baths, mineral waters, suggestion, manipulation, and, possibly, herbal drugs. These centers acquired a certain sanctity as mystic healings were reported.

Although homespun remedies for common ailments and simple repair of wounds had earlier been provided by traveling vagabonds and priests, a somewhat more rational care of the ills was introduced by the Greek practitioners who founded these health resorts. At these spas, physicians handed down their medical knowledge to their sons and a few chosen disciples. The most renowned of these cults were at the temples of Epidaurus, Rhodes, Cnide, and Cos.

The Greek Medical Clinic

It was into the guild at Cos that Hippocrates the Great was initiated as the son of a physician-member. His life is shrouded and even his very existence has been questioned by certain historians (Fig. 1-9). He was born on the island of Cos about the year 460 BC and grew up during the Golden Age of Greece. It is probable that Heraclides, Hippocrates' father, taught his son the elements of medicine. As was the custom, Hippocrates was instructed in astronomy, meteorology, mathematics, fine arts, and philosophy, which were considered to be the foundations of a medical education. To acquire the wisdom of other lands, Hippocrates traveled to Egypt and the countries along Asia Minor. At what point he returned to Cos, where he spent most of his life, is conjectural (Fig. 1-10). Even the date of his death, presumably 379 BC, is not known with certainty. No pictures nor statues of Hippocrates made during his lifetime exist. In fact, the tremendous adulation of his name did not occur until about a century after his death, when, as medical literature began to be collected for the library at Alexandria, the virtues of the writings of the

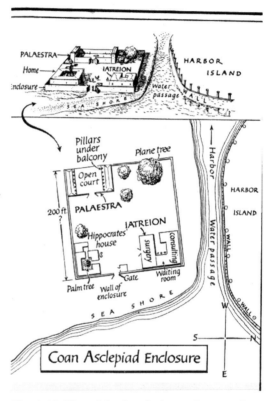

Fig. 1-10. Plan of the Aesculapian enclosure at Cos, where Hippocrates practiced the healing arts. (From the collection of A. Earl Walker)

physicians from Cos came to be recognized, and came to be known as the *Corpus Hippocraticum*. However, many manuscripts attributed to Hippocrates were probably composed by others, before or sometime after his death. In fact, manuscripts relating family or tribal practices in the time of Thales, as well as those of his contemporaries Empedocles and Democritus, were included in the Hippocratic *Corpus*. As a result, many writings attributed to him were probably the work of other physicians. In the treatises, not only were therapeutic practices discussed, but medical ethics, professional conduct, and instructions regarding the operating room, instruments, dressings, and bandaging of wounds were given. Of the extant manuscripts, only four, including *On the wounds of the head*, are with certainty from his pen. Unfortunately, many of the Hippocratic writings were lost and those remaining may not be a representative sample upon which to base an opinion of his concepts of the disorders of the nervous system.

The Hippocratic Oath

I swear by Apollo the physician, and Aesculapius, and Health, and All-heal, and all the gods and goddesses that, according to my ability and judgment, I will keep this Oath and this stipulation—to reckon him who taught me this Art equally dear to me as my parents, to share my substance with him, and relieve his necessities if required; to look upon his offspring in the same footing as my own brothers, and to teach them this art, if they shall wish to learn it, without fee or stipulation; and that by precept, lecture, and every other mode of instruction, I will impart a knowledge of the Art to my own sons, and those of my teachers, and to disciples bound by a stipulation and oath according to the law of medicine, but to none others. I will follow that system of regimen which, according to my ability and judgment, I consider for the benefit of my patients, and abstain from whatever is deleterious and mischievous. I will give no deadly medicine to any one if asked, nor suggest any such counsel; and in like manner I will not give to a woman a pessary to produce abortion. With purity and with holiness I will pass my life and practice my Art. I will not cut persons laboring under the stone, but will leave this to be done by men who are practitioners of this work. Into whatever houses I enter, I will go into them for the benefit of the sick, and will abstain from every voluntary act of mischief and corruption; and, further, from the seduction of females or males, of freemen and slaves. Whatever, in connection with my professional practice or not, in connection with it, I see or hear, in the life of men, which ought not to be spoken of abroad, I will not divulge, as reckoning that all such should be kept secret. While I continue to keep this Oath unviolated, may it be granted to me to enjoy life and the practice of the art, respected by all men, in all times! But should I trespass and violate this Oath, may the reverse be my lot!

Hippocratic Concepts of the Nervous System

In the time of Hippocrates, anatomy was not distinguished from physiology and both were included in the term "nature." Although Hippocrates taught that dissection of the human body should be the basis of medicine, at that time, anatomical exploration was forbidden as immoral and illegal. Hippocrates' knowledge of the structure of the body may have come from his father's instructions, in dissecting animals, or he may have learned some anatomy from repairing wounds. Most of the anatomical terms found in the Hippocratic writings were also used in Homer's history of the wars.

The structure of the skull and its contents were not well understood, although the Hippocratic physicians had acquired some knowledge from examination of head wounds and dissection of animals. They described the two membranes, an outer hard layer attached to the skull and an inner thin layer over the brain which encased the largely unexplored encephalon. The vessels of the brain were divided into veins, which were considered to contain blood, and arteries carrying air. The Hippocratic authors did not all agree upon the relationships of the veins; some considered them to originate from the brain, some from the liver, and still others from the heart, the rete, or the large veins along the vertebral column. These various concepts gave rise to bizarre ideas. The author of *The Nature of Man* describes two veins leaving the eyes, that from the left eye going to the right side of the body and that from the right eye to the left side.

The Hippocratic physicians did not differentiate the various fibrous cords of the body so that tendons, ligaments, aponeuroses, nerves, and other fibrous structures were grouped together. Their ideas of the workings of the heart and brain were crude. The brain was thought to be a gland which, like other glands, produced humors to be distributed to the various parts of the body. If these humors were altered by bile or phlegm, then upon returning to the brain, disorders such as apoplexy, epilepsy, delirium, and other untoward states resulted. If they were dispersed to other parts of the body, "catarrhs or fluxes" of disease ensued. Thus, disease might be ameliorated if the offending humor were eliminated from the sensitive glands, particularly from the brain. The author of On the Sacred Disease stated that when one draws a breath, the air goes first to the brain and then is dispersed to the rest of the body; however, the relationship of the air and blood is obscure. Some writers considered that the blood carried intelligence. The author of *Heart* wrote that intelligence of man is innate in the left ventricle, which gets its nourishment from a pure and luminous superfluity secreted in the blood. Hippocrates considered the brain to be the central organ—a gland containing humors which permeated all parts of the body.

> And men ought to know that from nothing else but thence (from the brain) come joys, delights, laughter and sports, and sorrows, griefs, despondency, and lamentations. And by this, in an especial manner, we acquire wisdom and knowledge, and see and hear, and know what are foul and what are fair, what are bad and what are good, what are sweet, and what unsavory; some we discriminate by habit, and some we perceive by their utility.

Obviously, the Hippocratic physician considered the brain as the seat of the sensations and the source of the motor activity, although the concept of these activities was quite bizarre.

With little knowledge of the anatomical structure of the brain, the physicians of that time had rather obscure notions regarding the basis of feeling. Although the brain was considered to be the definitive receptive organ, the pathways by which sensation reached that structure were highly imaginative. Vision was perceived from the images of the two eyes which passed through the bone in two veins separate from the brain. Sounds were carried by the bones of the ear through the meninges to the brain. The auditory canals passed the sounds to the tight, dry membrane which resonated to give rise to sound. Olfaction was transmitted by dry substances which carried odors to the cavities of the nose. Despite their meager anatomical knowledge, the Hippocratic writers gave a surprisingly clear clinical description of some neurological states.

Many commonly encountered neurological disorders, such as headache and dizziness, are described in almost modern terms. The physicians of Cos wished to know the character, location (whether in front or back or over one half of the head), and whether it was mild or severe and if it were caused by fever, otitis, overwork, exercise, venery, etc. Because the pain might be relieved by a nose bleed, they advised bleeding, cathartics, and even trephining. Different types of headache are described in the various books of the Hippocratic *Corpus*. In the seventh book of the *Epidemics* is a clear description of ophthalmic migraine. "It seemed to him to see a flash of lightening, usually in the right eye, then, after a short time, a violent pain occurred in the right temple and spread over the entire head and down the neck to the vertebral spines. If he attempted to move the head or open his mouth, he suffered a feeling of a violent contraction. Vomiting lessened or relieved the pain." What an excellent description of migraine.

In a number of the books, the clinical picture of meningitis, as the result of head trauma or otitis media, is presented. In *On Wounds of the Head*, the writer notes that as fever developed, the wound became discolored "like cured meat" and convulsions occurred usually on one side of the body. "If the wound is on the left side of the head, it is the right side of the body that convulses; if on the right, the left side of the body. Death comes in 7-14 days." In other accounts, the seriousness of head wounds was reiterated. Death in these cases was probably the result of infection. Hippocrates advised trepanning such cases, but cautioned that if the temple were incised, spasms might occur on the side opposite the incision. This pattern of events has been confirmed and elaborated upon many times by later writers. Souques considered that the ancient writer was describing what in common parlance is called "traumatic meningitis" and is characterized by fever, delirium, vomiting, focal seizures, and paresis of the limbs on the side opposite to the wound.

Hippocratic Concepts of Neurological Disorders

Many cases mentioned briefly in the Hippocratic writings might be attributed to clinical entities now commonly recognized, although on the basis of the history given, the diagnosis is not certain. This is particularly true of cases said to be meningitis, an all-encompassing term which may have included other disorders causing increased intracranial pressure, such as hydrocephalus, brain abscess, parasitic infestations, subdural hematomas, and brain tumors. The term "vertigo" is frequently used but not clearly described; in the *Aphorisms,* a condition is referred to as characterized by deafness, weight in the head, and vertigo with movements of the head and eyes.

The Hippocratic physicians were well acquainted with apoplexy, which they considered to be a sudden loss of consciousness with or without other concomitants. Premonitory signs and symptoms such as headache, ringing in the ears, dizziness, hesitancy in speech, numbness of a limb, seizures, or loss of memory indicated that a paralytic stroke was imminent. These premonitory symptoms are mentioned in several of the Hippocratic books (second book of *Maladies*), in which a description of the apoplectic state is well described—the speechlessness, paresis of the limbs, gurgling of the open mouth, and progressive coma. A sudden loss of speech was considered to be due to an excessive filling of the veins and, accordingly, a vein should be opened in the right arm. Certain factors such as old age, cold, and excess drinking predisposed to apoplexy. The writer stressed that such patients had fever and usually died in 3-5 days; if they should survive longer, they might recover. Severe sweating and embarrassed respiration were mortal, as was stupor with deviation of the eyes and forceful expirations.

A few delightful clinical vignettes are so clearly depicted as to be readily recognized. Epilepsy, for instance, may be identified even though it was thought to be of demoniac origin by many cultural and social societies. Even the name suggests the supernatural. The word "epilepsy" is derived from the Greek "epilambanein"—to seize or attack. Thus, the term would imply that the individual had been attacked or seized by a god or demon.

Although seizures are not uncommonly mentioned in ancient writings, few clear descriptions were given, probably because the attacks, being so unusual and frightening, were ascribed to supernatural beings which could not be defined.

Many ancient people considered epilepsy as divine or sacred, but some Hippocratic authors asserted it to be no more hallowed than other afflictions of the human body. These authors state that charlatans, impostors, and sorcerers deified epilepsy so that if their treatment was successful, they were venerated but if it was a failure, the responsibility would be upon the gods. In the Hippocratic treatise entitled *On the sacred disease,* the writer denied that epilepsy had a mystic origin and denounced the designation "sacred" for he considered the seizures as mundane as any other affliction. The disorder was explicitly stated to be a disease of the brain. The author of this treatise was unknown. In fact, some critics have questioned whether he was one of the Hippocratic physicians, although most historians concede that the treatise was a product of the Hippocratic school.

There is, however, no question but that the author was a physician who, like modern doctors, sought to clear up the superstitions regarding the epilepsies. The Hippocratic physicians considered epilepsy to be the same as any other illness to which man is heir and not as something quite distinct or sacred. The appellation "sacred" has been variously explained; early secular concepts of the condition considered the epileptic to harbor a god, devil, or demon which, during the attack, might leave the body and injure attendants or spectators. Later, the Latin term "morbus comitiales" referred to the custom of the assembly dispersing to prevent being contaminated when the individual had a seizure. Because the epileptic was considered unclean, people would spit to get rid of a sprite. This belief has persisted in some cultures; for even at the present time, certain races will draw a circle around a convulsing person to confine and prevent the evil sprite from affecting spectators.

According to the writer of *On the sacred disease,* many people regarded the epileptic as unclean and to be avoided. As a result, the superstitions of that time prohibited such afflicted individuals from engaging in a number of common activities (bathing and eating together), eating certain foods (fish, birds, veal, goat, deer, pig, and dog) and vegetables (mint, garlic, and onion), and from wearing black garments or goat skins. These proscriptions isolated the afflicted individual from contaminating other people. As well as these prohibitions, for the treatment of epilepsy, magicians and quacks used various orgies, incantations, and rites to cleanse the subject. Thus, drinking the blood of a gladiator and eating human bones (the atlas was considered to be particularly curative), mistletoe, and iron were prescribed. Some believed that an iron nail driven into the ground at the point where the epileptic had his first attack would transfix the responsible demon and rid the person of the disease. Amulets made of coral, peony, and roots of strychnos (if gathered at the time of the waning moon) hung around the neck would eliminate the condition. These ill-founded remedies were employed in various ways, often with diametrically opposed rationales so that some physicians forbid the epileptic to eat goat's flesh, while others advocated its consumption, particularly if it was parched in a funeral pyre. Although the Hippocratic physicians opposed these superstitious, magical, and religious forms of treating the epileptic patient, many healers used such supernatural therapies.

It is not difficult to see why all manner of healers (physicians and quacks) prescribed so many different means to dispel epilepsy. The condition is one which is periodic and its frequency may change depending upon many factors related to the physical and mental state of the individual. An epileptic patient having a seizure each day at home, when brought into the temple might be free of seizures for several weeks. Accordingly, a healer enthused with his form of therapy would be deluded into thinking that it was his treatment and not the patient's change of environment that was responsible for the alleviation of attacks. It might take a long time to establish that the condition was simply in remission and that the attacks would recur as before even though the treatment was continued. This led uncritical physicians to exalt their therapy.

Many clinical aspects of epilepsy were known to the physicians of the Hippocratic era. It was recognized that epilepsy tended to occur in early life, especially at the time of teething, and that after the age of 20, its onset was quite unusual. The writer of *On the sacred disease* implied that the condition had hereditary characteristics, but this may only be a reflection of his belief that all diseases were hereditary. The attacks were thought to occur more frequently in men than women and to be associated with sexual activity. Interestingly, the epileptic attack was likened to a sexual orgasm; both Hippocrates and Democritus wrote, "coitus is a slight epileptic attack." Along this line of reasoning, some physicians considered that intercourse would relieve the seizure, but others advocated abstinence from intercourse and even recommended castration. These ancient physicians assumed that the disease might cease at puberty; if it did not, it was considered incurable. In women, menstruation and pregnancy were thought to precipitate seizures—the frequency of attacks at the menstrual periods and with the eclampsias of pregnancies were pointed to as evidence.

Many environmental factors were considered either to cause or to precipitate seizures. The seasons, wind, and rain were all thought to be etiological factors. The routine acts of living, such as eating certain foods, were frequently cited as a cause of epilepsy. An alcoholic wet nurse might predispose the baby to epilepsy. Almost all human activities—exercise, sleep, and psychic disturbances of any kind—were considered capable of inducing seizures. Strangely, the ailments and diseases of mankind, with the possible exception of head injuries, were not commonly assumed to be responsible for epileptic attacks.

Hippocrates described the attack as when the patient is without consciousness and insensible to sound, sight, and pain, and his body drawn up and twisted to one side. In the motor phase, the hands became cramped, teeth clenched, face livid, eyes turned up, legs kicking, and foam flows from the mouth. The victim may suffocate and/or may pass urine or excreta, and profuse sweating may occur. Later writers elaborated upon this description of the convulsive seizure and described manifestations which warned of the attack. Upon such a premonition, the patient could isolate himself and lie down. The accounts of the major seizure included in vivid terms the details of a grand mal seizure, with which modern neurologists are well acquainted. In addition, some authors wrote of the confused state which followed as the individual began to regain consciousness—generalized weakness, heaviness of the head, distorted vision, and distended cephalic veins; in the postictal confusion some victims did not even recognize friends.

In the Hippocratic *Corpus,* a number of varied seizures are described, some of which are readily recognized and others which are unlike current attacks. Both the Hippocratic physicians and later the Roman attendants thought that night terrors and vertigo were related to epilepsy.

The Hippocratic physicians believed that if the seizures began before puberty, they might be cured, but if they developed after 25 years of age, they would persist *(Aphorisms,* 5th section). The author of *Premier Prorrhetiques* states that it is difficult to eradicate an epilepsy in those who acquire it in infancy or in the prime of life from 25 to 45 years of age. Moreover, they recognized that it is difficult to cure persons in whom the convulsions begin with a general spasm and do not have a focal beginning. They believed that if the attack began with a general spasm and in the side of the face, hand or foot, the epilepsy is easy to arrest, although attacks beginning in the face are most persistent and those starting in the hand or foot are less resistant to treatment.

The Hippocratic physicians knew that fever, especially that of quartian malaria, had at times cured epilepsy. But they were also aware that fever in children might cause convulsions. As in many other diseases, heredity was considered the main factor in epilepsy. Age was also thought to be important both in causation and in prognosis. They knew that small infants usually died if they had seizures; if they survived, they were likely to have a residual defect involving the mouth, eye, neck, or hand. Moreover, they were apt to have further attacks.

The Hippocratic writers were well aware that seizures followed a head injury. Such convulsions, they knew, often involved one side of the body. "If the wound is on the left side of the head, the right side of the body convulses; if the wound is on the right side, the left limbs are involved." In such cases, they advised an immediate trephination to the dura mater but cautioned incising the temporal region, especially the temporal muscle and temporal artery, lest convulsions ensue.

For spontaneously occurring seizures in young people, the Hippocratic physicians advised hygiene, diet, and change of place and kind of life *(Aphorisms,* 2nd section). Similar advice is given in *On the sacred disease.*

It was recognized that the majority of patients had the onset of their attacks in childhood and that the condition often disappeared at puberty, but if it continued, the attacks became worse over the years. The tendency for the attacks to have a rhythm, recurring at the full of the moon or only during sleep, was known to the Greek physicians. If the condition became chronic, the victim's personality became unsociable and sullen. Moreover, if an individual had been epileptic from youth, he or she might develop a mental state resembling that of extreme drunkenness. Older people were likely to succumb to a seizure; however, if they did not die, they might have no further attacks.

The dangers and complications of a seizure were recognized—death, injury, and certain visual changes such as squint or nystagmus. Moreover, as a consequence of the attacks, weakness of a limb might develop. Hippocrates wrote that if an individual with epilepsy reached old age, he or she might be paralyzed on one side.

Changes in lifestyle (particularly adolescence), in place and habits, might interrupt the sequence of the seizures. It was recognized that generalized seizures with no focal onset had an unfavorable outlook. On the other hand, if the attacks started in the hands or feet, there was a chance of recovery. It is particularly interesting that Hippocrates stated, "People who are seized by quartian fever are not seized by the great disease. If, however, they are seized first and quartian fever supervenes, they are released." It was even suggested that a patient might be given quartian fever to stop the epilepsy.

Although the Hippocratic writers maintained that the condition was not curable if a person with seizures was more than 20 years of age, some writers held that the epilepsy could be controlled. Souques commented that the writer was referring to infantile convulsions and fits due to teething. The Hippocratic writer attributed seizures in children to intoxications, environmental changes, and physiological factors such as amenorrhea and onset of menses.

If an attack was witnessed, the diagnosis of epilepsy was simple. In the interim between seizures, however, the diagnosis was more difficult. Yet it was of importance in Greece and Babylonia, because a slave might be returned and the sale price refunded if seizures occurred within 12 months after purchase. To provoke an attack artificially at that time, a potter's wheel was rotated before the eyes of the subject; if the slave became giddy or had a seizure, he was returned. This, of course, is an antecedent of modern photogenic epilepsy. Foul-smelling substances were also used to induce an attack.

Although the Hippocratic physicians affirmed that epileptic seizures should be differentiated from other convulsions, it is not clear how the distinction was made. Uterine disturbances as described at that time bore no relationship to what are now called "hysterical" episodes. Bizarre episodes apparently were differentiated from typical epileptical seizures. Psychomotor attacks seemed to have been considered as a form of mania. Consequently, although some seizures were genuine epileptic convulsions, many fits were difficult to classify, especially in view of the humoral, demoniacal, and other etiological factors believed at that time.

The Hippocratic authors present somewhat conflicting accounts of the pathogenesis of seizures. In *On the sacred disease,* it is stated:

> But if the air is cut off from the brain and the vessels, the person becomes dumb and unconscious; suffocation arises, which by violence makes the excrements pass.

The lung, being cut off from the breath, foams and causes frothing at the mouth. The small vessels of the eye beat vehemently, and so the eyes become distorted; in the legs the incarcerated breath causes cramp and pain and makes the patient kick; in the hands, however, the blood stands still and they become powerless and cramped.

Plato and some Hippocratic writers held that "when 'white' phlegm mingled with black bile disturbing its circulation, the 'sacred disease' resulted." In another Hippocratic manuscript, air mixed with the blood was said to obstruct the vessels so that the passage of blood was impeded and irregular, giving rise to a convulsion. Aristotle believed that food produced a vapor that rose into the brain, a process which also explained the phenomenon of sleep. In other words, sleep was an epileptic seizure, and for this reason, attacks often occurred during sleep. Aristotle also stated that epilepsy was a melancholic disease engendered by black bile. Perhaps this view was supported by the Hippocratic saying, "most melancholics usually also become epileptics and epileptics melancholics." Another view attributed to Praxagoras held that the phlegmatic humors forced bubbles that blocked the passage of the psychic pneuma from the heart and thus the body shook and convulsed. Other fanciful explanations for the seizure were propounded, only to add further confusion to the mystical subject.

Treatment by Hippocratic Physicians

The Hippocratic physicians were aware that effective treatment of persons with epilepsy was difficult. Since they recognized that long-standing cases were incurable, they advised early therapy. In young individuals, attacks starting in the hands or feet were considered to have a favorable outlook, but in older persons the prognosis was guarded. Attacks that began with a warning might be prevented from spreading by inhaling an offensive odor, tasting a bitter substance, or applying fomentations to the cold, stiff member. An attack beginning in an extremity might be confined by pulling or binding the limb to prevent the spread of the pneuma.

For generalized seizures, different treatments (many quite obnoxious) were advised. The basis of most therapies consisted of purging, diuresis, and exercise supplemented by various, often bizarre, activities or ingestants. Then the patient should exercise, drink vinegar and honey, and rest. In the evening, the patient should take a walk, rest, walk again, and then bathe. While resting and before eating, the patient should imbibe a concoction of hyssop containing vinegar and honey. If the attacks had a definite rhythm, a day or two before an attack was expected, the patient should be bled or given an emetic and, at the same time, a cathartic or enema. In addition to these physical measures, specific organs such as the brain of a camel, the testicles of a cock or goat, should be ingested. If these measures were ineffective, the surgeon might make an incision in the occiput in the form of the Greek letter "X," cauterize the scalp, or perforate the skull at the bregma with a trephine. Aretaeus advised that the bone be perforated to the diploë, and waxes and salves applied until the meninx separated from the bone. Eventually, after suppuration, the wound healed leaving a scar and "the patient . . . escaped from the disease." Many physicians were, however, doubtful and distrusted such surgical measures as arteriotomy, cauterization, and trephining. In the centuries after Hippocrates, the concepts and treatment of epilepsy changed little as the Romans displaced the Greeks as master physicians.

Of the works of Hippocrates, the book *On injuries of the head* is one of the most precisely written. The author first describes the sutures of the skull, the intervening bone, and the porous diploë containing thin vessels distended with blood. He then notes the varying thickness of the skull bones and their vulnerability to injuries, observing that the area about the bregma is the most easily injured. His conclusion that "more persons who are wounded in the back part of the head escape than of those wounded in the anterior part," suggests that the author gained his knowledge of the head from dissection of animal rather than human skulls.

The author gives quite detailed accounts of head wounds, especially of the state of the skull.

1. Fracture—a break of the bone which must of necessity be associated with contusion.
2. Contusion—an injury of the bone which seems to remain in its natural condition. This affliction is not clearly defined, for the unknown writer states that there are many varieties of contusion which are not apparent to the eye; in fact, immediately after an injury it may not be evident that the bone has been bruised.
3. Depressed fracture.
4. Dented injury.

The author observed that a different part of the head from that struck might be injured (contre coup).

Of these injuries, some require trepanning the contusion (whether or not the bone is bare), the fissure, and the indented (hedra) fracture with contusion (irrespective of the presence of a fracture). He stated that a depressed fracture rarely required trepanning, especially if it was broken up and depressed. An indentation (hedra) without fracture and/or contusion did not require trepanning. It seems obvious that the Hippocratic physician considered the state of the bone rather than the state of the brain to be significant. He was concerned with the danger of a contusion and/or fissure fracture of the skull which was thought to be potentially lethal. Just what the lethal factor was—invisible and late developing—is not clear. Possibly it was the coma from brain compression or infection. Because the trepan was not required in depressed, comminuted, and gutter (hedra) wounds, which usually accompany a scalp wound, the Greeks had apparently learned that a freely draining wound was not fatal. But if the continuity of the skull was disturbed, even if the scalp was intact, trepanation was imperative. Hence it was important to determine early if a linear fracture was present. Hippocrates wrote:

> . . . if you suspect that the bone is broken or contused, to see the truth of the matter, you must dissolve the jet-black ointment, and fill the wound with it when this dissolved, and apply a linen rag smeared with oil, and then a cataplasm of the maza with a bandage; and on the next day, having cleaned out the wound, scrape the bone with the raspatory. And if the bone is not sound, but fractured and contused, the rest of it which is scraped will be white; but the fracture and contusion having imbibed the preparation, will appear black, while the rest of the bone is white. And you must again scrape more deeply the fracture where it appears black; and, if you thus remove the fissure, and cause it to disappear, you may conclude that there has been a contusion of the bone to a greater or less extent, which has occasioned the fracture that has disappeared under the raspatory; but it is less dangerous, and a matter of less consequence, when the fissure has been effaced. But if the fracture extends deep, and does not seem likely to disappear when scraped, such an accident requires trepanning.

The trepanning is carefully described:

> . . . you must not at once saw the bone down to the meninx; for it is not proper that the membrane should be laid bare and exposed to injuries for a length of time, as in the end it may become fungous. And there is another danger if you saw the bone down to the meninx and remove it at once, lest in the act of sawing you should wound the meninx. But in trepanning, when only a very little of the bone remains to be sawed through, and the bone can be moved, you must desist from sawing, and leave the bone to fall out of itself. For to a bone not sawed through, and where a portion is left of the sawing, no mischief can happen; for the portion is now left insufficiently thin. In other respects you must conduct the treatment as may appear suitable to the wound. And in trepanning you must frequently remove the trepan, on account of the heat in the bone, and plunge it in cold water. For the trepan being heated by running round, and heating and drying the bone, burns it and makes a larger piece of bone around the sawing to drop off, than would otherwise do. And if you wish to saw at once down to the membrane, and then remove the bone, you must also, in like manner, frequently take out the trepan and dip it in cold water. But if you have not charge of the treatment from the first, but undertake it from another after a time, you must saw the bone at once down to the meninx with a serrated trepan, and in doing so must frequently take out the trepan and examine with a sound (specillum), and otherwise along the tract of the instrument. For the bone is much sooner sawn through, provided there be matter below it and in it, and it often happens that the bone is more superficial.

The Hippocratic writer gives a picture of the unfavorable case:

When a person has sustained a mortal wound on the head, which cannot be cured, nor his life preserved, you may form an opinion of his approaching dissolution, and foretell what is to happen from the following symptoms which such a person experiences. When a bone is broken, or cleft, or contused, or otherwise injured, and when by mistake it has not been discovered, and neither the raspatory nor trepan has been applied as required, but the case has been neglected as if the bone were sound, fever will generally come on before the fourteenth day if in winter, and in summer the fever usually seizes after seven days. And when this happens, the wound loses its color, and the inflammation dies in it; and it become glutinous, and appears like a pickle, being of a tawny and somewhat livid color; and the bone then begins to sphacelate, and turns black where it was white before, and at last becomes pale and blanched. But when suppuration is fairly established in it, small blisters form on the tongue and he dies delirious. And, for the most part, convulsions seize the other side of the body; for, if the wound be situated on the left side, the convulsions will seize the right side of the body; or if the wound be on the right side of the head, the convulsion attacks the left side of the body. And some become apoplectic. And thus they die before the end of seven days, if in summer; and before fourteen, if in winter. And these symptoms indicate, in the same manner, whether the wound be older or more recent. But if you perceive that fever is coming on, and that any of these symptoms accompany it, you must not put off, but having sawed the bone to the membrane (meninx), or scraped it with a raspatory (and it is then easily sawed or scraped), you must apply the other treatment as may seem proper, attention being paid to circumstances.

Although rabies was recognized by contemporary writers, the Hippocratic writers were vague and indefinite in their descriptions. Alcoholism in the Hippocratic era was uncommon. Three degrees were recognized; first, a slight intoxication causing some impairment of thought; second, a severe intoxication with coma; and finally, an alcoholic delirium. It was stated that if a person's hands trembled as the result of drinking, one could predict that delirium or convulsions would follow. Emetics, hot lotions and bleeding were advised, or as stated in the second book of *Epidemics*, "if after intoxication, there is headache, drink approximately a liter of pure wine."

The term "hysteria" was used to describe "uterine suffocation," a condition thought to occur in young women due to a displaced uterus pressing upon the liver. It is not related to the modern condition called hysteria.

The Hippocratic writers do refer to mania and depression, although not as cyclic events. They considered depression to be associated with psychothenia, hypochondriasis, compressive states, fear of heights, and various psychosomatic disturbances. These complaints were manifested by gastrointestinal upsets, bilious derangements, fatigue, trauma, and excesses of the environment. They might be brought on by unusual eating, undue exercising, or extreme changes in climate. Consequently, the measures for their relief were simple—diet, physiotherapy, and general hygiene. The Hippocratic physicians were more interested in prognosis than in diagnostic and therapeutic procedures. Unfortunately, their treatises on therapy were lost so that their results are unknown.

The precise instructions given for trephination would indicate that their surgeons had considerable experience in the use of surgical instruments. Assuming that the Greeks had surgical instruments similar to those found at Pompeii for procedures upon the head, their knowledge had greatly advanced since the time of the writers of the *Edwin Smith papyrus*. Probably they had learned the operations from the northern European races whose burial grounds provide evidence of craniotomies performed in the prehistoric era. Irrespective of the origins, however, the Greek surgeons had perfected the technique.

Although the writer of the *Edwin Smith papyrus* knew that paralysis resulted from spinal injury, some later philosophers, particularly Aristotle, confused the spinal cord with the marrow of the vertebral bodies. Plato believed that the spinal cord and brain constituted a unit, "the myelenencephalon covered by bones and surrounded by muscle which was divided into the encephalon, the home of the divine soul and the segmented spinal cord. From the latter passed the 'nerves' which connected the brain to the heart and liver." Plato located the amorous female soul in the caudal and the courageous male soul in the rostral spinal cord.

The Hippocratic writers had vague ideas regarding the structure and function of the spinal cord. If the section on the spinal cord which Hippocrates stated was being written had been preserved, perhaps the anatomy and functions of the cord might have been elucidated. Although the Hippocratic writers discuss spinal injuries in some detail, it is not clear that they understood the role of the spinal cord in the paralysis which resulted from vertebral injury. That they believed the spinal cord originated from the brain and was distinct from the bone marrow is not clear. It is the bony spine, the physicians emphasize, for "when the spine protrudes backward as the result of a fall, the dislocation is attended." Moreover, they related the loss of strength and torpor of the whole body when the upper vertebrae are displaced to the dislodgement of the vertebrae. They deny that such displacement can be reduced by succussion on a ladder or some other similar treatment. In addition, the Hippocratic physicians attributed paralytic conditions, which were probably infectious, to traumatic vertebral displacement. For example, they describe patients suffering from a sore throat, much phlegm, fever, dyspnea, paralysis of the face, mouth, and soft palate, and the inability to stand and who, in a short time, died in the same fashion as those having a dislocation. Souques presented cogent arguments that such persons were suffering from a post-diphtheritic paralysis; he pointed out that the authors were dealing not with an isolated case, but with an epidemic.

The clinical acumen and experience of the Greek physicians of that time were extraordinary. They were aware of contralateral paralysis, traumatic and otitic meningitis, amaurosis, cerebral apoplexy, generalized and focal epilepsy, migraine, tetanus, alcoholism, hereditary predisposition to mental disease, periodicity of certain psychoses, melancholic and hypochondriacal states, obsessions and phobias, paraplegia and quadriplegia, concussion and contusion of the spinal cord, diphtheritic paralysis, sciatica, and other spinal conditions. This is a storehouse of neurological treasures.

Alexandrian Practices

In the century between the death of Hippocrates and the founding of the Alexandrian School, the political situation changed in Greece. Philip of Macedonia attacked and conquered Thebes, Athens, and eventually Sparta. His son, Alexander (c. 356-323 BC), upon his accession, began an invasion of Asia with Greek forces. Under these circumstances, medicine had a low priority and, as a result, there were few physicians of note in this period. Praxagorus and Chrysippe are known from the writings of their pupils, Herophilus and Erasistratus.

This was the age of the philosopher Aristotle (384-322 BC), whose knowledge of the nervous system was scanty and faulty. If, indeed, he had seen the brain, it must have been in animals, because he describes it as situated in the anterior part of the head. He believed that the brain did not have veins nor contain blood and hence was cold; in contradistinction, the heart and lungs were warm and full of blood. The spinal cord was without blood but, unlike the brain, was hot. Aristotle thought that the heart was the *sensorium commune* (soul) of all organs. Because he could trace two canals to the heart, which he assumed subserved taste and touch, he concluded that all the other senses must have similar canals. Hence, the heart was the basis of life and the origin of the blood which the veins distributed to all parts of the body. It was the seat of reason, sensibility, intelligence, and voluntary movement. He denied that the brain was a sensory organ, as he believed that it had no connection with such sensory parts as the eyes, ears, or nose. Moreover, he considered it to be humid, cold, insensible, and without blood. Scientists have attempted to explain Aristotle's reasoning in various ways; perhaps the simplest is to attribute it to his lack of contact with the human brain.

After the death of Alexander the Great, his three principal lieutenants divided the Greek Empire. Egypt was given to Ptolemy, Athens to Pericles, and Alexandria (previously a small fishing village) to Ptolemy Lagus. Alexandria, being on the crossroads of travel and trade of the Mediterranean people, soon became a thriving capital. Ptolemy hoped to make it a second Athens and a cultural center to attract famous men of art and learning from all parts of the world. He collected and stored about 200,000 rare and precious manuscripts. For this library, many of the Hippocratic texts were copied. The members of the museum were distinguished and well-trained scholars of many disciplines (e.g., poets, historians, philosophers, physicians, mathematicians, and artists) presided over by a priest. It was to this scientific center that Herophilus came from Asia Minor. He was born, date unknown, in a town of Chalcedon where he was educated by a highly reputed Asclepian, Praxagorus of Cos. His associate, Erasistratus, was born on the isle of Ceos in 310 BC and grew up in Antioch. To follow in his physician father's footsteps, Erasistratus was educated in Athens and later gained medical experience at Cos.

Unfortunately, neither the works of Herophilus nor Erasistatus have survived. On the basis of fragments of their writings cited by later authors (Galen, in particular), an idea of their knowledge has been preserved. Unfortunately, Galen detested some of Erasistratus' analogies, such as the concept of the human body as a machine, so that his references to the latter's work may be biased.

The study of anatomy, previously prohibited, was revived when Ptolemy Soter authorized human dissection. In fact, Celsus, a few hundred years later, stated that Herophilus and Erasistratus were allowed to dissect living criminals who had been condemned to life imprisonment or death. Even without that dubious odium, Herophilus was severely criticized by some citizens who viewed his anatomical studies as butchering. Based on his dissections, however, he described the peripheral nerves, demonstrated their cerebral or spinal origins, and concluded that they had motor and sensory functions. Herophilus apparently sectioned the brain and, looking at its cut surface, noted cavities or ventricles. However, either he was unaware of the existence of fluid in them or, since it escaped as the cut was made, he ignored its presence.

Although Aristotle had noted cavities in the brain, Herophilus made a much more detailed description of the lateral, midline, and fourth ventricle; he referred to the fourth as the ventricle of the cerebellum. The caudal midline point of the fourth ventricle he termed the calamus scriptorius. He designated the two coverings of the brain on the basis of their consistency as dura mater and pia mater. Although he described (presumably in the ox) the rete mirabile as a vascular plexus at the base of the brain formed by intracranial portions of the carotid and vertebral arteries, he did not recognize its significance. He followed the cerebral veins and sinuses of the dura mater to their occipital collecting cistern or winepress which bears his name—"torcula Herophili." Finally, he studied the extension of the brain stem—the spinal cord—and demonstrated that it gave rise to motor and sensory nerves.

Erasistratus confirmed and elaborated upon the findings of Herophilus. He noted the origin of the cerebrospinal axis and the spinal nerves. For a time, he believed that the motor nerves alone came from the white substance of the cord; however, later he admitted the spinal origin of the sensory nerves. He did not clearly differentiate the motor nerves from the ligaments and tendons.

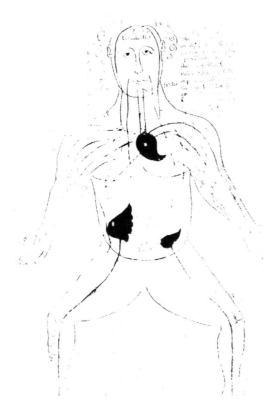

Erasistratus described the ventricular system of man and animals, noting the junction of the two lateral and midline ventricles, the latter much later referred to as the foramen of Monro.

The Alexandrians had rather primitive concepts of the nature of the nervous system (Fig. 1-11). Their philosophical reasoning led to curious conclusions; Erasistratus argued that the enormous volume of air respired must be to fill the arteries and that the veins must be the reservoirs for blood because "it was not possible that nature could create two sorts of vessels for the same function." During respiration, he thought that the air penetrated the trachea, the bronchi, and the lungs, and then through the pulmonary vessels reached the left ventricle of the heart. In this ventricle, it was transformed into

Fig. 1-11. Body schema from an Alexandrian manuscript of the 13th century. (From the collection of A. Earl Walker)

the pneuma vital. With each contraction of the heart, this pneuma was expelled into the aorta and transmitted to all parts of the body. The pneuma destined for the brain passed through the rete mirabile, finally reaching the central ventricles where it underwent a second transformation into a psychic pneuma. These pneuma (vital and psychic) were the "vital spirits" and "animal spirits" described by physicians until the Renaissance period. Erasistratus believed that the seat of the soul (the principle of life) was in the ventricles, particularly the fourth ventricle. It was there that the psychic pneuma encountered the particles and vibrations of external objects which produced sensation and awareness. They then passed in the motor nerves, carrying orders for muscular movement. The vital pneuma was conveyed by arteries to all parts of the body where it came into contact with the blood carried by the veins. The blood nourished, the vital pneuma stimulated, thus heat, energy, and life resulted from this encounter. In summary, animal life was dependent upon vital pneuma and intellectual life upon psychic pneuma. This theory of pneumas or spirits was held by physicians and philosophers without significant modification until the time of Harvey.

Erasistratus conceived of a very modern role for the cerebral convolutions. Because man, the wisest of the creatures, had the best-developed cerebral convolutions, he concluded that their complexity was related to intelligence. On the basis of the same logic, Erasistratus considered that the fine cerebellar convolutions or folia correlated with the rapidity and force of muscular action. This might be interpreted as indicating that he thought that the cerebellum played a role in the coordination of movement, an interpretation questionable from the available fragmentary writings of Erasistratus.

The Alexandrian physicians believed that paralysis resulted from injury of the dura mater, not of the spinal cord. Herophilus recognized that paralysis might be the result of lack of movement, of sensibility, or of both. He attributed sudden death without apparent cause to paralysis of the heart. Impaired neurological function was thought to be due to thick and gelatinous humors obstructing the canals of the vessels, thus stopping or impeding the flow of pneuma, particularly that transmitting motor orders.

Since Alexandria was the crossroads of the then-known world, specimens of plants, trees, and drugs were brought there from all lands. Herophilus considered them as possible medications, and tried them with the hope of finding a specific cure for each disease. When a single remedy was ineffective, he combined various drugs. Erasistratus did not share in this enthusiasm for multidrug therapy and used simple remedies, particularly vegetables, in very small doses. For example, for the treatment of a bilious dysentery, he prescribed three drops of wine. These two physicians, although often disagreeing, concurred in the value of hydrotherapy, gymnastics, and diet.

Herophilus had many more pupils and was better known than Erasistratus. He was more of an anatomist—describing the cerebrospinal system, the motor and sensory functions of the peripheral nerves, the cerebral ventricles, the choroid plexuses, and the venous circulation of the brain. On the other hand, Erasistratus was more of a physiologist; some have even called him the founder of physiology. Certainly, he suggested the function of the cerebral convolutions and, perhaps, guessed the coordinating role of the cerebellar convolutions. Between them, they created a working plan of the nervous system just 20 years after Aristotle's death. Without the support of an intelligent and liberal king who authorized dissection of cadavers, it might have been many centuries before the structure and nature of the nervous system was disclosed. Upon the death of these two great Alexandrians, however, the popular prejudices and religious tenets against dissection were reinstituted. Since the later Ptolemys no longer supported anatomists, dissection of cadavers was abandoned, although Alexandrian practitioners continued to make dissections and vivisections on animals.

In the centuries between the time of the Alexandrian physicians and Galen, neurological knowledge made little progress. With restrictions on dissection, anatomy of the nervous system continued to be based upon the treatises of Herophilus, Erasistratus, and the few anatomists who followed them. More attention was paid to the clinical and therapeutic aspects of medicine than to surgery. Hence, the popular Hippocratic works stored in the Alexandrian libraries formed the basis for most of the teaching. As Alexandria became the renowned school for that time, the writings of Hippocrates were more and more appreciated and venerated.

Roman Neurosciences

The health of Roman people before the Christian era was entrusted to uneducated practitioners and priests who prescribed such folk remedies as wines and herbs. However, midwifery was developed and laparotomies to save a living fetus were performed according to law ("lex regra") as early as 700 BC. As a result, a number of medical terms were in common use even before the destruction of Corinth in 146 BC brought the downfall of the Grecian states and the migration of Greek physicians to Rome. At that time, the native practitioners were poorly trained so that the well-to-do citizens and the "best" families welcomed the attention of Greek physicians, who in order to practice medicine were granted Roman citizenship. Even the Emperors of Rome appointed Greek doctors to their court rather than native practitioners.

As Alexandria declined and the power of the Roman Empire increased, Rome became the medical center of the world. In the military regime of the Romans, however, the physician came to play a lowly role, principally because there were no legal requirements in Rome; any individual, male or female, who wished to practice medicine could do so without special studies or examination. As a result, the healing art, taken up by slaves or liberated persons who plied their trade in the home or on the streets, was scorned by Roman citizens. Greek physicians with knowledge and experience in medicine came to occupy an enviable position in Rome.

Roman Practices

Perhaps the most noteworthy trend in the centuries between the height of Alexandrian and Roman medicine was the development of a number of sects of medical theory and practice. The founders of the Methodist school of medicine considered that the body was made up of atoms moving about in pores. Disease resulted from the interruption of this movement due to an excessively dry, tense, and stringent state becoming an unduly relaxed atonic state, or to an unnatural mixture of the two. As the diagnosis of these states does not require a knowledge of basic anatomy and physiology, the system could be learned in six months, so that all manner of uneducated artisans including the dregs of the populace could become physicians. Therapy consisted of restoring the normal tension either by relaxants or astringents; accordingly, the treatment was simple—massage, exercise, bathing, and small amounts of wine. One of the founders, Asclepiades of Prussia, by his kind treatment of patients gained the affections of the Romans. Instead of emetics and cathartics, he ordered simple medications and emphasized the value of walking, exercise, massage, and hydrotherapy. He was considered an astute diagnostician; it is said that one day in the street he met the funeral procession of a butcher, looked at the corpse, and exclaimed, "The man is not dead; extinguish the torches and release this butcher." The man returned to live a long life. Soranus, another highly respected Methodist, wrote of several neurological conditions, in particular, headache and epilepsy.

The Methodists, quite popular in Galen's time, were the most numerous and powerful medical group in Alexandria and Rome. Their influence persisted in the Middle Ages. Other schools of medicine emphasized, on the one hand, theory and reason (the Dogmatists) and on the other, pragmatic observation and experience (the Empiricists). The practical therapy of these two schools did not differ greatly. Other cults such as the pneumatists and encyclopedists had considerable, but fleeting, influence. Pliny, the best known and most prolific writer of these cultists, produced an encyclopedia which Durant described as "a lasting tribute to Roman ignorance."

Medical education in the Roman era was haphazard. Many teachers gave informal instruction, others were appointed by the city or state and provided a fixed course in medicine, philosophy, literature, and rhetoric. These professors, often political appointees, were not well versed in the practice of medicine although some renowned physicians gave courses in their special field. The best schools were at Alexandria, Athens, Constantinople, and Antioch; as a result, most Roman physicians spent some time in Alexandria. According to Galen, the instruction in Alexandria was quite superficial, consisting of the teacher reading the old treatises and making occasional personal comments. Apparently, the finest instruction was obtained by an apprenticeship to a well-established physician or surgeon.

Roman Military Medicine

To meet the needs of the Roman legions, a military medical service was developed with surgeons, ambulances, and hospitals stationed near the encampment. Although every soldier had a kit for taking care of minor injuries, more serious wounds of the legionnaires, such as those of the thorax or abdomen or those requiring amputation of a limb, were handled by a surgeon, often a Greek. Their hospital instruments were not unlike those used in the operating room of the early 20th century—spatulas, spoons, droppers, forceps, scarifiers, knives, curettes, stylets, gouges, extractors for foreign bodies, cauteries, needles, and cups for bleeding. Since probing rather than cutting was the practice, pointed steel or bronze instruments and grooved probes were used. The shears had springs rather than hinges. Trephines, hammers, and bone forceps were available for special cases. The wound was usually closed with a few loosely tied sutures. In spite of the skilled physicians, the mortality of battle, and even more the ravages of disease, scurvy, cold, plagues, and malnutrition decimated the ranks of the legions.

Roman Medical Practice

Although the military forces had excellent medical care, the Roman populace, except for the wealthy, were handled by less well-educated or untrained medical practitioners.

The best account of the medical practices of that time came to light when a manuscript entitled *De re medicina* was discovered in a European monastery. It had been written by a well-informed Roman scholar—Celsus, whose literary style was so pleasing that he was dubbed "the medical Cicero." A Roman aristocrat and sciences writer, Aurelius Cornelius Celsus lived in the 1st century BC, and wrote in Latin of agriculture, war, oratory, law, philosophy, and medicine. His writings were not mentioned until a century or so after his death when his text on medicine became popular, only to be lost with the inroads of the Moors. One of his manuscripts was discovered a thousand years later and was one of the early medical texts to be printed. According to Leonardo, Celsus' "anatomical knowledge . . . is not outstanding, his physiology is Hippocratic and his obstetrics is simple. His surgery, however, is excellent." In some matters, Celsus disagreed with the teachings of Hippocrates; for example, the latter advocated trephining for many types of skull fracture, but Celsus stated that only depressed bone should be removed.

Celsus' writings, being in Latin, were popular with the Romans who knew little Greek. They were annotated copies of Hippocratic writings with little neurological content. However, his many references to contemporary physicians and their practices gave a critical appraisal of Roman medicine as well as an account of the beliefs and philosophies of that time.

> At first, the healing art was viewed as a branch of philosophy; for both the treatment of diseases and the study of physics derived their origin from the same founders. . . . Therefore, [history teaches] that many of the philosophers were skilled in medicine, and that the most celebrated were Pythagoras, Empedocles, and Democritus. Hippocrates of Cos was the first to separate this study from that of philosophy. Next came Diocles, the Carystian; shortly afterwards Praxagoras and Chrysippus; and then Herophilus and Erasistratus, who were not merely practitioners, but the originators of different modes of treatment. At this time medicine was divided into three departments, one profession curing by diet, another by

medication, and a third by manipulation. To obtain knowledge of the body and its uses, dissections of the living or dead body was permitted. That dissection of the dead subject, for the thorough examination of intestines and other internal organs, is indispensably requisite; and [moreover] ... Herophilus and Erasistratus dissected such criminals alive, as were delivered over to them from the prisons by royal sanction; carefully observing before they had ceased to breathe, those parts which are by nature concealed ... no one can know the exact seat of an internal pain, if he has not previously made himself well acquainted with each organ and each intestine; that a diseased part cannot be cured by him who knows nothing about it; and that when internal parts are exposed by wounds, one who is ignorant of their healthy character, cannot know whether they are sound or unsound, and if unsound, cannot provide a remedy.

Celsus argued that even external remedies are applied with greater precision after examining the internal parts, and that "it is not cruel, as many assert, to search for remedies for the innocent part of society in all ages, at the expense of torturing a few of the guilty."

I know any person may ask me, how happens it, if the signs of approaching death may be relied upon, that patients given up by their physicians sometimes get well? And that some are reported to have revived, even during the funeral rites? Furthermore, Democritus, a man of well-merited celebrity, has asserted there are in reality no characteristics of death sufficiently certain for physicians to rely upon; much less did he concede, that there could be any sure prognostics of approaching death. In answer to whom, I will not avail myself of the argument that oftentimes cognate symptoms deceive not the skillful, but the unskillful physicians; that Asclepiades meeting a funeral knew that he was alive whom they were submitting to the ceremony of elation; and that the art ought not forthwith to be charged with the errors of its professors; but I will more temperately reply, that medicine is a conjectural art, and such the nature of conjecture, that although in the long run it may more frequently have turned out to be right, it nevertheless may sometimes be fallacious.

Celsus gave an excellent description of wounds of the head, much of which was copied from earlier writers, especially Hippocrates.

After a blow on the head, the immediate inquiry should be whether the person has vomited bile; whether he has lost his sight or his speech; whether blood has been discharged by his nostrils, or by his ears; whether he fell down from the blow; whether he lay insensible and comatose. These are symptoms which do not happen except in a fracture of the skull; and when they occur, we may conclude that an operation is indispensable, although dangerous. But if a torpor has also come on, if there be delirium—if paralysis or convulsion has ensued the probability is that the dura mater is injured, and the case is still more desperate. When, on the other hand, neither of these symptoms accrue, the existence of fracture may be fairly doubted; and our next consideration should be the nature of the weapon with which the blow has been inflicted; whether it be of stone, wood, iron, or some other material;—so again, whether it be smooth or rough, whether of a moderate or of a larger magnitude, whether the blow have been violent or slight; for the less violent the blow, the greater is the probability that the skull may have resisted it. The best plan, however, is to ascertain the fact by a surer sign. To this end, we must search the wound with a probe neither too small nor sharp, lest by entering into some of the natural sinuses, it should mislead us into an opinion of the existence of a fracture; nor should it be too thick, lest small fissures escape it. When the probe has come in contact with the bone, if it meet with a surface entirely smooth and slippery, such surface may be considered sound: if it meet with asperity, and especially if at a part where there are no sutures, it is a proof of fracture. Hippocrates has recorded that even he was deceived by the sutures: thus is it ever with the truly great, whose self-confidence is based on superior acquirements; for little minds dare not detract naught from their own merit, because they have none to spare; while the ingenuous avowal of real error is suited only to a transcendent genius, whose splendour is considerable enough to survive the sacrifice; especially in the performance of a task, which is to be handed down for the benefit of posterity as a beacon-light of truth to warn them against similar errors.

Hence, that we may not be deceived. The safest plan is to expose the bone; for, I have stated above, there is no certainty even in the relative situations of the sutures, and the same part may at once both be naturally joined by suture, and fissured by a blow; or it may have a fissure close by it. Nay, sometimes when the blow has been violent, although nothing have been detected by the probe, it is nevertheless better to expose the part. If no fissure be made evident even by these means, ink is to be applied to the bone, and to be afterwards scraped off with a chisel, for if there be any fissure, it will retain the dye.

The condition of the cranial bones seems to have been the main concern of Celsus and the Roman surgeons, for "cranial fractures, if not reasonably relieved, produce severe inflammation. . . . In all fissures and fractures of the bone, it was customary with the older practitioners to proceed at once to the use of instruments for excision. But it is far better, first to make trial of such plasters as are composed for the calvaria. . . . In this way, fissures are frequently filled up by a sort of callus, which serves as a cicatrix to the bone, and even more extensive fractures are agglutinated by the same callus. . . ."

The extravasation of blood and fluid was recognized as a serious complication. "Rarely . . . the bone remains entire while the internal rupture of some one of the veins of the cerebral membranes occasions hemorrhage (subdural), and the blood coagulating, excites severe pains, and in some cases, blindness." Thus, although the state of the bone was considered a prime factor, it was recognized that the presence of extravasations of blood or fluid within the intracranial cavity was a matter of serious consequence. However, Celsus did not mention the condition of the brain substance.

Surgery at that time was at a low ebb; operations upon the head and spine were rarely performed even by the few skilled surgeons. However, some physicians of that era were making interesting observations of neurological disorders, especially epileptic attacks. One was a celebrated pneumatist of the late first century, Aretaeus of Cappadocia, whose writings were so embellished and so repetitious of the Hippocratic works that they have been deprecated, but who nevertheless gives a colorful description of epilepsy.

> If the paroxysm be near, there are flashes before the eyes, as of purple or dark hues, or of all colours simultaneously blended "like the chequered bent of Iris' bow." The ears ring, there is a perception of heavy odours, an unusual irritability and wrathfulness. Some fall to the ground from mere prostration of mind, others from looking intently on a running stream, a top spinning round, or a wheel revolving; sometimes a disagreeable odour, as that of the gagate stone, over sets them. Occasionally the malady is fixed in the head, and that is the starting point of the paroxysm; in other cases it begins in the nerves, which are most remote from the head, and which sympathize with the part first affected.
>
> In these cases the thumbs or great toes become contracted; pain, torpor, and tremor succeed, and rush upward to the head. If the head be reached, the patient feels a crack as if from the blow of a stone, or a block of wood, and when he hath arisen he exclaims that he has been smitten.

One can recognize by putting this description in modern garb, the visual and auditory aura, photogenic precipitation of the attack, onset of the attack in the thumb or the great toe, abortion of the attack by peripheral stimulation such as tying a string about the twitching member, tonic spasm preceding the clonic phase, involuntary urination and defecation, profuse salivation and the eventual stupor when the spasms ceased. However, Aretaeus does end on a metaphysical note: "It seems to attack those who offend the moon and hence the disease is termed 'sacred' or it may be from other reasons, either from its magnitude [for what is great is sacred] or from the cure not being in the power of man but of God, or from the notion that a demon has entered the patient, or from all put together, that it has been so called."

Aretaeus clearly defined apoplexy as a paralysis of the whole body involving perception, understanding, and power of motion. Paraplegia was the loss of sense of feeling and power of motion of a part of the body. Loss of the sense of feeling, a rare occurrence, was termed "anaisthesia." Paresis was the inability to control the urinary bladder. Aretaeus clearly differentiated the types of paralysis resulting from spinal cord and brain involvement. "If any part . . . be attacked such as the covering of the spinal cord, continuous parts of the same name become paralysed, thus the right and left sides are involved as the right or left of the spine happens to be afflicted. If the attack originates in the head, the left parts become paralysed when its [brain] right side is affected . . . this is caused by the interlacement of the nerves, for those on the right side do not proceed in a direct line as far as the extremities, but uniting at their origin, each immediately attaches itself to one opposite in the manner of our letter X."

Aretaeus states that the nerves of the head have a different arrangement from those of the spine. If injured, they are likely to produce loss of sensation but not of motor power, a remarkable observation. He also noted the varying size of the pupil in disease, although he did not understand its significance.

In a chapter on headache, Aretaeus gives a clear description of migraine and hemicrania. Probably he is describing a case of subarachnoid hemorrhage when he asserts "the patient . . . has a sudden pain in the back of the neck as if smitten by the blow of a stick, has a feeling of nausea, vomits bilious matter, and falls down, and if the disorder gets worse, dies." This observant physician described many neurological conditions which modern writers have attributed to later authors.

Soranus, renowned for his work in obstetrics and gynecology, made some astute observations on neurological disorders. He considered epilepsy as arising from the meninges and wrote that Aesclepiades attributed epilepsy to "a blow, especially one which penetrates the membranes." Soranus noted that a bright light might bring on an attack. He treated the condition with diet, attention to the bowels, a peaceful routine, and avoidance of excesses and rejected the more drastic therapies of the times, such as diuretics and cathartics.

Soranus was aware of the manifestations of tetanus. He observed that it occurred when a wound was healing and was characterized by stiffness of the neck, clenching of the teeth, and difficulty swallowing. He gave an excellent description of hydrophobia—its inception 40 days after a mad dog bite with intense thirst but fear of drinking water, a rapid and feeble pulse, and fever and vomiting preceding death. He disparaged "those who suggest these futile and cruel treatments . . . for the disease is acute, swift, violent, and practically always continuous." Soranus recognized that sufferers from vertigo fell suddenly but got up immediately, thus differentiating it from an epileptic attack as the patient neither lost consciousness nor convulsed. However, some writers implied that there might be slight impairment of consciousness and referred to vertigo as "a little epilepsy." Paralysis, sciatica, apoplexy, and headache were all discussed much by the Hippocratic physicians.

In the writings of Aurelianus, the description of sciatica is excellent. After noting the many precipitating factors, such as exposure to cold, trauma, and excessive exertion, the author describes the clinical findings:

> These diseases occur in all ages, but more frequently among the middle-aged. In sciatica, there is pain in one or both hips; in the latter case many call the disease "double sciatica." There is also a feeling of heaviness and unusual difficulty in moving about; in some cases a slight numbness and a creeping irritation of the skin, sometimes with a severe pricking and burning pain which gives the patient the sensation of a creeping animal's tortuous motion. . . . The pain begins in the hip and then moves through the affected side; it reaches the middle of the gluteal region and the upper inguinal region, or passes to the bend of the knee and the

calf, and then even to the ankle and the extremity of the foot.

Later, when the disease becomes chronic, the whole leg becomes thin with the loss of nourishment. . . . It is accompanied by weakness in the leg and by a shortening thereof because of a contraction of the parts. . . . Some walk on tiptoe, others with body erect but with the back so arched that they are unable to bend forward; still others have their bodies drawn and bent.

Galenic Contributions to Neuroscience

The most outstanding and productive of the early Christian physicians was Galen, a Greek born in Pergamon, Asia Minor in 130 AD. Galen's father, an architect, was broadly educated and his mother was noted for her temper and violent speech. After a general education, at the age of 17, Galen began his medical training at the Esklepieion of Pergamon, after which he traveled to other centers eventually reaching Alexandria. He spent five not very stimulating years there. "The art of medicine was taught by ignoramuses . . . in long illogical lectures." While there, he compiled a five-volume dictionary of medical terms which unfortunately has been lost. Although he disliked the teaching, it afforded him ample time to study anatomy, especially of the abundant human bones.

At the age of 28, Galen returned to Pergamon. There he developed a method of repairing nerves and tendons, which in those days were not differentiated. The precise Greek description of his technique is not clear, but probably consisted of an aseptic or mildly antiseptic dressing made of flour cooked in oil and applied to permit the wound to heal by first intention. Previously, surgeons treating such wounds with hot water and a dressing cooked in oil and water had many wounds rupture and the patient die. As a result of his successful treatment, Galen attracted the attention of the Pontifex of the city and was offered the position of surgeon to the games held at the arena. This gave him the opportunity to treat many wounds, for the contestants in the gladiatorial bouts and chariot races often sustained serious injuries. Extensive head, limb, and abdominal wounds, which previously had been considered fatal, Galen repaired with his conservative technique and the victims recovered without inflammation or suppuration. He wrote that "even large ones [wounds] reach the stage of being practically healed in two to four days without inflammation." To repair a laceration of the quadriceps tendon, a wound that mounted gladiators sustained as the result of a transverse slash above the patella, Galen sutured the cut ends together. This unique repair was so successful that the victims recovered without the crippling disability that previous gladiators, if they survived such wounds, had suffered.

As physician to the gladiators, in addition to many abdominal and extremity wounds, Galen saw all types of head injuries. To render the victims unconscious so that such wounds could be closed, it seems probable that some anesthetic agent such as opium, mandragora or hyoscyamus was administered. Although Galen does not specifically so state, other surgeons of that time—Isadorus and Serpion—mention their use as anesthetic agents.

Apparently, Galen followed the Hippocratic treatment advocated in *On wounds of the head* and did not suture extensive scalp wounds, but dried them with soft linen soaked in freshly boiled wine (sapa). With this technique, he reported that many cases recovered.

For five sessions (about four years), Galen was surgeon to the gladiators at Pergamon. Then war with the Parthians took many of the young men to battle and put an end to the games. In early 163 AD, about a year and a half after the beginning of the Parthian War at a time when the Roman forces were driving the Parthians back into Asia Minor, Galen left Pergamon and went to Rome to practice medicine. At first, his critical comments regarding the teachings of several medical sects active in the city incurred considerable animosity; however, he rapidly gained fame and was appointed physician to the Emperor. In the next 30 years, Galen built a large practice and at the same time, carried on his writing and physiological experimentation.

When Galen was about to be given a royal appointment, which he feared would curtail his clinical and his investigational work in Rome, he returned to Pergamon. Shortly thereafter, the Emperors Marcus Aurelius and Lucius Verus requested that he return to Rome. He did not wish an appointment in the army, so he was assigned to attend Lucius Verus' son. In this capacity, he could continue his scientific work and writing. Although his reputation as a physician increased, he lost favor with many of the sectarians. Unfortunately, in 192 AD, while Galen was in the process of having his manuscript "published," a fire in the Temple of Peace destroyed the later books (XII-XV) of his works. Galen had the original notes for these books from which he made another revision before his death. This revision, which contained much neurological material, was available to the Arabs until the 9th century but then the text after the beginning of Book XI was lost until the 19th century, when two manuscripts of Hunain ibn Ishaq's Arabic translation (from Syriac) were found. An English translation was prepared by Duckworth.

Many books which appeared in Rome in Galen's name were probably spurious, but sufficient manuscripts in his handwriting have come down through the ages to establish their authenticity and his scientific stature.

Galen's anatomical knowledge was derived from dissection of apes, hogs, and other animals, although, in Alexandria, he may have dissected a human body. Certainly, while there, he had access to human skeletons so that he had a clear idea of the bones of the cranium and the vertebral column. Galen considered the cerebrospinal cavity to contain the noblest of the faculties, the animal faculty or the reasoning and the immortal soul. In the upper and anterior part of the cranial cavity was the brain, an oval mass gray on the surface but white inside. It was divided into two halves, or hemispheres, by a very deep longitudinal furrow. Beneath and behind the hemispheres was the cerebellum, or small brain, whose substance was scarcely a fourth of the whole brain. Connecting the two was a band of tissue which was continuous with the spinal cord. This description of the brain seems to be that of a lower animal, probably the ox, rather than that of man.

Galen noted that when a portion of the cranial vault was removed, the brain of a living animal alternately rose and fell, similar to the movements of the lung. Consequently, he thought that the brain expanded to draw in air and contracted to expel it. Thus, the atmospheric substance entered the cavity of the cranium through the cribriform plate and the excremental humors of the brain passed out through the nose and throat. But the air introduced into the cephalic cavity during inspiration was not entirely rejected by expiration; a portion insinuated itself into the anterior ventricles of the brain and united with the vital spirits which were carried there by the vessels of the choroid plexus. In this way, the animal spirits were formed and acquired their final attenuation in the fourth ventricle, which they reached through the round, narrow, vermiform tube (the aqueduct of Sylvius). The animal spirits entered the substance of the brain, the little brain, and the spinal marrow to be distributed by the nerves to all parts of the body, giving each region whatever was required for its activities.

Although Galen made brilliant studies of the functions of the spinal cord, his experimental techniques of sectioning were not so applicable to the brain; as a result, his knowledge of that structure and its coverings was little advanced from that of the Alexandrian scientists. His knowledge of neuroanatomy, based on the brains of oxen, barbary apes, and, perhaps, an occasional human corpse, encompassed the coverings of the brain, the gross configuration of the hemispheres, and its ventricles and their connections. He recognized seven pairs of cranial nerves and the nerves of the spinal cord with sensory and motor components. His most brilliant studies made on the spinal cord were the definitions of the motor and sensory deficits produced by transection of the spinal cord at various levels.

Although Galen had no agent to produce anesthesia and immobilize an animal, he found he was able to eliminate the squealing of the pig by cutting the recurrent laryngeal nerve. Thus, in peace, he could distinguish motor and sensory nerves and describe the physiological effects of sectioning the spinal cord at various levels.

Galen gave a precise account for removing the brain and a clear description of the cranial nerves recognized at that time. He described an "interlacement of the arteries" at the base of the brain, to form the rete mirabile. He noted that compression of the anterior ventricles produced only a slight stupor, but if the middle ventricle was compressed, the stupor was deeper, and if the ventricle at the nape of the neck was compressed, the animal developed a "heavy and pronounced stupor." Recovery was complete after anterior ventricular compression, but if the posterior ventricle was compressed or incised, the animal seldom recovered.

Although Herophilus had affirmed that the spinal cord, which was connected to the rhombencephalon, gave rise to the nerves, Galen first defined its functions. He wrote: "if the marrow did now wholly exist, one of two things would result; either all of the parts of the animal located below the head would be completely deprived of movement, or it would be absolutely necessary that a nerve descend directly from the brain to each part." Galen noted the protective coverings of the cord (bone, intervertebral discs, and pia mater) as well as the anterior spinal ligament, which he wrote was attached on each side to "the cartilage that lubricates the vertebrae. Both membranes of the cord resemble exactly the appearance of those that entirely envelop the brain, except that in the spine there is no space between them such as in the head; the differences are, therefore, that the dura mater touches and envelops all the pia mater and a very strong and very fibrous third tunic envelops them exteriorly." And Galen goes on, "in accordance with the sequence of the vertebrae, the nerves spring out on both sides of them, and the nerve roots pass out through perfectly rounded foramina, the width of each single foramen corresponding to the thickness of the nerve which passes through it."

To determine the use or function of the segments of the spinal cord, Galen cut the spinal cord at each vertebra and observed the state of the animal. He made the transverse cut between two vertebrae by rocking the knife to and fro in the "marrow" so as to leave no part of the spinal "marrow" undivided. He noted that "the capacity of sensation and the capacity of movement" below such a section were lost.

Galen wrote:

> The incision which is made behind the first vertebra paralyses the feet of the animal, and arrests the whole of its respiration. And this is found also with regard to the incision which is made behind the second, third, and fourth vertebra, when in making the cut you go to work thoroughly, so that you divide the nerve which springs off at its [fourth vertebra's] junction with the fifth. However, the first [i.e., upper] segments of the neck still move themselves in the animal on which the cut has been made in such a manner. Transection of the spinal marrow behind the fifth vertebra paralyses all the remaining parts of the thorax, and arrests their movements, but the diaphragm remains almost unscathed, and so also does a small portion of the upwardly ascending part of the musculature of the thorax. The transection which takes place behind the sixth vertebra damages in the same way the upwardly ascending thoracic musculature, and the diaphragm meets with less damage than that which followed in consequence of the preceding cut. But after the transection which takes place behind the seventh vertebra, and more particu-

larly after that made behind the eighth vertebra, the whole of the mobility of the diaphragm remains unscathed, and indeed in most instances still more so than is the case after the cut behind the sixth vertebra. Again the mobility of the upwardly ascending musculature, and the mobility of the whole neck will remain quite free from damage, but the intercostal muscles do not at the same time remain uninjured thereby. For the mobility of this musculature is destroyed and becomes totally lost when one imposes the cut upon any one of the vertebrae of the neck, and the whole hind-brain is cut off from the first thoracic vertebra. Amongst the proofs of that is the fact that the activity of the intercostal muscles becomes totally lost when one carries through the spinal medulla behind the first thoracic vertebra a cut which completely divides it, whereas a slight proportion of this activity stays retained when the cut takes place behind the second vertebra.

What precise observations! Moreover, Galen extended his studies to hemisection and longitudinal cuts of the spinal cord.

> Transverse incisions of the cord that reach only to its center do not paralyze all the lower parts but only the parts situated directly below the incision; the right when the right is cut, and the left when the left is cut.
>
> If one cuts the spinal cord along the median line from above downwards, there is no resultant paralysis of the intercostal nerves nor of those of the right or the left side, even in the lumbar region or in the legs.

Considering that he was making his studies on the pig, he may be forgiven for not examining the sensory disturbances after these cuts.

Galen followed the Hippocratic concept of "nature" or the inherent power of an object or person to cause it to act in a specific manner. As he conceived it, all matter was composed of four elements (earth, air, fire, and water) which might have any of four qualities (hot, cold, dry, or moist). The body had four humors—blood, phlegm, yellow bile, and black bile—which might be affected by any of the qualities. Thus Galen, once he had established the location of a diseased tissue, only considered qualitative and humoral etiological factors.

Galen's views on the causation and mechanisms involved in epilepsy were bound up in his concepts of humors and are of little interest. He distinguished three forms of epilepsy, one due to idiopathic or primary disease of the brain, a second the result of sympathetic involvement of the brain from the heart, and a third due to a disturbance of the brain in sympathy with another part of the body.

Galen described epilepsy as an impairment of consciousness associated with convulsive movements of the whole body. The attack might be initiated by a warning or aura consisting of various sensory and motor phenomena.

> It is a convulsion of all parts of the body, not continuous as tetanus, but occurring in an attack. There is loss of consciousness and of the senses which proves clearly that the site of the condition may be in the cerebrum.

Galen distinguishes those attacks which followed a primary affliction of the brain and those which were sympathetic. Although Aretaeus had described the spread of a focal (Jacksonian) epilepsy, Galen's description was more detailed. "The affliction begins in any limb, then ascends to the head clearly aware to the patient. A child related how the attack began in the leg, ascended the thigh, the side of the body to the neck and when it reached the face, consciousness was lost. This patient could not describe the sensation but another young man stated that it felt like a fresh breeze—the Greek term 'aura.'" Thus, Galen applied the term aura to all phenomena ushering in an attack.

Those seizures which involved only the limbs, Galen maintained, originated in the spinal cord, and those which involved the face arose in the brain. It is not clear from Galen's writings whether he knew of or believed in the contralateral influence of the cerebral hemispheres, although this concept was certainly known to Hippocrates whose teachings, in general, Galen accepted. The epileptic attack was considered to be due to a thick viscid humor or phlegm injuring the brain either by altering its constitution or by obstructing the psychic pneuma causing it to accumulate in the ventricles.

Galen advised different therapies for the various types of epilepsy. In the case of an ascending aura, he purged the patient, bound the affected limb, and applied a stinging medication such as mustard to the limb. In the case of sympathetic epilepsy, which originated from the heart, he prescribed a carefully prepared wheat bread to be taken in the morning with diluted and slightly astringent white wine. Two or three times a year the patient should be purged with bitter olives to relieve the stomach of excess material. In the case of the third type of epilepsy, the phlegmatic humor should be evacuated by purgative medications or bleeding. The patient was to lead a temperate life, avoiding excesses in eating and drinking. Although Galen scorned therapies based upon superstitions such as hare's rennet, ass' liver, or amulets made of stones found in the stomach of swallows at the waxing moon, he was not without gullibilities for he wrote that he knew of patients who were free of attacks for months when wearing a peony as an amulet and yet when it was removed immediately had seizures again. Accordingly, he stated, "it was not logical to assume either that certain particles of the root fell out, were sucked in by inspiration, and did thus heed the affected part—or that the air itself was tempered and changed by the root."

Galen did give a description of his operating conduct—the personal preparation of the surgeon, his clothing, fingernails, position of the patient and the surgeon, the lighting of the operative field, as well as the position of the surgical instruments. These included knives of different sizes, hammers, chisels with either a flat or curved cutting edge and a lenticular knob to prevent cutting through the dura mater, drills, trephines, elevators, and blunt dissectors. Although for opening the skull he preferred the mallet and a chisel with a knob to prevent plunging, occasionally Galen used the trephine or collared drill to avert penetrating too deeply. When fragments were depressed, he removed the loose pieces. In 196 AD, he stated that he had seen many compound fractures of the skull heal. That he had operated upon these patients is not clear for, in his later years in Rome, apparently he did little surgery. Most of his activities were at the Court and in writing.

Galen's comments about his contemporaries—surgeons and anatomists—were often uncomplimentary. He believed that their writings were "full of errors." This may have been the reason that his work was not acclaimed until some time after his death.

Galen wrote freely of his medical practice. Of neurological interest are several common disorders. Under the heading of melancholia, Galen included depressions, obsessive compulsions, neuroses, and phobias, all of biliary origin, but in some the bile involved all the blood and in others, only that of the brain. The differentiation was considered important, for if the entire body contained bilious blood, bleeding was indicated, but if only the brain had such blood, bleeding was not imperative.

Headache was considered to be of several types. Vertigo, a type of headache, was due to vapors and hot pneuma which ascended in the arteries to overfill the brain. On the other hand, migraine, provoked by odors such as incense and also originating from a hot pneuma and vapor, was a constant headache, difficult to relieve, during which the sufferer could not tolerate noise (even low voices), bright lights, or movements in the surroundings, but sought a darkened room. The pain felt like the blows of a hammer or, at times, was described as compressing or bursting the head. It might involve both eyeballs or be limited to one side of the head.

Hysteria, at the time of Galen, connoted a condition thought to arise from the uterus due to the retention of the female sperm. It was characterized by respiratory distress, sometimes referred to as uterine apnea, impaired motor power or sensation, faintness, and feeble pulse. Other than the name, the state had little in common with the "grande hysterie" of modern times. Galen's therapy, not specific for neurological disorders, consisted of sleep, work, food, baths, exercise, psychotherapy, and drugs acquired during his travels.

The remarkable neurological concepts of Galen, however, were marred by a few outstanding misconceptions of his day. These included: the failure to differentiate nerves and similarly appearing tendinous structures; the notion of a communication between the cerebral ventricles and the nasopharynx; and the misinterpretation of the role of the cerebral vessels.

Galen conceived of the blood carrying nutrients coming from the liver through the vena cava to the jugular vein into the dural sinuses and then to the brain. His description of the cerebral arteries was more accurate but he believed that they contained not nutrients, but only the pneumas which, passing through the rete mirabile, reached the ventricles and the nerves. A further misconception was his interpretation of the vascular system. He believed that the spirit or pneuma was drawn in from the world by respiration through the trachea, and passed to the pulmonary vein and the left ventricle of the heart. Through the aorta, the pneuma reached the liver, which formed venous blood from the chyle that had entered it from the portal vein. The liver was the center of the venous system and endowed the blood with a particular pneuma or natural spirit. The blood, charged with this natural spirit and with nutritive substances derived from the intestines, was distributed by the liver to ebb and flow throughout the venous system.

The venous blood also passed through the vena cava into the right side of the heart, where impurities were discharged through the pulmonary artery into the lungs and exhaled. The purified blood then ebbed back into the venous system. Part of the venous blood in the right ventricle passed through imperceptible small channels in the interventricular septum, where it came into contact with the air which had entered the left ventricle from the lungs through the pulmonary vein. Here, in contact with the pneuma which had been drawn in from the world spirit, it was transformed into the highly refined vital spirit which was distributed through the arteries. The cerebral arteries carried this vital spirit which, in the brain, became an animal spirit to be passed through the nerves to the various organs of the body. Diastole was considered as the active phase of the heart's action, systole the passive phase. During diastole, the heart drew air into the left ventricle and blood into the right, while, in systole, it collapsed and drove both air and blood outward.

Galen stated that all arteries arise from the aorta and that they contain not air but blood. He described the function of the heart valves correctly and noted that the pulmonary valves prevented the blood expelled by the right ventricle into the pulmonary artery from flowing back into the right ventricle. He stated clearly, that "not only may blood be transmitted from the pulmonary artery to the pulmonary veins (through the lungs), but then into the left ventricle and from there to the arteries." Galen was also convinced that there were anastomoses between terminal arteries and terminal veins, remarking, "If you will kill an animal by cutting through a number of its large arteries, you will find the veins becoming empty along with the arteries—now this could never occur if there were not anastomoses between them." Yet, he failed to understand the circulation of the blood.

Garrison noted additional Galenic misconceptions, the idea of "coction" or suppuration as an essential stage in wound healing, which prevented the introduction of primary repair of wounds. By his rather blunt and undiplomatic manner, Galen made many enemies among his contemporary physicians, so that his work was not taken very seriously during his lifetime, but his fame grew with time. It was enhanced when Emperor Julian had Oribasius edit and reproduce many of Galen's works, especially his therapeutics. That the church accepted his theories meant that his manuscripts were preserved, assuring that later generations would have the benefit of his genius. Moreover, the approval of the Church meant that any doubts cast on his concepts were considered sacrilegious and combatted with religious fervor.

In the years after Galen, the Roman Empire slipped from its exalted military position. During the 4th to the 7th centuries, few surgeons ventured to operate upon the head or spine. Oribasius at the behest of Emperor Julian wrote an encyclopedic work in Latin incorporating the teachings of the earlier physicians, especially those of Galen. This 70-volume treatise contained accurate extracts from many early medical writers and, although only a third was preserved, has served as a valuable source of material. Another critical compiler, Aëtius of Amida, born on the Tigris, was the first Christian physician to write on surgical subjects. He described paralysis of the soft palate following a sore throat, presumably post-diphtheritic paralysis. As Aëtius lived in the Eastern region, he was acquainted with a number of Chinese drugs such as cloves and camphor which he introduced to the western pharmacopeia. At about the same time, Alexander of Tralles, after acquiring an extensive medical experience in many lands, established a flourishing practice in Rome. He was perhaps the greatest physician of his time, but his extensive treatises, translated into several languages, did not advance knowledge of the nervous system. Although an erudite follower of Galen, he did not hesitate to prescribe, in desperate cases, magical remedies considered to have great curative powers.

Probably the most prolific writer of the Byzantine period was Paulus Aeginata, who lived in the 7th century. Although an experienced surgeon, Paul made sketchy references to trephining. Such evidence of the disrepute into which that operation had fallen was confirmed by the observation that few of the later great Arab surgeons knew how to trephine. Paul, who lived in Alexandria, wrote a compendium of the medical practices of the period which, although it added nothing original, was consulted for almost a thousand years. None of the late Roman physicians, although noted in their day, advanced either the knowledge of the nervous system nor the treatment of neurological disorders.

Yet this decline was not peculiar to medicine but merely an indication of the general corruption of the Roman Empire—a decay further evidenced by certain legal restrictions imposed upon physicians in the 5th century. The Visigothic Code decreed that "the physician . . . had to make a contract and give pledges and, if his patient died, he got no fee, if he injured a nobleman in venesection, he had to pay 100 solidi (about $225); if the nobleman died, the physician was turned over to the relatives of the deceased to be dealt with as they pleased. If he killed or injured a slave, he had to replace him by one of equal value."

As the influence of the Roman Empire declined, Byzantinum, a city on the Bosphorus founded about the 7th century BC, was selected by Constantine the Great to be the Nova Roma and in 330 AD was dedicated as the capital of the Eastern Roman Empire. Within two centuries, this beautiful, naturally fortified city, renamed Constantinople, became a metropolis of almost a million people. Although it developed into a cultural center with distinctive architectural motifs and attractive art, the city was frequently attacked by marauding tribes from the north and west which the Roman garrisons had difficulty repelling, especially when the Empire was disintegrating. Science and medicine could not thrive in such an environment and as a result it did not generate the medical advances nor outstanding physicians such as graced Rome earlier.

The Status of the Nervous System in Other Regions

During the Roman era, health care in remote parts of the world was at a primitive level. Little information is available of the medical practices in the Americas, Australia, Africa, and the South Sea Islands. Even the bones of people in these lands—especially the skull—give little evidence of the surgical prowess of these people and of the rationale for their medical practices.

2

From Galen Through
the 18th Century:
An Overview

Revival of the Medical Arts from
the 6th to the 13th Centuries

After the fall of the Roman Empire in the 5th century, communal life in Europe decayed. Except in major centers such as Rome, Constantinople, and Alexandria, where heads of state and the wealthy supported personal physicians, medical practice fell into the hands of poorly educated and inexperienced artisans. Consequently, the populace turned to the Church for the care of their common ailments. Since the available therapies—baths, herbs, exhortations to drive away the evil spirits, and minor surgical procedures—were simple, the clergy could take care of both the physical and spiritual needs of the people. But, as invading hordes of Ostrogoths from the north threatened the declining power of the military, the monks congregated in the monasteries of Monte Cassino, Benevente, and Squilace with medical manuscripts written in Latin scripts as well as in Greek and classical Latin. Later, when the Moslems invaded the Mediterranean coast, burning and destroying the art and literature in Alexandria and the East, these works were preserved in Church vaults and homes of the nobles. However, between the 5th and 14th centuries, there were several notable figures who introduced and carried on the practice of medicine.

As the conquerors craved to acquire the culture, literature, and health practices of their serfs, some Latin and Greek manuscripts were translated into Arabic and Syriac. Arab physicians, schooled in the ancient languages, translated and inserted the teachings of Hippocrates and some Roman physicians into their writings. In both the East and West, schools of translators were

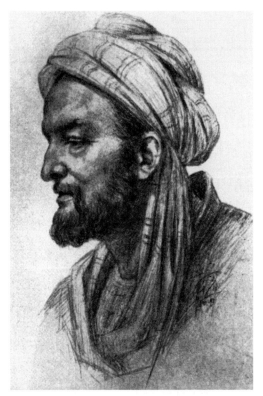

Fig. 2-1. The famous Arab physician, Rhazes. (From the collection of A. Earl Walker)

established to make the Greek and Roman writings available to cultured Moslems, thus preserving the treasures of the ancients.

It has been said that the Moslems had little knowledge of medicine, particularly of the basic sciences. Although dissection was banned and animal experimentation unlawful, the Arabs did know something of the workings of the human body. In the *Arabian Nights*,* a slave girl's account of the structure and functions of the brain exemplifies the learning of that time. In this tale, perhaps of the 10th century, the girl tells how man is made, the composition of the head, spine, and the ventricles of the brain; the latter were considered to subserve common sense, imagination, thought, perception, and memory. If this girl's knowledge of the nervous system is an indication of the Arabian understanding of the brain and spinal cord, it was more advanced than commonly thought.

A review of the Arab physicians of that time confirms the impression that the practice of medicine was not as decadent as some historians believed. After the Eastern caliphate was moved to Baghdad in 750 AD, Rhazes (Fig. 2-1), considered the greatest physician of that time, wrote a manuscript entitled *Liber continens* which contained some writings of Paul of Aegina, Hippocrates, Oribasius, and Aetius, along with an account of his own experiences. In it, Rhazes described his medical practices and, for the first time, referred to the use of mercury ointment for pediculosis, catgut sutures for closing wounds, and the cystic masses on the backs of infants, later termed spina bifida. His text was so popular that it was published when printing became available and editions appeared as late as 1886.

---

* A collection of about 200 folktales from Arabia, Egypt, India, Persia, and other countries. John Payne and Sir Richard F. Burton wrote English translations in the 1880s.

Following Rhazes, another great Persian sage, Haly Abbas, is well known because his system of medicine, written in Arabic, was translated into Latin by Constantinus Africanus without an acknowledgment of the author. Although it gives a clear and somewhat critical account of Arabic medicine at that time, it contains nothing of note concerning the nervous system.

At the turn of the millennium, another famous Arab physician, Ali al-Hussein ibn Sina, or Avicenna (980-1037), wrote prolifically in somewhat florid prose on many subjects, including medicine. Born near Bokara, he precociously acquired medical and ecclesiastical knowledge from reading in the Sultan's library. Later, Avicenna wrote 20 books on philosophy, theology, astronomy, and poetry, and many more on medicine, some of which have been termed "scribbling." However, he meticulously codified all aspects of medicine, except the inferior art of surgery, in a voluminous text entitled *The canon of medicine*, a work which served as the basis of medical teaching in European schools for 700 years. He described a number of neurological states—central and peripheral facial palsy, pupillary reactions, and facial pain—and differentiated between meningitis and meningism.

In western Europe at the beginning of the 8th century, Islamic forces under the Caliph Walid overran the Mediterranean coast of Africa, conquering Sicily and parts of Spain. The Moors established a Western caliphate in Cordoba, a small community which rapidly became a literary and scientific center with hospitals and a library of 125,000 Arabic manuscripts. A number of famous physicians and surgeons practiced there. Albucasis (936-1013), an outstanding Moslem surgeon, wrote a treatise divided into medical and surgical sections based upon the works of Paul of Aegina with the earliest, although rather crude, illustrations of surgical instruments (Fig. 2-2). He described operations on the cranium to treat fractures by removing fragmented bone using an elevator, lenticular, and spoon, or by making a series of small perforations in the skull and cutting the intervening bone with a curved saw so the fragment might be removed. In addition to discussing skull fractures, Albucasis wrote of spinal injuries, noting the resultant paralysis. His manuscript, composed in the early part of the 11th century, was the only surgical text of that period and was quoted by Italian surgeons until the time of Guy de Chauliac. When printing was introduced, the book went through a number of editions in several European languages.

In the 12th century, two other physicians, Avenzoar and Averroës, practiced in Cordoba. Avenzoar did some surgery, but Averroës, better known as a philosopher than as a physician, is remembered for his *Commentary on Aristotle*. The surgeons of Cordoba—Albucasis and Avenzoar—admitted that they did not trephine for depressed skull fractures as the Greek masters had advised. If the illustrations of their trephines are a faithful representation of the instruments available, their aversion is quite understandable. Also growing up in

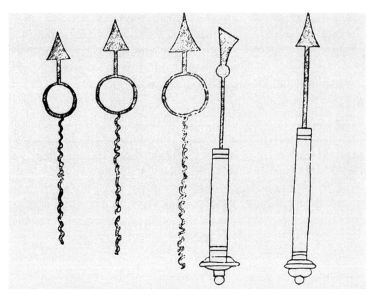

*Fig. 2-2. Instruments used by Arabic surgeons to treat skull injuries and to
perform trephination. (From the collection of A. Earl Walker)*

Cordoba in the 12th century was Maimonides, the greatest physician of the
medieval Jews. When he was 13 years of age, Maimonides and his family were
given the choice of conversion to Islam, death, or banishment, by a sect of
Mohammedans who had captured Cordoba. The family chose wisely and went
to Fez in Morocco. Later, they moved to Cairo, a city of culture, where Maimonides became physician to members of the Sultan's family. In spite of a busy
practice, he managed to write on medicine and other subjects in Arabic with
Hebrew characters. Perhaps this is why he is better known for his religious
commentaries, especially that on "mishra Torah," than his medical treatises.

Another Moslem physician, Ibn-al-Nafis, born in 1210 and educated in
Damascus, moved to Cairo and taught at Mansoury Medical School. In a
commentary on Avicenna's doctrines, Ibn-al-Nafis described in remarkably
clear language the lesser circulation, some 300 years before Michael Servetus
was burned at the stake for his heretical ideas on the subject.

It is also essential that there be in the heart of man, and other animals possess-
ing lungs, another cavity in which the blood is rarefied to be fit for mixing with air.
For if air were mixed with blood when thick, a homogeneous compound could not
result. This cavity is the right cavity of the two cavities of the heart.

After the blood has been rarefied in this cavity, it must of necessity pass to the
left cavity, where the animal spirit is generated. But there is no opening, as some
thought there was between these two cavities, for the septum of the heart is water-

tight without any apparent fenestration in it. Nor, as held by Galen, would an invisible opening be suitable for the passage of this blood, for the pores of the heart are not patent and its septum is thick. The blood, therefore, after thinning, passes via the vena arterialis [pulmonary artery] to the lung for circulation and mixes with air in the pulmonary parenchyma. The aerated blood gets refined and passes through the arteriavenalis [pulmonary vein] to reach the left cavity of the two cavities of the heart, after having mixed with the air and become suitable for the evolution of the animal spirit.

That Ibn-al-Nafis made experimental studies to verify his conclusions seems unlikely. If he had, perhaps his hypothesis would have been readily accepted.

Without anatomical dissection, the Arabian physician's knowledge of the structure and functions of the human body, especially the nervous system, remained at the Galenic level. Surgery was regarded by Moslem physicians as unclean, and as a result, even well-trained surgeons, believing that coction and laudable pus were essential to the healing process, avoided operating upon the head. However, the Arab physicians knew of numerous drugs acquired from the Chinese and Hindus—ambergris, camphor, cassia, cloves, myrrh, nutmeg, senna, and sandalwood oil—as well as the Western pharmacopoeia compiled centuries previously by Diskorides. The preparation of these medications was enhanced by the use of vehicles such as syrups, juleps, alcohol, and tragacanth. With these medications as well as splendid hospitals for the care of the sick and innovative methods of teaching students, the Moslem practice of medical care was quite advanced.

The Arabic schools of Spain introduced dialectic tournaments in which both students and teachers participated. This "scholastica disputatio" may have been the basis for the later formal defense of a dissertation. After the proposition had been stated, a negative reply was presented and argued on both logical and, particularly, religious grounds. This public debate in which both professors and students participated unquestionably brightened the previously dull medical lectures.

When freed from the Moslem yoke, Christian and Hebrew philosophers and physicians acknowledged the contributions of Islamic medicine. Through the translations of ancient medical manuscripts in Toledo, the Arabs, although hated by the masses for their cruelty, disseminated improved medical practices in Europe and fostered the medical talents of their subjects more than they are given credit. They contributed many new concepts of pharmaceutical and apothecary practices from China and India and constructed hospitals for the care of the sick and for medical instruction which were not improved upon for centuries.

In the countries outside of the Roman Empire, such as France, the low countries, England, and Germany, the medical practices in the 6th to 11th centuries—the Dark Ages—have often been considered barbaric. True, the care of the sick was based either upon supernatural healing by Christian saints, relics, charms, and magical incantations, or upon empiric herbals or surgical and dietary therapy. Yet this unscientific treatment for ailing young folks was often effective. Aside from blood-letting, performed by physicians in the Middle Ages before the time of barber-surgeons, operative procedures consisted of simple incision and bandaging—quite within the capabilities of the monks. Along the Mediterranean coast where the Roman influence still prevailed, monastery clerics, with a few herbals, diet, and blood-letting, took care of the common ailments of the peasants. When the Crusaders were active, medical practice began to advance.

On the shores of the Mediterranean Sea, bathed in sun and warm waters, spas and health resorts were established at the beginning of the 9th century. At Salerno, noted for its invigorating baths, fable has it that four physicians, a Greek, Latin, Arab, and Jew, formed a secular health clinic staffed by physicians from Spain, trained in Greek medicine somewhat tainted by passing through Arabic hands. The Crusaders from the East as well as prominent Romans came to Salerno for convalescent care. A medical school, quite independent of the Church, blossomed in the next century. Captured by Robert Guiscard in 1046, Constantinus Africanus brought medical manuscripts written in Arabic to Salerno. With some knowledge of Arabic, Latin, and Greek, he was able to translate the Arabic texts, many of which contained fragments of ancient manuscripts. His principal work was the translation into Latin of an Arabic treatise, presumably written by Haly Abbas, although the author is not mentioned, entitled *Pantegni [The Total Art]* containing many excerpts from Greek medical texts. The clinical section of the treatise emphasized the importance of examination of the pulse, body temperature, and naked eye urinoscopy at the bedside. This text gave the physicians of Salerno access to classical medical practice a century before other sources of ancient knowledge became available. Although Constantinus retired after a short time to the Benedictine Abbey at Monte Cassino, his productivity stimulated a number of Salernitan physicians to write on anatomy, medicine, and surgery. Some manuscripts were in verse to facilitate memorizing; a popular compendium known as *Regimen sanitatis* or *Flos medicine* provided physicians with clinical instruction and therapeutic advice for many centuries.

The study of anatomy, previously neglected, was revived as human dissection became lawful. Among the early anatomical works was a book by Mondinus in which there is a description of the gross appearance of the nervous system.

In the 10th and 11th centuries, the practice of minor surgery, under no regulation and ignored by the Church, was in the hands of barbers and itinerant surgeons lacking formal training. Only this type of homespun surgery was available until Roger Frugardi joined the Salernitans. Written in 1170, his text

Practica chirurgicae described the operative procedures of the Arab surgeons. Later, the practices of that time were incorporated in *The Surgery of the Four Masters*, a text used in surgical teaching for hundreds of years.

After the fall of Cordoba in 1235 and Baghdad in 1258, Arabic medicine declined. In the Mediterranean lands, stimulated by the Salernitan school and the advent of the universities, some trained surgeons began to practice in Italian cities. In the middle of the 13th century, Hugo da Lucci, a surgeon of Bologna and his pupil, perhaps his son, Theodoric, broke from the Arab practices of wound treatment. Hugo, physician to the city of Bologna, left no writings, but Theodoric wrote some time later, "It is not necessary, as Roger and Roland have written, that pus should be generated in wounds." Before Theodoric had penned this dictum, Bruno of Longoburgo, a professor at Padua, in 1252 wrote *Cyrurgia magna,* in which he clearly differentiated between healing by primary intention, "true union," and secondary intention, "union by a fleshy sarcoid or scar."

Noting that hair, oil, and salve hindered the healing of wounds, Bruno advised that lacerations be cleansed of all foreign materials, sutured, and covered with a dry dressing, a clear recommendation for aseptic surgery. Theodoric, who became the Bishop of Cervia, wrote a manuscript advocating his master's practices 14 years later, in which he borrowed generously from Bruno's text without acknowledging the source.

It is of interest to note that shortly after Theodoric's manuscript was written, a well educated and experienced surgeon of Bologna, William of Saliceto, produced a text entitled *Cyrurgia,* which Garrison called a landmark. In it, there is no reference to the dry aseptic surgery of Hugo and Theodoric. Nor did William of Saliceto's pupil, Lanfranc of Milan, who later lectured at the Collège de Saint Côme and wrote a superb text on head injuries, mention Theodoric's dry wound repair. In the latter part of the 13th century, however, Henri de Mondeville, a pupil of Lanfranc, who is acknowledged to be the founder of surgery at Montpellier, apparently had some contact with Theodoric and strongly advocated the dry treatment of wounds for they "dry much better before suppuration than after." He had his patients close their nostrils, blow out their cheeks, and thus get rid of debris from head wounds. Thereupon, he carefully washed the wound until clean, applied a dry dressing, and delighted the victims by prescribing wine. Henri de Mondeville's *Chirurgie* of 1306-1313 included a chapter on anatomy and 13 miniature illustrations depicting operations—the first to appear in a surgical text.

In the middle of the 14th century, the most erudite and influential surgeon of the period, often called the "Father of Surgery," Guy de Chauliac, disparaged the wine dressing of surgical wounds, accused Theodoric of "stealing all that Bruno said with some fables of Hugo of Lucca," and set back wound surgery some centuries.

The Renaissance Period

Surgery of the Nervous System

In the 14th century, most of the cutting for stone, trauma, and wounds was carried out by vagabonds. A few physicians, often educated as clergy, visited or apprenticed to a skilled surgeon to acquire experience. Such was the training of Guy de Chauliac (1300-1370). He was born in the small village of Chauliac, near Auvergnen, France. Apparently, he was educated in Montpellier, took Holy Orders, and became a cleric. Under the patronage of Chancellor Raymond de Molière, he completed a medical course based upon Arabic versions of Galenic medicine and the practices of Arabic and Italian physicians. He is said to have been a pupil of Henri de Mondeville, who practiced at Montpellier, but it must have been a brief encounter for Henri died when Guy was 20 years of age. By visiting the medical practitioners of Bologna and Paris, Guy gained both medical and surgical experience, so that upon his return to Lyon, he was recognized by church officials to be a professional, not a barber-surgeon. As the result of his close contacts with the Church, he was appointed physician to Popes Clement VI, Innocent VI, and Urban V during their reign in Avignon, France. This gave him access to Arabic medical manuscripts which contained extracts from Galen's writings. Based on these treatises, in 1363, he wrote a compendium of the medical practices of the 14th century, entitled *Ars chirurgica* in vernacular Latin. The text was translated later into classical Latin, French, Spanish, and other languages. When printing was developed, the text was published in 1478 and was reproduced from time to time as late as the 18th century.

Although many surgeons of the Middle Ages obtained their experience from treating war wounds, Guy's practice was based upon civilian activities and the writings of the great Arab physicians—Avenzoar, Albucasis, Rhazes, Haly Abbas, and Avicenna—all of whom relied upon Arabic versions of Galenic works. Brennan points out that these latter writings were practically unknown in Europe until the 11th century, when they were translated into Arabic long before the manuscripts of Hippocrates, Celsus, and Paul of Aegina. With his ecclesiastical background, it is not surprising that Guy composed a surgeon's code expressing much the same sentiments as the earlier Hippocratic Oath.

> The conditions necessary for the surgeon are four: first, he should be learned; second, he should be expert; third, he must be ingenious, and fourth, he should be able to adapt himself. It is required for the first that the surgeon should know not only the principles of surgery, but also those of medicine in theory and practice; for the second, that he should have seen others operate; for the third, that he should be ingenious, of good judgment and memory to recognize conditions; and for the fourth, that he be adaptable and able to accommodate himself to circumstances.

Let the surgeon be bold in all sure things, and fearful in dangerous things; let him avoid all faulty treatments and practices. He ought to be gracious to the sick, considerate to his associates, cautious in his prognostications. Let him be modest, dignified, gentle, pitiful, and merciful; not covetous nor an extortionist of money; but rather let his reward be according to his work, to the means of the patient, to the quality of the issue, and to his own dignity. (From the Introduction to the General Chapter, *Ars chirurgica*.)

Guy refers in his textbook to "first intention" healing when parts reunite without the medium of a foreign substance and to "second intention" healing when the divided parts were reunited by a foreign substance. He appreciated that persons with scalp and skull injuries sometimes survived; in fact, he had seen a man with a small superficial brain wound recover. However, he stated that "wounds of the brain and its tables are fatal because of subsequent lesion of the respiratory organ, as the result of which the good temperature of the heart is broken and so the whole animal perishes according to Galen."

As Salerno declined in influence, medical centers in other cities along the Mediterranean Sea developed. One of the earliest was founded at Montpellier, which until the 8th century had just been a stopping-off point on the road between Spain and Italy. After the victory of Charles Martel at Tours in 732 AD, it became a prosperous center. Freed of the religious and political restraints of many other cities, Montpellier grew into a commercial post where science and culture flourished as scholars from oppressed areas congregated there. A papal decree in 1280 raised the school to the status of a university. In medicine, the courses reflecting the Moslem influence were based upon the teachings of Avicenna, Johannitas, and Arabic versions of works by Galen and Hippocrates. A number of outstanding physicians and surgeons—Arnold of Villanova, Henri de Mondeville, and Guy de Chauliac—enhanced the academic fame of Montpellier.

The medical school of Montpellier prospered until the epidemics of the Black Death in 1348, 1360, 1372, and 1382 decimated the population. Guy de Chauliac, who lived through the first two epidemics, described two forms of plague—one a pneumonic type which occurred early in the epidemic and a second, bubonic form, milder, which was prevalent in the later outbreaks (Fig. 2-3). Guy recognized the contagiousness of the disease and that no measure—not even constantly burning wood—was an effective prophylaxis. Many therapies, including drugs, purgatives, bleeding, and various diets, were tried but to no avail.

The epidemics led to the decline of the medical school. Of more than 200 students and masters in the 14th century, fewer than 70 remained at the end of the 15th century. When civil riots broke out, students went to safer havens in Padua and Perpignan. In 1622, the French annexed Montpellier, ending contact with Spanish medicine, and the fame of the university faded.

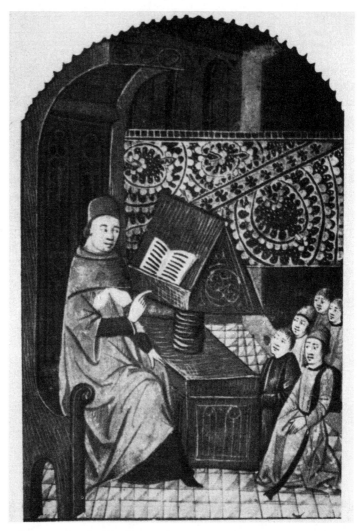

Fig. 2-3. Guy de Chauliac, erudite surgeon of the 14th century. (From the collection of A. Earl Walker)

Concepts of the Brain and Spinal Cord

Although the Egyptians of the 11th or 12th dynasty illustrated their writings with sketches and paintings of the body, none was of the nervous system. Nor did peoples of other lands who made cranial defects for various reasons leave any indication that they examined the brain. Indeed, the crude European sketches of the head and its cerebral contents were probably first made by the Salernitans in the 13th century and gave no specific localization of the functions they marked around the borders of the skull (Fig. 2-4). After that time, figures of a "disease man"—diagrams with cells indicating the site of presumed diseases in the head or body—became common. On the outlines of the head, the activities of the brain were marked in circular or quadrilateral cells identified by superimposed or adjacent labeling. The designated faculties were simple mental

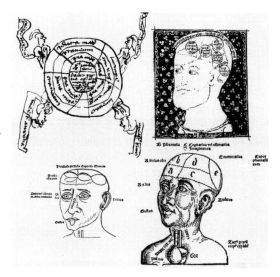

Fig. 2-4. Concepts of the brain depicted in medieval manuscripts. (From the collection of A. Earl Walker)

processes—common or general sense, image formation, imagination, judgment, thought, and memory. Their location was variously assigned, although usually the *sensus communis*, which was thought to receive data from all the special senses and general information from the body, was placed rostrally. Fantasy and imagination were located in the next cell, although occasionally judgment and thinking were assigned to this or an adjacent cell, and memory was consistently located posteriorly. In early times, these faculties were superimposed on the head, somewhat later were assigned within the cerebral ventricles, and finally localized to various superficial or deep structures of the cerebral hemispheres (Table 1). Clarke and Dewhurst have collected many of the schemes proposed

TABLE 1

THE LOCATION OF THE FACULTIES RELATIVE TO THE INTRACEREBRAL STRUCTURES

Faculty	Isolated Cell	Connected Cell	Total Schemas
Sensus communis	23	16	39
Fantasy	9	14	23
Imagination	23	18	41
Judgment	20	12	32
Mentation	17	18	35
Memory	26	18	44

during the Middle Ages; based on their findings, the relative frequency of the assignment of the faculties to various locations by the medieval writers is tabulated.

From time to time, surgeons reported wounds of the brain which did not give rise to the defects expected. Theodoric stated that his master Hugo da Lucci had treated a saddle maker whose fourth ventricle was completely void; yet he had an intact memory and plied his trade satisfactorily. Guy de Chauliac reported that he had seen a patient recover his memory after a wound of the posterior part of the brain that initially had caused memory impairment. Massa described another patient completely aphasic as the result of a halberd cut to the base of the skull, who, after the depressed and penetrating bone was removed, commenced to talk to the astonishment of his assistants. These isolated cases, not anatomically verified as autopsies, were illegal but did suggest that the faculties were represented more widely in the brain.

The 16th Century: The Nervous System

The 16th century was a time of change in the political, social, economic, and health status of the people of Europe. In the medical field, advances were being made in both the basic and clinical sciences.

Anatomy was the earliest science to be recognized by law. Although a few bodies had been dissected earlier, Mondinus in the 13th century was usually considered to have made the first public anatomical demonstration (Fig. 2-5). He read from a Galenic text as the prosecutor pointed out in the cadaver the part being described. Such a public dissection was held periodically at many European centers in the following centuries. Probably the first anatomist to break the ritual

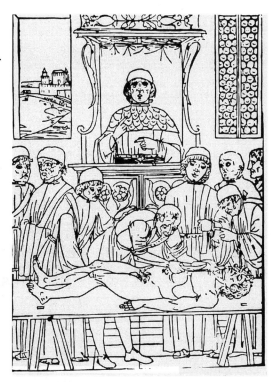

Fig. 2-5. Mondinus, a 13th century physician, said to have performed the first public anatomical dissections. (From the collection of A. Earl Walker)

by taking the knife in his own hand and demonstrating the viscera was Vesalius (1514-1564). Although a devout follower of Galen, Vesalius noted mistakes in Galen's anatomical descriptions, many of which stemmed from the fact that Galen had dissected apes and pigs, whose cerebral structure was not comparable to that of humans. Vesalius had artists make sketches of his dissections; a few, he drew himself. These beautiful illustrations of the human anatomy, both accurate and pleasing to the eye, formed the basis for his masterpiece *De humani corporis fabrica*, printed in 1543.

In the introduction of this classic, Vesalius discussed the practice of medicine, which in his day was divided into three schools—the logical, the empirical, and the methodical. The first followed a rational dietary system, the second a pharmacological system, and the third was surgical intervention. Vesalius bemoaned that the doctors of Italy were becoming ashamed to work with their hands, but had servants perform autopsies while they stood alongside and watched. Similarly, the physicians no longer prepared prescriptions but had pharmacists compound the medicine, and the surgeons had the barbers do the cutting. He noted that the writers of that time only abridged the opinions of Galen that "deviated more than 200 times from the correct description."

By the 15th century, examination of the dead was pursued in practically all European countries to dissect the normal anatomy as well as to examine diseased organs. As a result, the structure of the nervous system was disclosed. Gabriele Fallopius, a pupil of Vesalius, described a number of neurological structures—the chorda tympani, sphenoid sinus, and the course of the trigeminal, auditory, and glossopharyngeal nerves. Costanzo Varolio (or Variolus) visualized the structures at the base of the brain by removing the head and dissecting the base of the skull.

Postmortem examination of the human body was performed not only to ascertain the relationship of anatomical structures, but also to determine the cause of death. Such examinations had been prohibited by the Moslems. Although Morgagni referred to necropsies carried out in Byzantium in the 6th century AD to determine the cause of the plague, the first legal postmortem examination was made in Bologna by William of Saliceto in 1275. Singer has reproduced a scene depicting a 14th-century autopsy in which the head does not appear to have been examined. By the next century, necropsies were common. Antonio Benivieni of Florence regularly requested permission to perform such examinations. However, his brief descriptions of the findings suggest that the examination was confined to the site of the presumed disease and was not a complete autopsy. Shortly thereafter, Berengario da Carpi (1470-1550), a renowned surgeon of Bologna, examined the entire body and made illustrations of the brain. Fernel, "the French Galen," who in his clinical studies distinguished between symptoms and signs, reported on the naked-eye appearance of diseased organs, noting, in particular, nodular growths which he defined as granulomas, and polyps, and fleshy tumors which he called sarcomas. He noted that the latter growths involved the medulla oblongata and compressed the spinal cord.

In the early part of the 16th century, an outspoken, egotistical Swiss physician, Aurelius Theophrastus Bombastus von Hohenheim (1493-1541), the son of a chemist, conceived that disease, which he thought to be of astral origin, produced autointoxication resulting in psychic and corporeal dysfunctions. For these mystic ailments, he had many therapies, including mineral baths, tinctures, and especially one of the base metals (mercury, lead, arsenic, copper, or potassium). "Paracelsus," as he called himself, made a pilgrimage throughout European countries, from the British Isles to Greece, Alexandria, and Sweden, denouncing older forms of treatment as medical nostrums and extolling the virtues of his doctrine of specific therapies. However, his ranting verbiage concealed the wisdom of his teachings. In 1536, he wrote a manuscript in Swiss-German on the treatment of wounds, in which he maintained that injuries, even of the head, were not dangerous if bleeding was arrested and the wound cleansed. But he wrote that the care of wounds was not taught in universities, although it could be learned from gypsies! His teachings and therapies, in some ways quite modern, were so interspersed with mysticisms (such as weapon salves and signatures) that they were ignored and, like Mrs. Malaprop, he is remembered more for his mistakes than the introduction of therapeutic pharmacology. Yet, in his day, he was highly regarded, for Shakespeare refers to Paracelsus and Galen in *All's Well That Ends Well*. Although acquainted with some disorders, in particular epilepsy, paralysis, aphasia, and the dancing mania, Paracelsus advanced neither understanding of their pathogenesis nor their treatment.

Surgery in the 16th Century

As the European people emerged from the so-called Dark Ages, the practice of medicine improved and three classes of medical practitioners evolved— physicians, surgeons, and barber-surgeons. As a result, some legal restrictions were placed upon the practice of medicine, although the inferior art of surgery was not regulated. This left the better trained surgeons competing with barber-surgeons and itinerant operators. Consequently, surgical practice was looked upon with disdain. In England, the guild of barbers, skillful in the cutting art, gained favor so that with the approval of Henry VIII, they and the surgeons united to form the United Barber-Surgeon Company. In France, where the medical groups were similarly divided after the founding of the College of St. Côme, the surgeons followed the example of the physicians, and with their square caps and long robes assumed the role of examiners of the barber-surgeons. The latter, who learned their trade on the battlefield or as dressers in the hospitals of Paris, often had a better practical knowledge of surgery than the haughty surgeons of the long robe. This led to much rivalry and bickering among the three types of practitioners. In the low countries and Germany, physicians were considered "bleeders" and the care of the sick was often in the hands of itinerant quacks. Consequently, the medical and surgical care of the head-injured and neurologically impaired was left to nature and the blessings of the saints.

Until the 16th century, an obstacle to the development of surgery had been the fact that most treatises were written in Greek or Latin, languages which the barber-surgeons, who only spoke in the vernacular, did not understand. To aid the barbers, some surgeons wrote treatises or translated the ancient writings into the native tongues, a departure frowned upon by many physicians but favored by others. Harken to the words of Jean Canappe, physician to King Francis I of France, who translated his lectures on the works of Galen and Guy de Chauliac into French:

> I make bold to state that I have known many surgeons, unequipped with either Greek or Latin, but tireless in applying their minds to matters germane to their art, who were comparable, if not superior, as gauged by results, to hosts of other men, who look upon themselves as quite the thing in letters Greek and Latin.

In spite of vehement opposition, Ambroise Paré in 1545 wrote his surgical treatises in French. Even with this assistance, the barber-surgeons had difficulty training some illiterate apprentices. Candidates who knew little or were obviously quacks were barred from practice; however, many barber-surgeons continued to gain training on the battlefields of Europe. Eventually, the practices of the surgeons and barber-surgeons diverged. The barbers, prohibited by law from bloodletting, dressed the hair, shaved, applied salves, plasters, and poultices, and occasionally pulled teeth. The surgeons did venesection and operative surgery, but no longer practiced the tonsorial arts.

The Contributions of Ambroise Paré

The use of gunpowder in 1346 at the battle of Crecy introduced a new type of wound which at first was considered to be poisonous and to be treated by promoting suppuration. Accordingly, the army surgeons, including da Vigo, Brunschwig, and Gersdorff, applied boiling oil or the cautery to counteract the poison. But some surgeons decried such harsh treatment. In 1551, Maggi of Bologna showed that such wounds healed in experimental animals with a simple cleansing; 12 years later, Thomas Gale also advocated a plain dressing.

It was Ambroise Paré who gave the "coup de grâce" to the barbaric treatment of wounds (Fig. 2-6). Born in France between 1509 and 1518, he began his medical career in the early 1530s as an apprentice to a barber-surgeon in Paris. He learned to shave men, comb hair, prepare lances, dress wounds, and treat

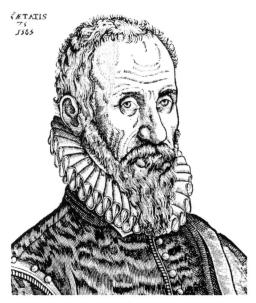

ÆTATIS
7$
J585

Fig. 2-6. Ambroise Paré, 16th century French army surgeon who originated modern concepts of the care of head wounds. (From A History of Neurosurgery. *Greenblatt SH, Dagi TF, Epstein M, editors. Park Ridge, Ill: American Association of Neurological Surgeons, 1997, p 356)*

nonoperable tumors and ulcers. He probably read the text of Guy de Chauliac, from whom he quoted freely in his later writings. He served an internship for three years at the Hôtel-Dieu in Paris, after which he entered the French Army in 1537 as an infantry surgeon. His fame came primarily from his rejection of the cruel burning-oil treatment of wounds and his adherence to soothing dressings. Apparently he treated many head wounds with "an oily cloth as the ancient surgeons had taught." Paré recognized, as had Guy de Chauliac and others, that brain wounds were not necessarily fatal: "many persons with cranial wounds of small size die; others with larger wounds and loss of substance sometimes survive." However, he wrote, "wounds of the brain and membranes [were] very often mortal because frequently, they abolish the action of the thoracic nerves and the others serving respiration so that death follows."

Paré classified head injuries as scalp wounds with or without fissure, fractures, contusions, depressions, incised wounds, contrecoup, and concussion injuries. His treatment was simple. If the wound was confined to the scalp, Paré cleansed the area, shaved around it, and sutured the lesion. An open wound was packed and allowed to granulate in. If the bone was involved overtly, or presumed to be injured, it was trephined to remove spicules of bone, blood clots, or debris (sanies) and to apply medications. However, Paré stated that the trepan was contraindicated if bony fragments were loose or the fracture was over a suture or at the base of the skull, bregma, fontanelle, or temple. For an unconscious head-injured victim, Paré recommended bleeding from a cephalic vein and the application of cataplasms and clysters. He emphasized that no head injury should be neglected, especially if a fracture were present. However, he recognized that if there was free movement of the dura mater, the outlook was favorable. Paré mainly used trephines, saws, chisels, and, if necessary to remove crushed or broken bone, elevators.

Although a barber-surgeon without formal medical training, Paré wrote of many afflictions of the brain and spinal cord. Hydrocephalus, Paré stated, was due to water between the scalp and pericranium, the pericranium and cranium, bone and dura mater, or within the ventricles. The first two types, he considered, might be treated by incising the scalp and draining the fluid. Ventricular hydrops, which had been described by Vesalius and Albucasis, was considered untreatable by Paré. He described three types of spasms of the nerves and muscles—tetanus, opisthotonos, and emprosthotonos—but he mentioned no cures. Paralysis was the result of softening of the nerves producing sensory or motor impairment of a part or the whole body; the latter was termed apoplexy. Syncope was defined as a sudden loss of the faculties which might result in death; if due to hemorrhage or loss of spirits, it might produce pallor, sweating, cessation of movement, and fainting. Paré attributed delirium to bad spirits. He ascribed scotoma or vertigo, which might be associated with noises in the ears, to a vaporous spirit passing up the arteries to the head moving the spirits in a confused or turbulent manner as if the body had had too much wine. He stated that Paul of Aegina had recommended cutting the arteries behind the ears for relief. Paré described migraine or hemicrania as pain in the temple or at the vertex of the head caused by local disease of the sinuses, arteries, meninges, or brain, or the result of general disturbances such as gastric upsets. He mentioned a number of medicinal therapies as well as, in serious cases, cutting the temporal artery. Obviously, he had acquired considerable folk medicine as well as many practical remedies, although he knew little of their rationale. Paré's surgical skill and courage on the battlefield led to his recognition as the greatest surgeon of the time. Moreover, for his kindness to his patients, he was beloved and venerated. As a result, his services were in great demand by the nobility and royalty until his death in 1590.

In Europe during the 16th century, most of the cutting for stone, hernia, cataracts, and infections was shamelessly and brutally done by disreputable vagabonds. Garrison lists only seven competent surgeons in all of Europe, several of whom did not operate upon the nervous system. In Italy, Giovanni della Croce, the teacher of Fallopius (1523-1562), wrote a treatise so clearly depicting the instruments and operations of that time that Adams, 300 years later, copied them to illustrate his translations of the Hippocratic writings.

The 17th Century: The Birth of Neurology

The great medical centers of the 17th century were in Leyden, Paris, and Montpellier. At that time in most European schools, anatomy was taught by lecture, although in France, Vieussens made 600 dissections, and in Holland, Dutch artists depicted the anatomies attended by elaborately dressed physicians. It seems that the brain was superficially examined, for Steno remarked in 1669 that of "its inner substance, you are utterly in the dark." His statement that it had "two substances, one grayish, the other white, which last is continuous with the nerves distributed all over the body" confirmed his conclusion.

Thomas Willis' Account of the Brain

The structure and function of the brain was being elucidated by English investigators known as the Invisible College. The master was a stimulating young man educated at Oxford between the years 1642 and 1646. An imaginative and brilliant thinker, Thomas Willis began his practice in Oxford but moved to London in 1660 where he acquired a fashionable clientele (Fig. 2-7). He had the ability to attract clever young men, some of whom later founded the Royal Society. They included Robert Hooke (an inventive physicist and microscopist), John Locke (a physician philosopher), Richard Lower, Thomas Millington (President of the Royal College of Physicians and, later, Willis' successor as Sedleian Professor of Natural Philosophy at Oxford), and Christopher Wren. Some critics have implied that Willis exploited his associates. Certainly, Lower skillfully dissected many of the brains which Willis used to illustrate his book. Without the help of such talented associates, Willis could never have carried on his busy practice and done his writing. Yet his critics' caustic remark that his associates did the experiments and that he merely philosophized seems unwarranted, for Feindel asserts that his collaborators appreciated his stimulating influence and were quite content with his acknowledgment of their cooperation.

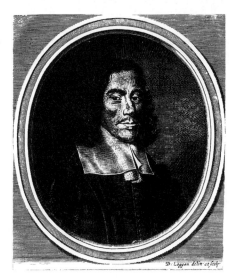

Fig. 2-7. Thomas Willis (1621-1675). (From A History of Neurosurgery. *Greenblatt SH, Dagi TF, Epstein M, editors. Park Ridge, Ill: American Association of Neurological Surgeons, 1997, p 113)*

Thomas Willis' claim to fame rests upon a number of fundamental studies as well as his exposition of the vascular supply of the brain. His description of the gross morphology of the brains of humans and lower animals, his classification of the cranial nerves, and his vivid clinical observations of neurological disorders and their pathological correlates all contributed to his renown (Fig. 2-8). Willis was one of the earliest scientists to use comparative studies to elu-

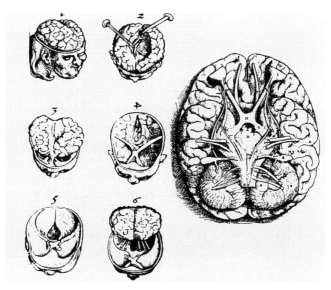

*Fig. 2-8. Willis described many aspects of cerebral anatomy.
(From the collection of A. Earl Walker)*

cidate brain function in his writings. He
refers to the anatomy and function of
the nervous system in 15 different mam-
mals and in other creatures such as birds,
fish, oysters, lobsters, and earthworms.
Previously, the brains of humans and
animals had been observed after removal
of the calvarium and being sliced *in situ*
from above—a procedure which did not
disclose its base. Willis' technique of
"cutting" the nerves and arteries at the
base of the brain and turning it over
allowed him to examine the basal structures and their relationships. Moreover,
he probably used a fixative such as wine
to harden and preserve the configuration
of the brain. Wren's drawings of Willis'
preparations have a more natural
appearance of the cerebral cortex than
those of earlier anatomists (Fig. 2-9). In
addition, Willis "traced by the help of

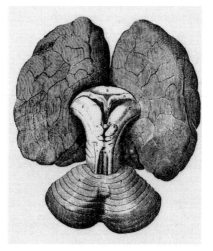

Fig. 2-9. Illustration from Willis' The
Anatomy of the Brain *drawn by
Christopher Wren. (From the collection
of A. Earl Walker)*

glasses" the finer details of the cortical markings.

Willis' designation of the cranial nerves was followed until the time of von Soemmerring. Willis identified the first six nerves as they are now known. The facial nerve was not clearly differentiated from the auditory nerve, although Willis did note that there were two types of fibers entering the internal acoustic meatus. The eighth cranial nerve included all of the fibers—glossopharyngeal, vagus, and spinal accessory nerves—which entered the jugular foramen. The ninth cranial nerve was the hypoglossal, and the tenth was the upper cervical rootlets. His detailed account of the spinal accessory nerve led to its being named after him. The autonomic nerves, which Willis called "intercostal" nerves, were described more accurately than previously. He noted the nerves to the aortic arch, to the blood vessels, and to the heart.

Undoubtedly, Willis' outstanding contribution was his demonstration of the arterial supply at the base of the brain. That vasculature had been noted by many previous anatomists, but the design was confused by its differing structure in humans and some animals in which a plexus of vessels—the rete mirabile—covered the base of the brainstem. However, when human dissection became legal in the 15th century, some physicians were unable to find a rete at the base of the brain. Berengario da Carpi denied its existence. Vesalius in 1543 pointed out that Galen had been describing the brain of oxen, in which there is such a basilar vascular plexus. But the rete mirabile was not forgotten, for Varolio in 1573 described "a plexus of vessels crossing one another which anyone may, if he wishes, call the rete mirabile." Massa in 1536 also accepted the concept of a rete although he thought that the choroid plexus of the lateral ventricles produced the animal spirits as excrement. In the next century, Wepfer described the cerebrovascular tree and ridiculed the idea of a rete. At about the same time, Thomas Willis, in his superb account of the cerebral circulation, wrote of "the vessels that cover the base of the brain and constitute the rete mirabile." However, the cerebral circulation was being more critically examined by injecting the arteries with various substances—warm water, air, colored solutions, and ink. Willis injected a dye into the carotid artery to mark its passage from the base of the brain to the cerebral vessels. A few anatomists had described somewhat earlier the vascular channels of the brain. Although the illustrations of Vesalius were fanciful and erroneous, the sketches of the cerebral vessels by Vesling and Casserius in the 17th century were much more exact. That of Vesling is a rather crude representation of the base of the brain with the neural structures diagrammatically depicted. The vascular pattern is correctly shown, although the vessels at the base are disproportionate and lack the posterior cerebral arteries and the cerebellopontine arteries. Each anterior cerebral artery passes along the callosal gyri without joining its mate. The drawing by Casserius more accurately depicts the arteries, but lacks a left posterior communicating and right posterior cerebral artery. Many of the cranial nerves as well as the branches of the basilar artery are not shown. Recognizing these discrepancies, one would have no doubt that Willis' illustrations were more precise than those of his predecessors. Certainly, he had a better concept of the anastomoses and of their relevance in providing collateral channels if one were occluded. Unquestionably, Willis pointed out the significance of the "mutual conjoynings" of the major arteries at the base of the brain. This arterial system, termed a circle by von Haller, has provided a mechanism by which the most important part of the brain may have a blood supply even if one link of the polygon is occluded.

Although Willis considered that complex activities were carried out in the basal ganglia and cerebral cortex, he had unusual ideas regarding their functions, namely that the sensory nerves carried the spirits to the corpora striata—the sensorium commune—and then, to produce further effects, to the corpus callosum and the cortex. The effector motor animal spirits followed the same path but in the reverse direction. They passed through the corpus striatum, which Willis conceived as an important organ of movement as well as of sensation.

Such fanciful concepts were received skeptically by many of Willis' associates and later critics. Foster stated that "Willis . . . loved words and looked upon an illustration as an argument . . . an analogy as a proof." Critical scientists did not accept his theories. Regardless, his anatomical and clinical observations were astute and compensated for his bizarre ideas of the workings of the nervous system.

The clinical acumen of Willis is well exemplified by his observations that a deaf woman could hear only when a drum was beating (percussis). This remarkable ability to relate minor phenomena to functional principles permitted Willis to define clinical syndromes recognizable as modern pathological entities. From his many bedside descriptions, a few examples are of interest.

In his rather long discourse on headache, Willis noted that the pain may be due to structures within or outside the skull, but he asserted that the skull was not as sensitive as the meninges and that the brain, cerebellum, and their medullary dependencies "are free from pains because they want sensible fibers." Migrainous headaches were well known to Willis although he added little to the brilliant descriptions of the Romans. Another patient had headaches due to increased intracranial pressure. This woman about 50 years of age suffered from severe pain in the head for 6 months and fell into a lethargic state from which she recovered but still suffered headaches. She again became stuporous and died. Upon opening her skull, a scirrhous tumor was found occupying the space between the dura mater and the pia mater.

Two of Willis' cases probably were subdural hematomas. A young man had, for a fortnight, severe pain in the head which was made worse by fever. Later he had convulsive movements and talked irrationally. Upon his death "his skull being opened . . . the blood presently rushing forth flowed to the weight of several ounces above half a pint; further, the membranes themselves being distempered throughout the whole, with a fiery tumor appeared discolored; these coverings being taken away, all the infoldings of the brain and of its ventricles, were full of a clear water, and its substance being too much watered was wet, and not firm." In a second case, the collection of blood was described as being under the temporal suture. Willis' treatment of headache was not particularly imaginative—abstention from eating, rest, and evacuation of the bowels by an enema—so that the "matter be suffered to evaporate from the membranes of the head." Sometimes he applied blisters to the back of the head. He apparently had little use for surgical intervention, for he stated that, in some cases, trephination had been advised, but he knew of no one who had been willing to submit to it. In fact, he doubted that opening the skull to the air would cause a swelling, abscess, or scirrhous tumor to evaporate.

In his discussion of lethargy, Willis may have referred to a subdural hygroma. However, he was acquainted with hydrocephalus for he stated that he had found "interior cavities swelled with water, and the whole frame of the brain overflowed with a dropsy." He recognized that lethargy does not necessarily arise from the interior ventricles of the brain, for he had seen them overflowing with water and distended with blood, and yet "the sick patient, while he lived, was free from coma or great stupidity."

Apoplexy, discussed at some length by Willis, was considered to be a loss of consciousness, although the causes were not defined, for he wrote, "extravasated blood, the breaking of an imposthum, and a great flood of serous humor plentifully flowing forth, are wont to affect the greater breach of the unity within the brain." He describes how, in an autopsied case, he had found "the right carotid rising within the skull plainly bony or rather stony—its cavity almost wholly shut up." He also commented, that it was "wonderful that he had not died of apoplexy." Moreover, Willis states that "I have known sometimes those distempered, to be stiff and cold, pulse and breathing to be thought quite gone, and to be indeed esteemed quite dead, and put into their coffin, yet after two or three days to have revived again; but whoever awakes out of this fit, whether it be a short or long continuance does not for that reason fall into a palsy or half palsy of one side, as those for the most part do, who are distempered with the apoplexy." Although Willis stated that apoplexy usually occurred quite suddenly, he noted that occasionally it was gradual. He vividly described what we now refer to as "stuttering hemiplegia" in these words: "At first they are exercised only with light skirmishes, but after some time, they become more grievous, and of which at last for the most part, they die."

Willis was aware that palsies may be due to a number of causative factors. It is quite possible that he knew of the post-epileptic palsies, for he stated that "the Spasm or Cramp or Convulsion, doth sometimes bring in the Palsy." He described a spurious palsy in this fashion: "The persons, in the morning, able to walk firmly . . . before noon . . . they are scarcely able to move hand or foot." Referring to a garrulous woman suffering from this disorder, he noted that after speaking "long or hastily or eagerly, she is unable to speak a word, but becomes as mute as a fish." It is not difficult to recognize this classical description of myasthenia gravis.

Willis described another clinical condition so vividly that again the medical student will recognize it immediately. "They eat and drink well, go abroad, take care well enough of their domestic affairs, yet whilst talking, or walking, or eating, yea, their mouths being full of meat, they shall nod, and unless roused up to others, fall fast asleep." Where could one find a more delightful account of narcolepsy?

Willis was interested not only in the organic neurological syndromes but also in the disorders of the mind. He stated that short distemper is called delirium and the long or continued distemper is called a "phrenzie" or psychosis. It is to be feared that Willis allowed his theoretical musing to override his reason at times, for he related how he was sent to cure a maid who was strong but with fever raging and had to be bound to her bed. This continued for seven or eight days and was associated with a continual request for cold water. Willis had the woman taken in the middle of the night, put in a boat, her clothes removed and then thrown into the river, with a rope tied about her middle. Immediately, the maid fell to swimming and after a quarter of an hour, came out sober and was quite well. Willis comments that "the cure succeeded so happily and so suddenly for as much as the excess of both the vital and animal flame being together immanently increased, was taken away by a proper remedy for the more intense fire; to wit, by the moistening, and cooling of the water." A somewhat overzealous rationalization!

One might interpret Willis' many clinical descriptions as referring to recently described disease entities. For example, Feindel believes that Willis gave the first description of temporal lobe epilepsy, but too much should not be read into the writings of this imaginative 17th century clinician.

It would seem appropriate that the man who named a special branch of medicine should be recognized. Thomas Willis introduced the term neurology, although as might be expected, he defined it in a somewhat different frame of reference from what is used today. In the 1681 edition of Willis' work, the word appears in the text with the notation "The doctrine of the nerves." It is also listed in "the table of . . . hard words." It is of interest that the root of this term, "neuro," although given in modern dictionaries as derived from the Greek "neuron," originally had the connotation of a "sinew, tendon or bowstring," structures which were confused by early anatomists with the nerves. Willis' limited definition of the term was not expanded to include the spinal cord and brain until a century later.

It is difficult to evaluate the place of such a brilliant, but self-sufficient

TABLE 2

TERMS USED BY RIVERIUS AND WILLIS

Current Names	Riverius	Willis
Apoplexy	apoplexia	apoplexia
Brain abscess	abscessus cerebri (spacelus cerebri)	
Cataplexy	catoche sei catalepsi	
Catarrh	catarrhus	
Coma	comate, soporosis, caro, lethargo, apoplexia, coma vagile	comate, caro, lethargo, sommelantia, comate vigile, comatis, pervigilio
Convulsion	convulsivo	convulsivo
Delirium	phrenitis	deliria (agitatio, confusio)
Epilepsy	epilepsia (inf. & puer.)	morbus convulsiones (falling sickness)
Headache	cephalalgiae (dolor cap.)	cephalalgia (dolor capitis)
Hypochondriasis	hypochondriacea	hypochondriacea
Hysteria	hysterica	hysterica
Mania	mania	mania
Melancholia	melancholia	melancholia
Nightmare		incubus
Paralysis	paralysis	paralysis
Phrenitis	phrenitis	phrenitis (long delirium)
Sciatica	ischiadicus	
Feeble-mindedness		stupiditas
Syncope	syncope	syncope
Tremor	tremor	
Vertigo	vertigo	vertigo

physician as Willis in the development of the neurological sciences. He made little reference to contemporary or previous writers in the field. Yet, he must have known of the many anatomical works which had been published in the 15th and 16th centuries. The revolutionary and beautifully illustrated book by Vesalius is not cited. It is perhaps understandable that Eustachius' plates, although made in 1552, were not known to Willis for they were not printed until 1714. But the illustrations of the base of the brain by Varolio and Casserius should have been available. Even Riverius' text on nervous diseases is not mentioned. Willis' and Riverius' books cover essentially the same subjects (Table 2). Although Riverius' text was written 10 years before that of Willis, it

seems likely that Willis was unaware of the writings of the Montpellier professor. If that was the case, knowledge of neurological disorders was probably
poorly disseminated in academic circles. At that time, the parentage of neurology might not have been so clear.

Undoubtedly, Willis' contributions to anatomy carved a niche for him in
the neurological hall of fame. His clinical and pathological correlations introduced a scientific approach to the study of the nervous system for the first
time. On the basis of these fundamental investigations, Willis surely has a just
claim to the title of "founder of neurology." Since there is no other contender
for the paternity, it seems quite justified to designate Thomas Willis as the
"Father of Neurology."

Other Contributions in the 17th Century

Lazarus Riverius (1589-1655) made many contributions to the knowledge
of neurological disorders. He was born in Montpellier where he obtained his
education and graduated in medicine in 1611. Eleven years later he became
professor of medicine at that university. He was a famous physician throughout the south of Europe and was offered the chairs in Toulouse and Bologna,
both of which he refused. He was known for his descriptions of chicken pox,
purpura, and endocarditis.

Riverius' textbook on medicine in Latin was published in 1665, 10 years
after his death, by his pupil, Bernhard Verzaschae. In the first section, Riverius
described the various impairments of consciousness—stupor, coma, lethargy,
and apoplexy. It is of interest that he mentions brain tumor as a cause of coma,
for at that time intracranial tumors were a rarity. Convulsions, he says, are
involuntary nervous contractions which may be the result of causes other than
epilepsy according to Hippocrates, Galen, and Averroes. He referred to paralysis following a convulsion, an observation credited to Bright, Todd, and Hughlings Jackson 200 years later. In the chapter on epilepsy, he divided seizures
into idiopathic and symptomatic epilepsy. He discussed hereditary factors,
especially in infancy and childhood seizures. Vertigo was considered to be
caused by flatulence which, as vaporous material in the ventricle and choroid
plexus, agitated the animal spirits. Tremor was described and said to be cured
by paralysis—a phenomenon also discovered in the 19th century. Phrenitis,
mania, and melancholy were recognized as a kind of delirium without fever.
Their therapy was unsatisfactory. In the short chapter on brain abscess, gangrene and suppuration were described but Riverius had no better treatment
than that of Galen. Finally, a chapter on headache ended with the statement
that arteriotomy will cure hemicrania.

Another physician of that period interested in neurological disorders was
Thomas Sydenham (1621-1681), who followed the tenets of Hippocratic
medicine. Bedside observation was the basis of his teachings. Called the "Eng-

lish Father of Medicine," Sydenham revived the manual practices which had been discarded in the enthusiasm for medical theorizing and experimentation. In the preface of his book on medicine, Sydenham wrote, "in describing any disease, it is necessary to enumerate both the peculiar and constant phenomena, or symptoms, and the accidental ones separately; of which kind are those which differ occasionally by reason of the age and constitution of the patient, and the different method of cure." Of neurological interest are his clear accounts of hysteria, hydrophobia, and palsy. His succinct description of St. Vitus' dance, which he considered as a kind of convulsion attacking children of both sexes, reads as a classic. "It manifests itself by halting or unsteadiness of one of the legs, which draws up after him like an idiot. . . . Before a child who hath this disorder can get a glass or cup to his mouth . . . he does not bring it in a straight line thereto, but his hand being drawn sideways by the spasm, he moves it backward and forwards, till at length the glass accidentally coming nearer his lips, he throws the liquid hastily into his mouth, and swallows it greedily, as if he meant to divert the spectator."

As in the 16th century, the surgical advances in the 17th century were minor. In Italy, Cesare Magati held as Paré had, that gunshot wounds were not poisonous and should be dressed with bandages saturated with plain water. In France, little surgery of the head was practiced. The "Father of German Surgery," Wilhelm Fabry, whose portrait shows him with a skull on which he is pointing out a lesion, was a barber-surgeon whose practical surgical teachings were quoted for more than two centuries. His writing was reminiscent of the Roman teachings—avoid injury to the temporal artery, lever up depressed fractures or in infants pull the sunken fragments up by a string attached to a plaster cast on the depressed bone. Although he knew that brain wounds might cause mental disturbances, he did not consider them to be lethal, and he made no attempt to remove intracranial bullets or foreign bodies.

In the middle of the 17th century, England was engaged in conquest, civil strife, and combating epidemics of plague, dysentery, influenza, and smallpox. During that time, an army surgeon named Richard Wiseman (1621-1676) treated more than 600 head wounds, many of which he never saw after the primary dressing. He wrote a treatise on surgery of the head, "the noblest member of our body," in which he states that the "brain is of itself insensible; that such symptoms which accompany those wounds proceed from the pain which the meninges, dura and pia mater suffer." Wiseman described cerebral concussion and contusion and noted that the wounded brain caused "convulsions, howling and a dispatch of the patient." Although he never expected a cure unless the dura mater was intact, he admitted that occasionally patients with minor cerebral wounds did recover. Wiseman advised trephining if the extent and nature of the wound were not evident, to elevate depressed fractures, and to evacuate "sanies" but "not at the full of the moon" because the vessels were turgid then. He washed out epidural clots; although he removed bullets from the brain, he had no hope that the person would recover. For closed head injuries, he bled and purged the patient.

Wiseman discussed hydrocephalus and encephaloceles, both of which he considered deadly. Although a skillful and prudent operator—the best in England—he was not in the mainstream of the exciting explorations of the nervous system and so his imprint on evolving neurosurgery was covered by the shifting sands of time.

The 18th Century:
The Beginning of Medical Specialization

Although Garrison wrote "the medicine of the 18th century is as dull and sobersided as that of the Arabic period," changes were being made in the organization and practice of the art. A detailed medical history and physical examination were replacing the medieval inspection, palpation of the pulse, and urinoscopy. The introduction of percussion gave new physical evidence of some internal organs. The legal autopsy made it possible to verify a clinical diagnosis. The advances in the practice of clinical medicine tended to have physicians confine their activities to a single system of the body. Thus, many of the leaders in medicine, such as Stahl, Herman Boerhaave, Albrecht von Haller, van Swieten, Auenbrugger, Giovanni Morgagni, the Monros, Lind, Heberden, William and John Hunter, Jenner, Stephen Hales, and Mesmer, were confining their practices largely to one class of disorders.

Anatomical knowledge of the nervous system was advancing. Pacchioni described the bodies lying along the vascular sinuses of the brain which were later named after him. Vicq d'Azyr, physician to Queen Marie Antoinette, is best known for his neuroanatomical works published in 1786. Unfortunately, Emanuel Swedenborg's timely observation of the significance of the cerebral cortex was lost for more than a half century. He asserted that the cortical substance of the brain was the *sensorium commune,* since the impressions of the external sense organs were referred to it. The cortical substance was also the *motorium voluntarium,* for it initiated and executed whatever actions determined by the will were to be mediated by the nerves and muscles.

In the physiological laboratory, Robert Whytt (1714-1766), the foremost neurophysiologist of his time, was studying the functions of the spinal cord, being "careful not to indulge his fancy in wantonly framing hypotheses, but . . . to proceed upon the surer foundations of experiment and observation." As a result, he demonstrated that the entire spinal cord was not necessary for certain actions, but that a segment sufficed. Moreover, he showed that the spinal cord could not function during shock and inhibition. In 1764, he described two types of peripheral nerves, one under voluntary control, and the second involuntary or not requiring central nervous stimulation. The latter system he called sympathetic, implying a sympathy between tissues or organs. Later it became a part of the autonomic nervous system.

In Germany, Albrecht von Haller (1633-1714) was propounding his ideas that sensibility and irritability were the fundamental properties of nervous and muscular tissues. In 1788, Samuel von Soemmerring presented a classification of the cranial nerves which superseded that of Willis. Both of these scientists illustrated their works with superb artistic plates.

3

The Evolution of Encephalization

Although the gray covering of the cerebral cortex was recognized by the early anatomists as different from the intrinsic white matter of the cerebral hemispheres, the investigators of the 17th century were unable to define their fine structure. Using the simple lenses available, Malpighi in 1686 described the structure of the cerebral cortex as "an assembly and congeries of most minute glands." The fibers that van Leeuwenhoek (Fig. 3-1) saw conveying spirits in their canals were equally obscure. In fact, not until 1781 did Fontana give a reliable description of the primitive nerve fiber. Forty years later, Dutrochet, noting that the nerve fiber was attached to a nucleated body, called the unit a "nerve cell." In 1833, Ehrenberg, using the newly developed achromatic microscope, described "pearls" covering a fiber which connected with a cell body in the cerebral cortex. Other naked fibers were called organic or primitive fibers, and later termed the fibers of Ranvier. Many were sympathetic nerves originating from the nucleated, globular cells of the sympathetic ganglia.

The relationship of the nucleated body and the fibrous strands in the white matter was not resolved. Valentin in 1836 described in detail the nerve cell as being simply apposed to

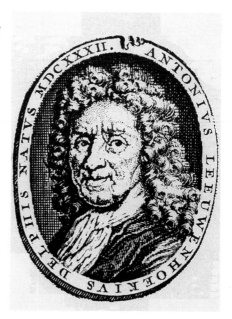

Fig. 3-1. Anton van Leeuwenhoek explored the cerebral cortex with his microscope. (From the collection of A. Earl Walker)

a fiber; however, Schwann in 1839 defined the cell and nerve fiber as a unit. Adolph Hannover, a Dane working in Müller's laboratory, stated that the cell membrane was continuous with that of the nerve fiber. Von Kölliker's classical paper of 1849 seemed to confirm the view that the ganglion cells were connected with the nerve fibers.

A question arose when Franz von Leydig observed in the spider a nervous organ of interlacing fibers. A few years later, von Gerlach, discussing the central nervous system of vertebrates, described a somewhat similar rete which formed a diffuse plexus giving rise to axons. In 1872, von Gerlach stated that the medullated nerve fibers could arise from the cells or from the network. Later, Golgi, using gold to impregnate individual nerve cells, described two types of ganglion cells in the cerebral cortex: namely, one with nerve extensions giving off only a few lateral filaments before changing into the axis cylinder of a myelinated nerve fiber, and a second with nerve extensions subdividing and losing their identity in a network intertwining in all layers of the gray matter. Even when awarded the Nobel prize in 1906, Golgi had not entirely abandoned the latter concept. Paul Ehrlich, who introduced intravital staining with methylene blue, thought axis cylinders terminated upon the cell but did not fuse with the cell cytoplasm. The net concept was denied by His, who found in embryonic life each nerve fiber originating as a process from a single nerve cell. A Spanish

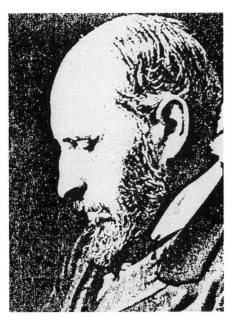

Fig. 3-2. Santiago Ramón y Cajal (1852-1934). (From the collection of A. Earl Walker)

histologist, Santiago Ramón y Cajal (Fig. 3-2), observed that the cells of the molecular layer of the cerebellum formed baskets around Purkinje cells coming in contiguity but not in continuity; thus, he determined that transmission by contact was the more complete system. After reviewing the evidence, Wilhelm Waldeyer (Fig. 3-3) in 1891 concluded, "The nervous system consists of numerous nerve units (neurons) connected with one another neither anatomically nor genetically." Although, as Ramón y Cajal bitterly remarked, this was in essence only "a resumé of my research and the creation of the term 'neuron'," Waldeyer was credited with formulating a new concept.

From time to time, the controversy was revived until the issue was settled in 1908 by Harrison, who grew in tissue culture neurons which developed nerve fibers. Other observations also supported the neuron theory. Waller, an English physician, had demonstrated that when a peripheral nerve was cut only the myelin sheaths of the fibers in the distal segment underwent granular degenerative changes; the proximal segment was little altered. Waller concluded that "the central nutrition of the sensory spinal fibers was to be found in the intervertebral ganglia" and the trophic center of the motor fibers was in the spinal cord. Franz Nissl, using basic aniline dyes, selectively stained the cell contents and observed pathological changes within the cell, termed "primary irritation" or "chromatolysis" after axonal injuries which he thought would not occur unless there was unity of the cell and axon. Thus, by the end of the 19th century, the evidence was conclusive that the neuron was the functional unit of the nervous system.

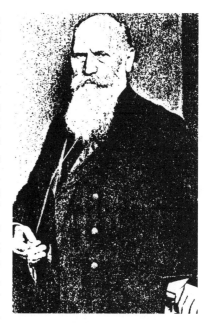

Fig. 3-3. Wilhelm Waldeyer (1834-1921). (From the collection of A. Earl Walker)

With the early microscopes, all cells seen in the nervous system were considered to be related to nerve fibers. With better magnification, however, small elements without long processes such as characterized nerve cells were seen. Virchow described these small cells, which he presumed to have arisen from the lining of the cerebral ventricles and to have been insinuated among the nervous elements, as a sort of glue; for this reason, he called them neuraglia or glia. They were not, however, all alike—at times, some smaller ones distended with fat globules; he referred to these as microglia. Other larger glia of varied shape had to await silver impregnations to be defined.

Cerebral Localization of Function

As the cell concept gained acceptance in the early part of the 19th century, the idea that the cells in different parts of the cerebral cortex might have varied functions was gaining credence stimulated by a pseudoscience—phrenology. One of its proponents, Franz Gall (1758-1828), had noted that some students with a remarkable memory for words had prominent eyes. Gall reasoned that the overdeveloped faculty for memory, if responsible for the proptosis, must lie above and behind the orbit. If that was the case, would not other mental faculties be associated with bumps or prominences on the surface of the skull? Upon this premise, he proceeded to draw a cranial map of the organs of the mind. However, this mosaic arrangement of the psyche drew the scorn of critics, who noted in a satirical vein the craniological association of such alien domains as pugnacity and friendship.

Phrenology gained a popular following, however, and stimulated physicians to reconsider their concepts of cerebral function. Some previous experimental work had suggested that the cortex might provoke motor activity. In 1760, Zinn and Haller had noted convulsions as the anterior part of a dog's forebrain was being excised. Sixty years later, Cabanis pricked certain parts of the cerebrum, inducing convulsive movements. De Renzi observed that the forelimbs moved as the forebrain was being cut. These mechanically induced motor responses were confirmed when Aldini and Rolando applied electric current to the cere-

bral cortex. Rolando's observations of limb movements as one conductor of a voltaic pile was being introduced into the cerebral hemisphere of a pig were the first clear descriptions of a muscular response. Although he also saw violent muscular responses when the cerebellum was stimulated, Rolando concluded that the fibers of the cerebral hemispheres produced voluntary movements.

Somewhat contrary to these results were Flourens' experiments in 1823 (Fig. 3-4). Upon exposing a dog's hindbrain, he explored the limits of excitability of the brainstem by pricking it successively more rostrally until a point was reached at which muscular contractions no longer occurred. In another dog, he stimulated the anterior parts of the brain extending caudally until a point was reached at which twitching resulted. The common point of

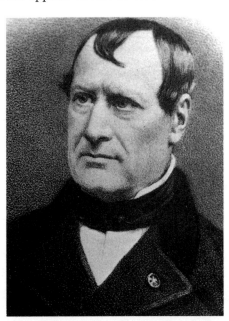

Fig. 3-4. Pierre Flourens (1794-1867). (From A History of Neurosurgery. Greenblatt SH, Dagi TF, Epstein M, editors. Park Ridge, Ill: American Association of Neurological Surgeons, 1997, p 135)

change was in the region of the quadrigeminal plate, which Flourens assumed demarcated the limits of the excitable lower brainstem and the inexcitable rostral cerebral structures. When questioned, he maintained that the contractions produced by Rolando were due to a spread of current to adjacent muscles.

Flourens' concept of the motor system was accepted by many physiologists and clinicians. Todd, known for his elucidation of focal postepileptic paresis, wrote of the volitional motor centers: "I would say that the centre of volition is of very great extent; it reaches from the corporata striata in the brain down the entire length of the anterior horns of the grey matter of the spinal cord, and includes the locus niger in the crus cerebra, and much of the vesicular matter of the mesencephale and of the medulla oblongata."

Clinical evidence was accumulating to indicate that the cortex had specific functions. Within a year of Flourens' report, Bouillaud described speech disturbances as the result of lesions involving either orbitofrontal lobe. He concluded that the loss of speech followed damage to the anterior lobes of the brain and he offered a reward to anyone who could show otherwise. Dax further observed that speech disturbances resulted from lesions of the left frontal lobe. In line with these observations, Bouillaud pointed out that a number of highly coordinated acts, such as writing, were preferably performed by the right hand, which was innervated by the left cerebral hemisphere.

By the mid-19th century, the localization of cerebral function was in a state of flux, with many physicians favoring Flourens' concept of a unified activity of the cerebral hemispheres, but some investigators believing that certain functions were carried out in discrete parts of the cerebral cortex. In 1861, Broca presented a paper to the Société d'Anthropologie in Paris in which he concluded that a lesion of the left inferior third frontal convolution produced a loss of the faculty of speech but not a paralysis of the muscles involved in phonation. The crucial brain upon which Broca based his theory of "aphemia" had a left frontal softening but, when examined many years later, also had quite extensive subcortical softenings. Broca proclaimed: "We now know that all parts of the brain have not the same function, that all the convolutions represent, not a single organ, but many organs or groups of organs and that there are large distinct regions of the brain which correspond to the regions of the mind." The validity of this dictum was debated for the rest of the century.

Spencer, a philosopher, had argued in 1855 that the seat of the higher psychical activities must be in distinct parts of the cerebral hemispheres. One of his associates, John Hughlings Jackson, seeking the locus of motor activity, concluded that a focal disability implied a local, not a diffuse, lesion and accordingly postulated that the striatum was the center for initiating movements of the contralateral face, arm, and leg. In 1885, Jackson, with a change of mind, wrote, "I had for years assumed that convolutions contain processes representing movement and impressions."

Little was done to advance the knowledge of cortical physiology until two young doctors began to investigate the basis of some observations they had made. One, Gustav T.F. Fritsch, had noted some years previously that the contralateral limbs twitched while dressing a head wound. His companion, Eduard

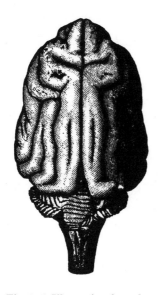

Fig. 3-5. Illustration from the fundamental work of Fritsch and Hitzig (1870). (From the collection of A. Earl Walker)

Hitzig, when stimulating the canine temporo-occipital region, had observed eye movements which he thought might be due to cortical excitation or spread of current to the quadrigeminal plate. To resolve these assumptions, they anesthetized a dog's cortex and applied platinum electrodes attached to a voltaic pile, which produced a current of about one milliampere and not more than 11 volts. Stimulation of the anterior region of the dog's cortex produced muscular contractions of the contralateral limbs; stimulation of the posterior part of the cerebral cortex caused no responses (Fig. 3-5). Using weak currents, the muscular responses were quite discrete; with stronger stimuli, the responses became widespread, even involving the ipsilateral muscles. To confirm the existence of such excitable cortex, Fritsch and Hitzig, after defining the zone producing movements of the right forelimb, excised the cortex in two dogs. Upon recovery from the anesthetic, the animal walked by raising the right forelimb awkwardly, at times placing it upon the dorsum of the forepaw, or, if correctly planted, slipped on it. When sitting with the limbs resting in front of its body, the animal would tend to fall to the right. Thus, in a Berlin home, both by cortical stimulation and ablation, the doctrine of localization of cerebral function was established.

These findings, although confirmed by Ferrier, were not universally accepted (Fig. 3-6). Burton Sanderson assailed the conclusions because he thought that the results were due to spread of current to the striatum, which was considered a motor ganglion. Similar experiments by Carville and Duret in France, Ferrier in England, and Luciani and Sepalli in Italy, however, confirmed the existence of a cortical motor area in the dog and monkey. The demonstration of its presence in man only awaited a fortuitous occasion and a courageous physician.

In 1874, Roberts Bartholow of

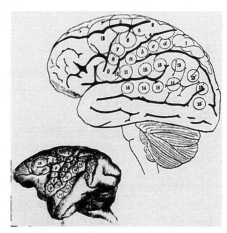

Fig. 3-6. Illustration from David Ferrier's work on cortical localization (1873-1876). (From the collection of A. Earl Walker)

Cincinnati, Ohio, obtained the consent of a feeble-minded servant girl dying of a malignant, purulent ulcer of the scalp to insert fine insulated wires through the granulating tissue over the dura mater in order to stimulate the underlying cerebral cortex. When the electrodes (presumably in the left postcentral convolution) were activated, muscular contractions were produced. The right arm was thrown out, the fingers extended, the leg kicked, and the head turned to the left. When a stimulating needle was inserted further into the left cortex, muscular contractions occurred and a strong, unpleasant tingling was felt on the right side, particularly in the arm. The study was terminated when, upon increasing the strength of the current, a generalized seizure developed lasting five minutes. Unfortunately, two days later, the patient became right hemiplegic, comatose, and died within a day or two. At autopsy, the sagittal sinus was thrombosed and a thick layer of greenish pus extended over the whole of the left hemisphere. Bartholow's report of his experimentation upon the human brain drew intense and heated criticism both in the United States and Europe.

In the meantime, physiologists stimulated the cerebral cortex of many animals under a variety of conditions. Ferrier carefully mapped the cortex of the monkey, noting the excitable precentral convolution, parietal lobe, and superior temporal gyrus. Horsley explored with Schäfer the cortex of monkey and orangutan, finding both precentral and postcentral convolutions excitable. In contrast, Grünbaum and Sherrington reported that using unipolar faradization to stimulate the cortex of 16 anthropoids, the excitable areas (with the exception of the eye fields) were confined to the precentral convolutions (perhaps related to the depth of anesthesia). Finally, Krause stimulated the human cerebral cortex and demonstrated a topographical orientation within the precentral gyrus.

Cortical stimulation, however, also produced negative effects. In 1881, Bubnoff and Heidenhain reported that powerful contractions of the extensor muscles of a dog could be relaxed by weak stimulation of the motor cortex. About the same time, Brown-Séquard found that excitation of the nonmotor cortex of dogs and rabbits abolished the excitability of the motor cortex for minutes. These inhibitory reactions were further studied and their mechanisms investigated by Sherrington, who previously had demonstrated reciprocal innervation of antagonistic muscles.

The increasing interest in the cerebral cortex from the time of Willis may be followed in the illustrations of the hemispheres. The crude representations of the cerebral convexity in the 16th and 17th centuries were gradually replaced by accurate sketches and, finally, by photographic illustrations.

Observations of the sensory function of the cerebral cortex were being made by ablating cortex and observing the animal's deficits—a task often technically difficult both to perform and to interpret the results. Consequently, the sites of appreciation of the primary sensory modalities were often controversial; many animals seemed to appreciate sensation both subcortically and cortically. Goltz observed that a dog deprived of its cerebral hemispheres, after the initial effects of the operation had receded, behaved as a normal animal. However, if the thalami were damaged, a dog sat motionless and died of starvation. Goltz's notable observations were made upon so-called "brainless" dogs, two of which he managed to keep alive for 57 and 92 days, and a third dog for 18 months. The latter had no structures above the tentorium other than a markedly shrunken left anterior quadrigeminal body, a small, soft, grayish mass representing the left corpus striatum and thalamus, an atrophic right thalamus and corpus striatum, and a small amount of the cornu ammonis. For a few months after the cerebral ablation, the dog had a severe malnutrition which Goltz attributed to restlessness. The dog's sleep cycle was shorter than that of a normal animal. The dog walked on its paws; however, on a smooth floor it would slip, although usually recovering itself. When a limb was injured, the dog trotted about on three legs, holding up the injured member. If the limbs were placed in an abnormal posture, the position would be corrected. If irritated, the animal turned its head sharply in the direction of the annoyance and snapped but seldom bit. Its sense of touch seemed to be blunted. Taste was intact, at least for very bitter objects. Hearing was much reduced, although the blare of a trumpet would rouse the animal from sleep. Vision was so impaired that the animal did not avoid objects in its path, although it did respond and turn away from a bright flash. The pupils contracted briskly to light. The dog was indifferent to caresses and threats. If a dish of milk were placed near its nose it would lap, chew, and swallow with apparent satisfaction; however, it did not seek food nor show any sexual interest. Other investigators also were to keep decorticated animals alive for some time. Rothman's brainless dog lived for over two years; Karplus and Kreidl maintained two monkeys for approximately two weeks.

Visual Representation in the Cerebral Cortex

Circumscribed injuries or ablations were required to localize sensory representation in the cerebral cortex. The earliest investigations of the effects of lesions, both in man and lower animals, were made of the visual representation. Flourens' report of decorticated pigeons suggested that vision had a cortical representation. De Panizza, in 1855, traced the visual pathway in the raven and a number of other animals from the optic nerves to the occipital cortex, but his observations were ignored until Ferrier and others studied the problem. Munk confirmed de Panizza's observations and extended them, showing that parastriate lesions produced psychic blindness or visual agnosia and that the entire occipital lobe had to be excised to cause blindness. This concept, contrary to Ferrier's conclusion that the visual center was in the angular gyrus, caused considerable debate but eventually prevailed. The precise projection of the retina upon the striate cortex was the contribution of Henschen, who studied the brains of patients with lesions of the visual pathways. He asserted that the primary visual field coincided with the striate cortex, although he thought that the macula was represented anteriorly, rather than at the occipital pole. A few years later, Minkowski corrected the location of the macular representation in the occipital cortex or "cortical retina" as Henschen had termed it, and described the crossed and uncrossed retinal projections upon different cell layers of the lateral geniculate body.

Prefrontal Lobe Syndromes

Ablations rostral to the excitable motor area carried out in the dog, cat, and monkey by Hitzig, Horsley and Schäfer, and Ferrier resulted in no definable motor or sensory deficits; however, a change in behavior characterized by hyperactivity was described by all observers. Hitzig noted that an animal deprived of its frontal lobes would neglect its food, exhibiting "a poor memory." Goltz reported a stupid, fixed expression on the animal's face and a lack of normal fear. Associated with these ablations, Bianchi described behavioral disturbances and an attention hemianopsia which gradually regressed.

Perhaps the earliest example of a human frontal lobe lesion was the famous "crowbar" case reported by Harlow in 1848 and again in 1868. A previously quiet citizen sustained a brain wound when a crowbar passed through his orbit and out the left temple. After this insult, the peace-loving citizen became a profane, impulsive man unable to plan his activities in an orderly fashion. Other such frontal wounds, reported by Welt in 1888, Jastrowitz in 1888, and Oppenheim in 1898, all produced severe behavioral and personality changes with impaired judgment. Oppenheim referred to the mental changes following frontal lobe lesions as "Witzelsucht" or "Moria" (wisecracking); although general intelligence and memory were preserved, psychological tests later demonstrated a number of personality and intellectual changes. Phelps attributed the defective control to involvement of the left prefrontal region.

Parietal Lobe Function

Although the cortex of the parietal lobe is extensive, it received little attention until the Elizabethan anatomists. Sylvius de la Boë described the lateral fissure in 1663, although Caspar Bartholin had mentioned it in 1641. Leuret named the central fissure after Rolando, an earlier anatomist who had described the convoluted cerebral surface in man. Finer divisions of the cerebral hemispheres were made by L.P. Gratiolet, professor of zoology at the University of Paris. Gratiolet included the precentral gyrus in the parietal lobe, but both Turner and Ecker in the 1860s-70s placed its anterior limit at the central fissure. The precise functional localization, however, was uncertain. Fritsch and Hitzig's excitable motor cortex subserved both sensory and motor functions. Munk maintained that the entire cortex was sensory and that the motor responses resulted from the sensory impulses activating lower motor centers. Schäfer, however, believed that cortical paralysis could result without sensory loss. Other investigators considered the entire peri-Rolandic cortex to be sensorimotor. Sherrington's later studies seemed to settle the issue that the motor area was confined to the precentral cortex.

The localization of cutaneous and deep sensibilities in the cerebral cortex was difficult to determine for, in the 19th century, the modalities of sensation were not clearly established—in fact, the sensory status of pain was questionable. As a result, tactile sensation was variously localized in the hippocampal region (Ferrier), the Rolandic cortex (Hitzig and Munk), and even more diffusely.

Both in animals and man, the effects of parietal lobe stimulation and ablation were being studied. Munk noted that light touch or pressure on the skin was not appreciated after cortical ablation, whereas stronger tactile stimulation might elicit responses. In 1909, Cushing confirmed that electrical stimulation of the parietal cortex in an unanesthetized patient produced responses of a tactile nature. As the result of head wounds in World War I, much more of the cerebral sensory representation was demonstrated, but the precise sensory representation of the parietal cortex was not disclosed until much later.

Temporal Lobe Syndromes

Perhaps the earliest evidence of localized function in the nervous system, although not recognized as such, came from the varied manifestations of epilepsy. The Hippocratic writers knew that some seizures consisted of generalized convulsions, some of focal muscular jerkings, and others of unconscious, complex behavior. The overt manifestations of these latter bizarre epilepsies took many forms. Hallucinations and automatisms which could be construed to be seizures were described in the writings of Hippocrates, Galen, Aretaeus, and Celsus. More elaborate accounts appeared after the Middle Ages. John of Gaddesden in 1314 described an attack in which "the patient would rub his back . . . or sit down and hold his forehead with his hands and rub his face. . . . Then, the patient himself stood up and recited the Lord's prayer and spat once and threw off the paroxysm." In 1667, the Commissioner of Health of the Kingdom of Bohemia, in a book on the nature, origin, and cause of epilepsy, stated that "epileptics are not only those whose principal brain functions cease . . . while their entire body is convulsed during the access, but also those whose lips alone are deliriously convulsed; also, the sick who turn steadily in a circle like a spinning top or a trundling hoop; also, the girl who was running backward and forward for half an hour must be counted among epileptics." Richard Bright wrote that his patient "became delirious and wandered in the street without hat or coat, walking in a state of complete unconsciousness from Clapham Common to Shoreditch and was between four and five hours on the road." Falret, the director of an insane asylum, described "a kind of intellectual aura, which precedes the convulsive attack by a few minutes only and, which in some manner, constitutes its first symptom." He noted incomplete or aborted attacks in which "the patients, who have no rapport with the external world, utter certain incomprehensible sounds or articulate a few incoherent words. In these incomplete attacks . . . the patients also have only partial convulsive movements, such as involuntary contractions of certain muscles of the face, or of the limbs, automatic movements of swallowing, chewing etc." Griesinger also refered to automatic movements. Falret emphasized that the automatisms might result in homicide or arson of which the person had no or very vague awareness. Griesinger's pupil Höring reported a patient who "falls into a state of deep dreaming and stretches his hands in front of him. . . . At other times he runs away during the attack and talks gibberish, or he searches, as in a dream, in all his pockets, as if he were missing something . . . then, has no idea of what happened."

Herpin studied 300 epileptics and found 61% to have incomplete episodes. He described a "cerebral onset" which began with a sensation, hallucination, intellectual disturbance, or impaired consciousness. One patient with "partial delirium" stated: "I can still read words but I no longer grasp their meaning . . . it seems . . . that one part of my intellect witnesses the disorders of the other." Herpin also described fugue states as an epileptic manifestation of cerebral origin.

That these episodes came from cerebral structures was established as Hughlings Jackson and others reported autopsy findings. Hughlings Jackson collected the reports of patients whose fits started with an intellectual aura or "a sort of dreamy state coming on suddenly" followed by an unconscious, complex automatism. Anderson in 1886 wrote of a patient whose attacks began with a "rough, bitter sensation" and, at times, a childhood scene. At necropsy, a tumor was found at the base of the temporal lobe; Anderson reasoned that the tumor initially affected the tip of the gyrus uncinatus, where Ferrier had located the centers of taste and smell. This was the first autopsied case of a dreamy state. Shortly thereafter, Hughlings Jackson published more such cases to substantiate the site of origin of this "uncinate group of epileptic fits." These attacks characterized by an initial dreamy state were variously designated as psychomotor, epileptoid, incomplete epilepsies, absences, grand mal intellectuel, epileptic madness, or delirium. To convey the concept that they were in lieu of a convulsion, the terms "psychical or epileptic equivalent," "psychic variant," and "psychic seizure" were introduced early in the 20th century. Psychomotor epilepsy gained favor among clinicians. When Fuster and Gibbs showed that the electroencephalographic concomitants of such attacks were temporal lobe discharges, however, their term "anterior temporal lobe epilepsy" was accepted in the United States, but the attacks were classified as "complex partial seizures."

When the cerebral cortex was being explored in animals, the large temporal lobes were stimulated with minimal results. Even the localization of audition presented problems due to its bilateral representation, its broad spectrum, and its inadequate means of testing experimental animals. Ferrier noted that monkeys and a number of lower animals pricked up their ears and made contraversive head movements when the superior temporal gyrus was stimulated. Moreover, if this region was extirpated bilaterally, the animal did not even respond to loud noises. Consequently, Ferrier called that area "the centre of hearing." Luciani and Sepalli in 1885 and Brown and Schäfer three years later concluded, however, that audition in animals was not exclusively represented in the temporal lobe.

Brown and Schäfer did report marked behavioral alterations after removal of the superior temporal gyrus and adjacent tissue (the extent of the ablations was never confirmed). They stated, "it is, in fact, more easy to produce a condition of semi-idiocy in monkeys from extensive bilateral lesions of the temporal lobes than from complete severance of the prefrontal region; an operation which may, indeed, be affected without producing any very obvious symptoms." Little attention was given to these findings at that time, so it remained for Klüver and Bucy to rediscover the marked behavioral changes following bilateral temporal lobectomy.

The Corpus Callosum

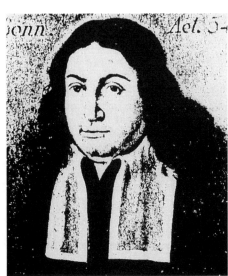

The term corpus callosum as used by Galen probably referred to a much more extensive subcortical area than that occupied by the midline white commissure. He seems to have included much of the white substance of the hemisphere. This usage was followed by most authors for centuries, until Vesalius limited the extent of this commissure. Note that Malpighi (Fig. 3-7) in 1664 wrote "regarding the marrow of the brain or the corpus callosum." Willis stated that the corpus callosum "forms almost the whole roof of

Fig. 3-7. Marcello Malpighi (1628-1694) described the corpus callosum. (From the collection of A. Earl Walker)

98

the ventricles." Using the scraping techniques which de Vieussens had originated, subsequent investigators were able to trace fiber tracts quite accurately.
Vicq d'Azyr, in 1781, gave a precise account of the arrangement of the fibers
from the posterior, middle, and anterior parts of the corpus callosum. Using a
better means of hardening the brain, Reil described it and its connections in
quite modern terms.

In 1760, Zinn and Haller sectioned the corpus callosum of dogs and noted
no motor or sensory disturbances. In the following 200 years, a number of investigators studied the results of lesions of the corpus callosum with inconstant
results. Clinical disorders of the corpus callosum such as infarction, Marchiafava-Bignami disease, and agenesis, although generally causing some impairment of higher mental activity, did not produce a typical syndrome. Lesions
of associated midline structures, such as the cingulate gyrus, septum pellucidum,
and fornix, although usually accompanied by mental dysfunction, did not produce a consistent picture. The demonstration of the integrating function of the
corpus callosum was not to come until well into the 20th century.

Disturbances of Communication

The interchange of ideas is best developed in man, who has elaborated language as a means of communication. This is a complicated system, however,
and is easily disrupted by disease of the brain. As language has many component parts (e.g., visual reading, auditory comprehension of sounds, or tactile
interpretation of the feel of objects), disease of any one part may produce a distinct disturbance affecting predominantly one or many components. An artificial classification of these afflictions has evolved largely based upon the sensory
modality that is most disturbed (e.g., aphasia and agnosia). This discussion will
be based upon the generally accepted classification of speech and language disorders.

Aphasia

Although it has been known from ancient times that loss of speech could
result from a head wound, modern views date from the latter part of the 18th
century. Gall, who was interested in cases which would support his concept of
cerebral localization of function, described a young man who, after a fencing
wound that penetrated the left nasal fossa and entered the left anterior lobe of
the brain for a distance of approximately 2 cm, had a transient right hemiplegia
and loss of memory for names. It is not clear, however, whether this deficit was
due to a speech defect or an anomia. A second patient had a cerebrovascular
accident causing a severe inability to express himself appropriately. Although
able to speak only an occasional spontaneous expression, he could move his
tongue freely and could make himself understood by gestures. Had Gall been

more interested in analyzing the language disability and locating the diseased parts of the brain in these patients, the understanding of speech might have been advanced many years. As it was, he only concluded "that the principal lawgiver of speech is to be found in the anterior lobes of the brain."

Bouillaud, who accepted this concept, pointed out that a number of highly coordinated acts were performed by the right hand and deduced that such special functions, including speech, should be represented in the cerebral hemisphere. In 1839, he reaffirmed his position and suggested that the faculty of speech resided in the anterior lobes of the brain. In the meantime, Marc Dax, a physician in Montpellier, presented a paper in which he correlated the loss of speech with lesions of the left hemisphere. His manuscript was not recognized until March 24, 1863, the very day on which Pierre Paul Broca (Fig. 3-8) filed his stimulating work on the localization of speech, which he had presented to the Société d'Anthropologie in Paris two years previously. Broca's premise rested mainly upon his experience with two patients. One was a right hemiplegic patient named Laborgue, who for years had only been able to say "tan" and to curse. Broca pointed to a cystic cavity occupying the posterior part of the left third frontal convolution, adjacent precentral and second frontal gyri, ascending parietal gyrus, insula, angular gyrus, and first and part of the second temporal gyri, as well as a softened striatum.

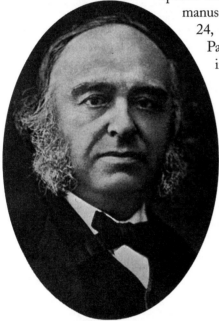

Fig. 3-8. Pierre Paul Broca (1824–1880). (From The Founders of Neurology, *2nd ed. Haymaker W, Schiller F, editors. Springfield, Ill: Charles C Thomas, 1970)*

A second patient described by Broca was an 84-year-old man with a fractured femur, who 9½ years previously had lost consciousness and upon regaining his senses was able to speak only a few words. Twelve days after sustaining a femoral fracture, he died. His brain had a collection of fluid, 1.5 × 2 cm in diameter, over the posterior end of the third left frontal gyrus and generalized convolutional atrophy. Had these two brains been sectioned at that time, the history of aphasia might have been quite different, for years later when Laborgue's brain was examined by computed tomography, an extensive left parieto-occipital softening was found.

In 1874, Karl Wernicke (Fig. 3-9) published a book on aphasia. After discussing Bouillard's and Broca's theories and his own findings in 10 aphasic patients, two of whom were autopsied, Wernicke formulated a scheme of the speech mechanism. He described cortical speech centers and connecting fiber tracts, on the basis of which he outlined four types of aphasia: 1) motor aphasia (Broca's aphasia, due to the inability or impaired ability to activate the speech musculature); 2) conduction aphasia (Leitungsaphasie), which results from sectioning the connections between the auditory and motor cortices; 3) sensory aphasia, due to the destruction of the left superior temporal gyrus producing nonunderstandable speech, hearing being intact; and 4) total aphasia, the result of destruction of both centers so that the understanding and expression of speech are lost. Although Wernicke had a complex mechanism for speech, other neurologists formulated elaborate diagrams to indicate circuits postulated for the production of speech. However,

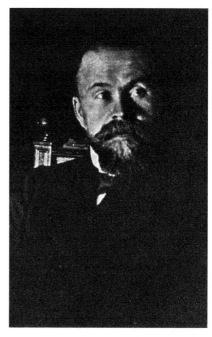

Fig. 3-9. Karl Wernicke (1848-1904). (From The Founders of Neurology, *2nd ed. Haymaker W, Schiller F, editors. Springfield, Ill: Charles C Thomas, 1970, p 532)*

some clinicians questioned such diagrams. Pierre Marie in 1906 denied that the third frontal convolution had a special role in the function of language. He insisted that every aphasic patient had some defective intelligence and impaired understanding of spoken language which could be brought out if sufficiently difficult tasks were given. Thus, Marie assumed that Wernicke's aphasia was simply an anarthria with some mental impairment. Marie held that pure anarthria was the loss of speech, the result of a lesion in the lenticular zone of either hemisphere—an area including the insula, claustrum, caudate and lenticular nuclei, and the two medullary capsules. Dejerine maintained that Broca's and Wernicke's aphasia, as well as the "subcortical" pure aphasias (pure motor, pure word-deafness, and pure word-blindness) were generally accepted. He criticized Marie's concept of anarthria and the lenticular zone.

Although Hughlings Jackson studied the problems of linguistic communication for years, his observations, so painstakingly written, were too complex for many associates and international colleagues to understand. Hughlings Jackson divided language into intellectual (propositional) and emotional (interjectional) speech. He recognized that these expressions were preceded by an internal proposition, the whole producing speech. Hughlings Jackson postulated that a lesion might produce both positive and negative effects, the positive being the released functions of other centers and the negative being the destroyed function. Thus, imperception involved defective formation of images, the symbolization or their precursors. He stated, "To localize the damage which destroys speech and to localize speech are two different things. The damage is in my experience always in the region of the corpus striatum." Later, Hughlings Jackson proposed a more psychological basis for aphasia without specific localization in the left frontal lobe. He emphasized that aphasia was more complex than a loss or defect in speech; as pantomime was frequently impaired, there must be a defect in symbolization or formulation of ideas. Nevertheless, some writers failed to understand such concepts and defined aphasia, as Trousseau did, as an abnormality of vocalization and not as a defect in the processes underlying propositional speech.

Agnosia

The story of agnosia began in the physiological laboratory, where Munk observed that dogs with partial removal of the occipital cortex could perceive objects as things or entities but without meaning—a condition Munk termed "mind-blindness." Finkelnburg in 1870 termed a similar state in man "asymbolia," and Hughlings Jackson called it "imperception." In 1891, Freud used the term "agnosia" to describe this defect. The term, generally accepted, has been qualified by the modality examined, although it was recognized that other modalities were involved to some extent.

The inability to recognize an object by sight was described by Lissauer in 1890 as visual agnosia. Tactile agnosia was described by Puchelt in 1844, but the term had several meanings. "Astereognosis" was used in the 1880s by Hoffmann. Other terms have been suggested, but astereognosis has survived in spite of its limited spatial definition of an object. Auditory agnosis implies the inability to appreciate the significance of a sound that can be heard.

Apraxia

Apraxia is a disturbed execution of a motor task although its elements are intact and carried out normally. This disordered action, usually due to a left hemisphere lesion involving the dextrad anterior corpus callosum was termed "apraxia" by Steinthal in 1791. The classical example presented by Liepmann in 1900 related to a patient who was able to use the left limbs normally; although he knew what he wanted to do with his right limbs, they performed quite awkwardly. Pick in 1892 described a somewhat similar case with bilateral difficulties in carrying out purposeful acts. He termed this impairment "ideational apraxia"; the impairment described earlier was called "ideomotor apraxia." These disturbances have been analyzed in a number of spheres of activity and, on that basis, subgroups such as constructional apraxia have been formulated.

Agraphia

Writing is a complicated means of communication, from ideography to the various languages of the world. Aberrant writing by persons in a diseased state of the brain was observed in the 19th century.

Marcé in 1856 analyzed writing processes, but Benedikt, nine years later described aphasia and related disturbances in greater detail and introduced the term "agraphia." At about the same time, Hughlings Jackson was discussing writing and reading abnormalities. A year later, Ogle divided writing difficulties into amnemonic (letters written but used incorrectly) and agraphia (letters unable to be written). In 1873, Pitres classified the agraphias as agraphia by reason of word-blindness, agraphia due to word-deafness, and agraphoplegia or motor agraphia, in which writing spontaneously from dictation or copying is impossible. Wernicke, adhering to his classification of aphasia, divided agraphia into cortical, subcortical, transcortical, and conduction types.

Benedikt was the first to suggest that writing and speech, while not individually localized in the brain, were composed of discrete elements. A number of early neurologists, including Wernicke, noted that writing was a late and acquired skill and denied that it had a specific center in the brain, while others, such as Exsner and Henschen, placed a writing center in the left frontal lobe. Dejerine and others rejected the concept of such centers. Miraillié concluded that the disturbance was of "inner speech" and noted that writing was only a means of exteriorization similar to showing blocks or typing. Herrmann and Potzl stated that the writing centers are bilateral in more cases than the speech centers. The complex mechanisms of writing and their cortical substrates were not resolved in the 19th century, and in fact are still being investigated.

Alexia

Alexia is the inability to understand written or printed language. As this implies that the person previously had the ability to read and was literacy was rare centuries ago, it follows that the condition would be uncommon. Perhaps this accounts for the few examples of alexia before the modern era. Valerius Maximus in 30 AD wrote of a man who, being struck on the head, lost his memory for letters but otherwise seemed to be normal. More than 1500 years passed before Mercurialis in the 17th century reported that a man, after a convulsion, could write but was unable to read what he had written. In the 17th century, a German after a stroke was said to have more trouble reading that language than Latin, which he had acquired later. In the following centuries, isolated cases were reported (Gendrin, Trousseau, Broadbent, and Kussmaul). Both Gendrin and Trousseau note with amazement that their patient "cannot read what he himself has written, although it is written correctly enough."

Charcot discussed many of the early references to acquired disturbances, but it was Joseph Jules Dejerine (Fig. 3-10) who first critically reviewed the disorder. Dejerine had a 63-year-old patient who, after a stroke causing right-sided weakness, right hemianopsia, and verbal paraphasia, was totally unable to read or to write anything but his name. The alexia and agraphia persisted until his death six months later. On autopsy, an old infarct involving most of the left angular gyrus and extending posteriorly to the occipital horn of the lateral ventricle was found. A year later, Dejerine encountered another case with two lesions. An old lesion, apparently responsible for the isolated alexia, was a yellow, scarred infarct of the medial and inferior parts of the left occipital lobe which involved the splenium of the corpus callosum. Dejerine argued that the occipital infarct had produced the

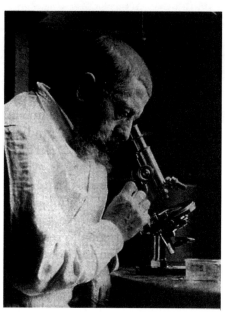

Fig. 3-10. Joseph Jules Dejerine (1849–1917). (From The Founders of Neurology, 2nd ed. Haymaker W, Schiller F, editors. Springfield, Ill: Charles C Thomas, 1970, p 427)

right homonymous hemianopsia and the callosal lesion had interrupted the connections between the two visual areas, isolating the left parietal cortex from its usual visual input. He considered a recent lesion of the left angular gyrus to be responsible for the agraphia which appeared after the second insult.

Based on these cases, Dejerine concluded that lesions of the inferior parietal lobule with or without involvement of the first temporal and angular gyri of the dominant hemisphere, produced alexia. If the lesion were isolated, writing skills might be preserved or impaired to varying degrees. The ability to read music might or might not be affected by lesions producing alexia. Reading numbers is likewise inconstantly affected. It is interesting to note that if letters or figures are traced in the palm of the hand, the alexic patient may be able to recognize them.

Amusia

Music in many civilizations and of many types, often associated with danc-ing, has been an integral part of social, religious, and medical activities. Until the Middle Ages, music was thought to be appreciated in the ear. Willis placed the center for the appreciation of music in the cerebellum. Gall, who assigned many functions to the brain, thought music was appreciated in the cerebral cortex. The disorders of speech, so thoroughly studied in the last century, only occasionally involve musical capacity. Proust and Tillaux described a musician who after a stroke was unable to read musical symbols. In 1871, Steinthal used the term "amusia" to describe a state in which a person cannot read or express music, a condition elaborated upon by Knoblauch 17 years later. In the same year, Oppenheim referred to a patient who was able to sing words that he was not able to pronounce.

Ballet in 1888 called attention to the similarity of aphasia and amusia. He attempted to fit the latter into a diagrammatic schema for aphasia, but the principal elements in amusia (rhythm, pitch, and the ability to perceive music emotionally) were ill-fitted to the aphasic schema. The basis of the apprecia-tion of music has been studied in detail in the 20th century.

Acalculia

The ability to manipulate numbers may be affected independently or in varying degrees with other forms of communication. Calculating was learned later in life than talking and was often done with the fingers. More complex mathematics, such as multiplication tables and monetary transactions, even as simple as making change, were still later acquisitions. Accordingly, it is quite understandable that cerebral disorders affect calculating in various ways and to different degrees. The location of lesions causing such disorders is varied; per-sons with acalculia have been reported to have lesions in the occipitotemporal and/or parietal regions of one or both sides.

Body Schema and Its Disorders

The unity of the human body must have been appreciated by philosophers in bygone ages. Certainly, the unique entity of the corpus was apparent to the sur-geons of the Renaissance period, who not uncommonly disrupted the image by amputating a part of the body. After removal of an arm or leg, the amputee still experienced intensely the missing member and could describe in vivid terms the cramped position of the phantom; however, the concept of a body image was not fully developed until the studies of Bonnier and Demy and Camus. To indi-cate the awareness of one's own body, Wernicke in 1906 coined the term "somatopsyche" and Holmes and Head used "postural scheme." The unappreci-ated or denial of the presence of a neurological impairment was recognized at the beginning of the century; its various manifestations were shortly described in a considerable body of literature. These clinical phenomena include unilateral, conscious, or unconscious anosognosia, hemiasomatognosia, neglect syndromes, autotopagnosia, right-left disorientation, Gerstmann's syndrome, asymbolia for pain, macro- and microsomatognosia, and autoscopia. One might include the out-of-the body experiences occurring in near-death situations as a unique conscious dismemberment.

These disruptions of the normal body schema are usually accompanied by other neurological disturbances of the sensory-motor system, higher mental functions, and/or special senses.

Disorders of Memory and Sensation

Amnesia

Memory from earliest times has been located variously within the body. With the acceptance of the encephalic cell doctrine in the 4th or 5th century, memory was usually placed in a posterior cell. Thus, damage to the back of the head was considered well into the Renaissance to be associated with memory disturbances. Willis was one of the earliest writers to suggest that the cerebral cortex was involved in the storage of memory. He wrote: "then, if the same fluctuation of spirits is struck against the cortex of the brain, which, when it is afterwards reflected or bent back, raises up the memory of the same thing."

Several centuries passed, however, before substantial evidence of its cortical locus was present. In the early 19th century, Gall observed that persons with prominent eyes had a good memory, and so concluded that the faculty must reside in well-developed frontal lobes to have pushed out the orbits. Although erroneous, the assumption stimulated the search for the localization of mental functions.

In the last quarter of the 19th century, physicians in England (Lawson), Germany (Strümpell), and France reported that chronic alcoholics had a poor memory, at times simulating dementia. In 1889, the condition was more fully described by S.S. Korsakoff as a profound amnesia greater for recent events than remote happenings and associated with confabulation, agitation, confusion, apathy, depression, and a peripheral polyneuritis. The syndrome was ascribed to various lesions of the nervous system: atrophy of the mammillary bodies (Gudden), destruction of the third ventricular walls and hypothalamic nuclei (Bonhoeffer), degenerative changes in the mammillary bodies, the posterior and at times the anterior quadrigeminal bodies (Gamper), and, later, lesions in the thalamus, brainstem, and cerebral cortex.

In the meantime, Wernicke in 1881 had described "hemorrhagic polioencephalitis," a syndrome of drowsiness, confusion, unsteady gait, and extraocular muscle impairment in three patients, two of whom were drinkers. At first glance, this would seem to have little to do with Korsakoff's alcoholic patients. Yet, as more cases accumulated it became evident that the two drinkers described by Wernicke suffered from an early stage of the polyneuritic amnesia subsequently described by Korsakoff. Later, Bonhoeffer on clinical grounds and others on the basis of pathological findings concluded that the two syndromes were actually different stages of the same disorder, which Bonhoeffer termed "Wernicke-Korsakoff syndrome." Some time later, it was shown that both syndromes were due to a deficiency of thiamine associated with chronic alcoholism.

Interest in this subject has exploded in the latter part of the 20th century as psychologists have analyzed the elements of the memory process with sophisticated techniques.

Spatial Organization

One's spatial organization is developed early and in adult life is well established. However, cerebral disorders, especially motor and sensory, are often associated with some degree of spatial disorganization, and often overlooked as the result of the more obvious motor or sensory disruption. Consequently, few cases were reported in the early literature.

In 1886, Hughlings Jackson described an adult woman who one day was unable to find her way to a park she had been visiting daily for years and which was only a short distance from her home. One night a few weeks later, she suddenly developed a left hemiplegia. Her mental state and hemiplegia cleared somewhat, although she suddenly became comatose and died. A large gliomatous tumor was found to occupy her right temporosphenoidal lobe. Two years later, Badal reported upon a young woman who complained of difficulty finding her way about her home and locating objects a few weeks after an eclamptic episode. She even had trouble meandering about the neighborhood in which she had lived for years. She could read numbers and letters but was unable to spell or to estimate distance, direction, or the location of objects to either side of the fixation point. Although her central vision was normal, she had bilateral inferior hemianopsias and constricted superior fields. She had difficulty drawing simple designs. In 1936, Foerster reported a similar case with bilateral hemianopsia but preserved central vision. His patient had no sensory or motor disturbance, could read, write, and recognize pictures but was unable to remember the arrangement of furniture in the room in which he had lived for years. Street maps and geographical locations were difficult to plot. At autopsy some years later, bilateral occipitotemporal softenings were found.

Extinction

A normal individual feels equally pinpricks or tactile stimuli such as wisps of cotton applied at the same time to symmetrical points on the two sides of the body. Certain lesions of the brain impair the simultaneous appreciation of two symmetrical points on the body, usually suppressing the appreciation of stimuli applied to the impaired side, although when singly applied, the stimuli are considered of equal quality. This disparity was described by Loeb and also by Oppenheim in 1885; Oppenheim termed the phenomenon "double stimulation." The irritant may be visual, tactile, somesthetic, auditory, barognostic, stereognostic, or gustatory. A somewhat similar disturbance impairing the recognition of the side stimulated was described by Obersteiner as alloesthesia, which may be related to tactile, visual, or olfactory stimuli.

The Internal Brain

Although the configuration of the human brain was known to Erasistratus, subsequent writers, basing their descriptions upon gross examination of animals' brains (monkeys, oxen, and lower forms), gave confused accounts of the cerebrum. The Alexandrian physicians knew of the irregular appearance of the surface of the brain; in fact, Erasistratus likened it to the coils of the intestine and suggested that such a configuration was related to superior intelligence. The internal structure was usually poorly preserved, so that only the ventricles attracted attention. Galen noted the masses lying on either side of the midline ventricle and called them the thalami nervorum opticorum. He described the corpus callosum (a firm body), which he thought extended bilaterally into the white matter of the cerebral hemispheres. But of the large masses of white and gray matter of the hemispheres, neither he nor early anatomists had much to say. In the 15th century, Mondinus D'Luzzi referred to the thalami, or as he termed them, "anchae." Not until 1586, when Piccolomini gave an account of their relationships, were they further delineated.

In the 16th century Vesalius, with the help of Calcar, described and illustrated the configuration of the brain but added little to the structure of the central gray masses.

In the next century Willis, studying brains that had been hardened in alcohol, described the quadrigeminal bodies of the upper brainstem, noting their configuration and connections. Using the same technique as Willis, Raymond de Vieussens of Montpellier dissected 500 fixed brains, layer by layer, to display the internal structures, particularly the thalamus and basal ganglia with their connecting tracts.

The lower brainstem was also being explored. In an essay on apoplexy in 1709, Mistichelli described a fibrous band, which resembled a woman's tress of hair, traversing the medulla oblongata with its roots in the meninges. A more explicit account of these tracts in the pontine region was given by a military surgeon, Pourfour du Petit, who produced a contralateral hemiplegia by cortical wounds in dogs. He clearly described the fibers of the pyramid originating in the corona radiata, passing through the pons, and decussating in the pyramidal body of the medulla oblongata. In 1769, Nicolai Saucerotte, also experimenting with dogs, confirmed the crossing of the pyramidal fibers. He described a somatotopic organization of the motor cortex based upon the observation that anterior lesions of the cerebral cortex produced weakness of the contralateral hind limb and posterior lesions produced paresis of the forelimb—a concept soon forgotten.

A few years later, Vicq d'Azyr, by slicing the brain in several planes, was able to trace the commissures which "establish sympathetic communications between different parts of the brain." He referred to the white cords running from the mammillary bodies to the anterior tubercles of the thalami—tracts later named after him.

As the structural characteristics of the internal gray masses of the cerebral hemispheres were delineated, investigators explored their functions. Saucerotte destroyed parts of the thalamus and observed circus movements. His crude techniques probably damaged adjacent structures, as had other investigators of the early part of the 19th century who reported motor activity after thalamic injuries. In the first monograph on the thalamus, written in 1834 as an inaugural dissertation for a doctorate at the University of Copenhagen, S.A.W. Stein concluded, however, that the optic nerves took origin from the thalamus, anterior quadrigeminal body, or the brainstem, depending upon which was the most perfectly developed. In higher primates, he concluded that the optic nerves arose from the thalami and that fibers passed to the entire cortex. He did not suggest that the thalamus might subserve other functions.

A few years later, Richard Bright wrote of a thalamic lesion: "in this case, the more remarkable symptoms displayed themselves in connection with vision and the sense of touch, as exercised by the fingers; and the lesion of the brain was most decided in the optic thalamus; corresponding, therefore, with our preconceived notions of the influence exerted by this portion of the brain."

Although Gall and Spurzheim were ridiculed for their phrenological scheme, Gall contributed significantly to the knowledge of the fiber connections of the cerebral hemispheres, which he believed were made up of two systems of fibers, one "afferent," which converged (rentrant), and one "efferent," which diverged from the thalamus. This novel concept was to be accepted and elaborated upon as more became known of the structure and functions of the cerebrum.

Up to this point of time, the nervous system had been examined with the naked eye. As methods of fixing brain tissue, staining, clearing, and mounting sections on glass slides were developed in the latter half of the 19th century, with the achromatic microscope the fine structure of the cerebrum could be seen and graphically demonstrated. In 1869, Meynert wrote of the six-layered cerebral cortex and its cellular arrangement. Two years later, he published an account of the fiber connections of the sensory pathways. Although the description of these systems was crude, it did emphasize that there was an organizational plan of the cerebral cortex, which previously had been considered a homogenous covering of the white matter. As this new concept was developing, other methods were being developed to study the fiber arrangements. In 1859, Gudden sought a means of identifying changes in a neuron whose processes had been injured. He removed a sense organ, such as the eye, in newborn kittens, and after some time examined serial sections of the brain which he stained with carmine. He found that some cells were shrunken; he presumed that these cells had axonal connections with the ablated cortex. These cellular changes were easily identified and stimulated further investigation of the connections of the cortex and subcortical nuclei. Based on this technique, von Monakow explored the thalamic connections of kittens. He concluded that the middle and anterior thalamic nuclei subserved a motor function and the lateral thalamic nucleus a sensory function. There was, however, some overlap of the connections.

Paul Flechsig devised another method of tracing fiber tracts by observing the myelination of the developing nervous system. He was able to follow the corticospinal tract from the pyramids to the cerebral cortex—a path which Gudden had identified as the cortico-capsular link.

On the basis of morphological studies, Luys in 1865 concluded that the thalamus was the "sensorium commune" with four centers—an anterior concerned with olfaction, a medial with vision, a median with somatic sensation, and a posterior with audition. Eight years later, Fournié injected zinc chloride into various thalamic nuclei to destroy them and concluded that all sensory systems converged upon the thalamus, from which other fibers projected to the cerebral cortex. Veyssière, who repeated these experiments in 1874, maintained that the sensory disturbances resulted from injury to the internal capsule; he thought that the sensory fibers passed directly to the cerebral cortex. In 1873, Nothnagel produced thalamic lesions in rabbits and other lower animals, causing only lasting defects of vision and abnormal postures of the limbs. At the end of the century, Sellier and Verger produced electrolytic thalamic lesions and noted that pain sensibility was diminished but not completely abolished on the contralateral side of the body. As no motor impairment was observed, they concluded that the thalamus was concerned with sensory perception. These physiological studies, handicapped by the failure to make discrete lesions and the inability to test sensory deficits in animals, were amplified by clinical investigations.

William R. Gowers (Fig. 3-11), in his textbook of 1888, stated that the function of the basal ganglia, including the thalamus, was unknown although paralysis, mobile spasm, and choreiform movements had been reported. He concluded that there were no sensory or motor palsies; he considered any transient sensory disturbances to result from coincidental capsular damage. A few years later, Mills described the fiber connections of the thalamus, although he was uncertain they were related to sensory or motor activities. Charcot, without anatomical confirmation, attributed choreiform or hemichoreic movements occurring after a stroke to thalamic involvement.

At the beginning of the 20th century, French neurologists clarified the functions of the thalamus. In 1906, Dejerine and Roussy described the thalamic syndrome as a slight hemiplegia rapidly regressing, a persistent superficial hemianesthesia at times followed by a cutaneous hyperesthesia, but always

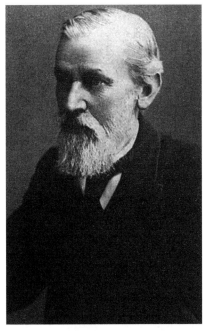

Fig. 3-11. William R. Gowers (1845-1915). (From The Founders of Neurology, *2nd ed. Haymaker W, Schiller F, editors. Springfield, Ill: Charles C Thomas, 1970)*

accompanied by a marked and persistent disturbance of deep sensibility, slight ataxia, and severe astereognosis. These cardinal symptoms were occasionally accompanied by paroxysmal or persistent intolerable pain and choreoathetoid movements on the hemiparetic side. Foix and Hillemand and L'Hermitte later amplified the syndrome.

Basal Ganglia Disorders

Although the function of the thalamus was being explored in the latter part of the 19th century, the adjacent basal nuclear structures, separated by the internal capsule, were retaining their secrets. True, various investigators had studied these ganglia earlier and attributed diverse functions to them—"tendencies to track motion without reflection over descending pathways," "to provide specific limb activation," "to integrate the motor responses of the various centers which are differentiated in the cortex," and "to initiate and execute movements." The striate bodies, however, proved to be inexcitable and their destruction caused no significant motor or sensory disturbance. Yet isolated clinical reports of lesions suggested that they played a role in motor activity. In 1881, Pölchen reported in carbon monoxide intoxication the loss of consciousness, pink color of the skin, and a progressive Parkinsonian syndrome as well as various cortical defects such as paresis, spasticity, reflex changes, and abnormal movements. Typically, the globus pallidus was necrotic. Softening of the subthalamic nucleus produced a coarse flinging of the contralateral limbs termed hemiballismus. Westphal in 1883 described a choreic muscular disorder, which Wilson in 1912 showed was associated with hepatic sclerosis and necrotic lesions of the lenticular nuclei. As these disorders became better defined and their pathological basis clarified, a number of basal ganglia syndromes were recognized.

Choreatic Syndromes

Involuntary movements are so obvious, especially if they involve the face, that observers as well as the afflicted are quite conscious, even embarrassed, by their occurrence. In Greek and Roman times, "saltus" and "spasms" were the terms used to describe such movements. Asclepiades held "that extension and contraction alternate more frequently in tremor than in saltus and quite infrequently in spasm; also that the amount of extension and contraction is small in cases of tremor, greater in saltus and very great in cases of spasm." However, saltus was also used to refer to the pulsations of the heart and vessels. The term "chorea" seems to have been derived from the Greek word for chorus, which was applied to the singing and dancing accompanying their dramas. Centuries later it was again brought into fashion to describe the fanatic dancing of the people of Strassburg, who in long processions sought aid at the chapel of Saint Vitus in Zabern. Sporadic episodes of dancing mania must have occurred in the next 300 years before Sydenham observed another choreiform outbreak in children. "This disorder is a kind of a convulsion which seizes children of both sexes, from the tenth to the fourteenth year; it manifests itself by a halting or unsteadiness of one of the legs, which the patient drags after him like an idiot. If the hand of the same side be applied to the breast, or any other part of the body, the child can't keep it a moment in the same posture but it will be drawn into a different one by a convulsion, not withstanding all his efforts to the contrary. Before a child who hath this disorder can get a glass or cup to his mouth, he useth an abundance of odd gestures, for he does not bring it in a straight line thereto, but his hand being drawn sideways by the spasm, he moves it backwards and forwards, till at length the glass accidently coming nearer to his lips, he throws the liquor hastily into his mouth, and swallows it greedily, as if he meant to divert the spectators."

The motor dyskinesia called "chorea minor," characterized by involuntary, jerky movements, particularly of the peripheral parts of the limbs, was one of a number of later conditions in which muscular contractions were prominent—

Huntington's chorea (muscular jerking predominantly of the trunk muscles), tetanic chorea (slow movements of the limb), dystonia (slow writhing contortion of a limb), fibrillary chorea (muscular fasciculation), muscular unrest or restless legs, habit chorea, or tic—but which would not be considered chorea at the present time.

Parkinson's Disease

One of the earliest and most obvious disorders of mankind is the deranged movement resulting in shaking or jerking of the limbs. Galen observed that shaking might occur while a person was at rest or when the individual was carrying out a muscular act. He referred to the former as "tremor" and the latter as "palpitatio." In medieval times, the tremor was recognized to accompany intense emotional states such as fear. Sylvius de la Boë, in the Elizabethan era, pointed out that the tremor developing with the limb at rest differed from that which occurred during voluntary motion. Other features were noted which would be described later as part of the Parkinsonian syndrome. The flexed posture and festinating gait were pointed out by Gaubius. In 1763, de Sauvages de la Croix wrote of the peculiar gait due to a "want of flexibility in the muscular fibers" (rigidity). But such isolated accounts of the clinical picture of the Parkinsonism syndrome were rarely found prior to the 19th century.

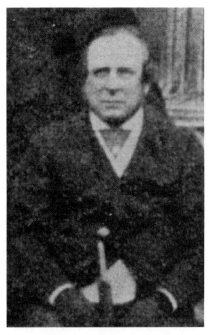

James Parkinson's (Fig. 3-12) description of the afflicted individual is a classic. "Involuntary tremulous motion, with lessened muscular power, in parts not in action and, even when supported; with a propensity to bend the trunk forwards, and to pass from a walking to a running pace; the senses and intellect being uninjured." Parkinson differentiated the tremor of his patients from the shaking of epileptics, the tremulous movements of the alcoholic, the excessive tea or coffee drinker and the elderly. He noted that if a patient had a stroke involving the shaking limbs, the tremor ceased but might return as the strength was regained in the limb.

Fig. 3-12. James Parkinson (1755-1824). (From Classics of Neurology. Huntington, NY: Krieger, 1971)

Charcot, in a detailed description of "paralyse agitante," as he termed the shaking palsy, pointed out the rigidity or stiffness of the muscles of the extremities, limbs, and neck, which he believed had been overlooked by earlier writers. Charcot noted the general stiff state of the patient which, at times, was present in the absence of the tremor—"formes frustes."

Parkinson's disease attracted little attention until the epidemic of encephalitis lethargica in 1915-20, when many cases developed as a result of that disorder. After a few years, the majority of cases seemed to have no specific etiological agent unless it was the aging process. Although various degenerative changes—pigmentary loss in the substantia nigra as reported by Blocq and Marinesco in 1893, diffuse cortical atrophy and progressive increase in ventricular size—may occur, as shown much later, it is dopamine deficiency that produces the Parkinsonian syndrome.

Kernicterus

Jaundice of the newborn has been known for ages, but that it might involve the brain was recognized little more than a century ago. In his doctoral thesis of 1847, Hervieux discussed icterus neonatorum and noted the staining of the basal ganglia, but neither he nor Orth, who recognized the pigment as bile deposits, knew its significance. Just after the turn of the century, Schmorl observed that the pigmentation was confined to nuclear structures and called the condition "kernicterus." The clinical concomitants—hypotonia, lethargy, and decreased sucking followed by fever, spasticity, opisthotonus, and a high-pitched cry—were described five years later by Esch. If the infant survived, a few weeks later, athetosis, gaze palsies, hearing loss, and dental dysplasia developed and the previously pigmented neurons of the subcortical nuclei lost their pigment, dropped out, and were replaced by gliosis. The Rh factor is not always the pathogenesis of the condition.

Huntington's Chorea

Although only recognized since the first half of the 19th century, the hereditary chorea known as Huntington's chorea probably has afflicted the human race for ages. Progressive dyskinesia and dementia were known to the natives of New York state as "magrums." Typically, several adult members of a family developed increasingly severe convulsive-like movements, became demented and died.

At the middle of the 19th century, Gorman in his inaugural dissertation at Jefferson Medical College, Philadelphia, described "a form of chorea, vulgarly called magrums." In 1863, I.W. Lyon of New York noted that hereditary chorea called "migrims" and traced through generations might occur in a juvenile. It was in 1872 that George Huntington presented his paper on chorea minor and referred briefly at the end to a hereditary chorea occurring in adult life and associated with mental disturbances, a condition which he considered "a medical curiosity." Unknown to Huntington, Lund, a Norwegian physician, had published a series of papers in 1859, 1863, and 1868 in which he gave a masterful description of "twitches" (aykka) beginning in late adult life and leading to a fatal dementia. The characteristics of this hereditary disease were clearly described in several Norwegian journals. In the latter part of the 19th century a number of other cases were mentioned in the European literature. In addition to Lund, in 1880 Harbinson from Lancaster and others reported on the condition. Yet it was Huntington's comments, based upon remarks by his father and grandfather, that stimulated not only interest in hereditary chorea but in other hereditary conditions.

Dystonia

Bizarre muscular movements of the limbs have been referred to as dystonia since Oppenheim and Vogt used the term in 1911. Oppenheim stated that the muscles might rapidly reverse from a hypotonic to a hypertonic state and that the tone of antagonist and agonists might be dissimilar. Although he used the term in describing the motor signs of dystonia muscularis deformans, the concept was shortly applied to the changing tone of muscles unrelated to pyramidal tract involvement. Thus this appellation was applied to a number of states differing from the condition originally described by Schwalbe in 1908.

This was further confused by the inability to find a consistent pathological substrate for dystonia muscularis deformans. As experience accumulated, it became evident that dystonic movements might be symptomatic of many brain disorders—prenatal brain injuries, degenerative, vascular, inflammatory, traumatic, toxic (drug), and surgical neurological disorders. Even hysterical manifestations might be of a dystonic nature. As a result, the designation "dystonia musculorum deformans" was reserved for a specific dystonic complex.

Dystonia Musculorum Deformans

In a doctoral thesis in 1908, Schwalbe of Ziehen's clinic described the clinical course of a condition characterized by tonic spasms with hysterical manifestations. In his cases, the disorder began insidiously in childhood, often with an inversion spasm of a foot or hand cramps spreading to involve the entire limb and trunk, thus producing grotesque postures and an awkward gait. Since three patients were siblings and one had three children, two of whom were afflicted with the same disorder, he postulated a genetic factor.

When Schwalbe's report became known, a number of earlier cases were recalled. Probably the earliest case was reported by Destarac in 1901. The patient was a 17-year-old girl who had torticollis, writer's cramp, and spasmodic talipes equinovarus.

In 1904, Leszynsky reported a case of hysteria which was subsequently examined by Fraenkel and Ramsay Hunt, who established the diagnosis of dystonia. In 1911, Oppenheim gave a clinical description of the disorder and named it dystonia musculorum deformans. In the same year, Flatau and Sterling reported two brothers with a similar disorder which they called progressive torsion spasm. Subsequently, various terminologies (e.g., tortipelvis, torsion dystonia, and Ziehen-Oppenheim disease) were suggested, but dystonia musculorum deformans retained its place.

Hepatocerebral Degeneration

In 1912, S.A.K. Wilson (Fig. 3-13) described in great detail a rare hereditary affliction manifested by involuntary movements, rigidity, and dysarthria which was associated with a peculiar form of hepatic cirrhosis. All but four of his patients had familial traits. Wilson does mention six previously reported cases, the earliest being that of Gowers, entitled "Tetanoid chorea associated with cirrhosis of the liver" in which no definite lesion was found in the nervous system. In 1906, Gowers referred to this case again, noting that a brother and three other relatives had died of "chorea." At that time, a sister who had developed a similar affliction was found on postmortem examination to have cirrhosis of the liver. Two previous publications, one by Westphal in 1883 and one by Strümpell in 1895, were referred to as patients suffering from the same condition. Westphal's cases, however, had neither lenticular lesions nor cirrhosis of the liver, and Strümpell's cases had no specific changes in the brain although in one person there were early signs of cirrhosis of the liver. It is doubtful that these reports of involuntary movements should be included as variants of lenticular degeneration. In 1921, Hall emphasized the hepatic changes and designated the disease as hepatolenticular degeneration.

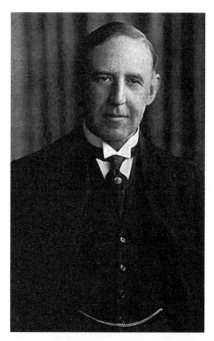

Fig. 3-13. S.A. Kinnier Wilson (1878-1937). (From The Founders of Neurology, *2nd ed. Haymaker W, Schiller F, editors. Springfield, Ill: Charles C Thomas, 1970, p 536)*

A somewhat inconstant feature of the disease was a greenish-brown or yellow ring of pigmentation near the limbus of the cornea. Although first reported by Kayser in 1902 in a patient diagnosed with multiple sclerosis, 10 years later Fleischer recognized its significance. His patient had the ring with signs of motor incoordination and hepatic cirrhosis.

Although for years the brain has been known to have metallic constituents, notably copper, it was Haurowitz who confirmed an increased copper content in formalin-fixed brains of two patients with Wilson's disease. A few other cases had been reported before Cumings in 1948 gave a detailed account of the copper in three patients with Wilson's disease and controls. He affirmed that the condition was due to a disturbance of copper metabolism causing impaired ceruloplasmin synthesis, as the result of which copper was deposited in subcortical ganglia and some other parts of the brain.

The Cerebellum

The small brain was rarely mentioned in ancient literature. Even the early Alexandrian anatomists left no description of what Herophilus referred to as the "parencephalis" and Erasistratus as the "epenkranis," terms which included those neural structures below the tentorium that gave rise to the cranial nerves and the spinal cord. Erasistratus astutely observed that the convolutional patterns of both the cerebrum and cerebellum were progressively more complex in ascending phylogeny. He concluded that this augmented complexity was related to man's greater mentality and the development of the limbs. Other Greek and Roman authors until the time of Galen paid little attention to these structures.

Following the example of the early anatomists, Galen included the lower brainstem as part of the cerebellum. Consequently, his belief that it was the source of the motor nerves and the spinal cord is quite logical. Additionally, his idea that the vermis acted as a valve to regulate the ventricular flow of animal spirits was not entirely irrational. He stated, "since all the nerves of the body that are distributed from the head to the lower parts must arrive either from the parencephalon or from the spinal cord, this ventricle of the cerebellum must be of considerable size to receive the physic pneuma elaborated in the anterior ventricles." However, Galen denounced the suggestion of Erasistratus who, he stated, "claims that the cerebellum and with it, the cerebrum, is more complex in man than in other animals because the latter do not have an intelligence like that in man, it does not appear to me that he is reasoning correctly, since even asses have a very complicated cerebellum although their imbecile character demands a very simple and unvariegated cerebrum."

In the next thousand years, physicians reiterated the concepts of Galen. Even Andreas Vesalius, who described the cerebellum of man, oxen, dogs, and sheep, made only passing reference to the cerebellum's assumed role in memory and intelligence. He noted that the convolutions of the cerebellum were not as deep as those of the cerebrum, so that the former were more accessible to the ventricle.

Whereas Galen, Vesalius, and the early anatomists viewed the brain in situ with the skull-cap cut away, Varolio removed the brain from the calvarium. This enabled him to see the structures on the undersurface much better than previously. Varolio wrote, "On each side of the cerebellum near the trunks . . . there arises a process which is carried transversely forward and downward; by means of this process, the cerebellum enfolds the anterior part of the spinal marrow. . . . Since I have observed the marrow to be carried under this transverse spinal process in the same way that a flowing channel is carried under a bridge for the sake of clearer meaning, I shall call it a bridge (pons) of the cerebellum."

By hardening the brain, Willis could get a better view of the external appearance of the cerebellar structures. After acknowledging that the ancient writers did not have a satisfactory explanation of the function of the cerebellum, Willis postulated, "The duty of the cerebellum, however, seems to be to supply animal spirits to certain nerves by which involuntary actions take place." As the involuntary functions were the same in all species, he considered that the constant configuration of the cerebellum was related to involuntary activity, and the fluctuating voluntary functions such as imagination, memory, and locomotion were assigned to the cerebrum, in which the convolutions varied greatly in the animal scale.

Willis described the cerebellum as resting below on the medulla oblongata and above affixed to two peduncles. Between these, the cavity of the cerebellum, commonly called the fourth ventricle, was bounded by the three cerebellar peduncles. "The first of these issued from the orbicular protuberance and ascends obliquely; the second descending directly from the cerebellum and running across the first, circles around the medulla oblongata; the third process descending from the rear of the cerebellum is inserted into the medulla oblongata, and, like an additional cord, augments its trunk."

In 1684, Raymond de Vieussens made the next contribution to the knowledge of the cerebellum in his book *Neurographia universalis*. After a precise account of the internal appearance of the cerebellum, including the anterior medullary velum, known for some time as the valve of Vieussens, he described the external features of the cerebellum. He referred to a soft membrane which is joined to the anterior vermiform process, to the processes (superior cerebellar peduncles), and to the tectum so that "this membrane lines the anterior part of the cavity of the fourth ventricle and closes off the aqueduct at the rear, hence, we assert it acts like a valve."

Perhaps the most precise account of the cerebellum came in 1819 from the pen of Malacarne, an anatomist and surgeon, who eventually became professor of the theory and practice of surgery at Padua. He noted the folial structure of the cerebellar cortex, its parallel furrows of varying depth, the deeper ones dividing the hemispheres into lobes, which he named anatomically as tonsil, pyramid, lingula, and uvula—names that are still in use. This detailed description of the cerebellum was, however, little recognized at that time.

It remained for the German anatomist Reil to elaborate upon the descriptions by Malacarne and to illustrate the cerebella of hare, sheep, ox, and horse in 1795. Reil designated the parts of the vermis in geographical terms which were less appealing than Malacarne's names and accordingly were soon forgotten.

French surgeons were also interested in the role of the cerebellum. Lorrey made unilateral cerebellar lesions and noted that cats had weak and awkward movements of the extremities on the injured side. Abnormal jerkings of the eyes—"nystagmus"—were seen after cerebellar lesions. Saucerotte referred to them as "une agitation continuelle" and Méhee de la Touche as "convulsive movements of the eyes."

Willis' idea that the cerebellum was the seat of vital activities was still held. In the early part of the 19th century, Gall and Spurzheim, without foundation, suggested that the cerebellum controlled sexual functions. Luigi Rolando removed the cerebella of a number of animals (including goats and rabbits) noting as he "excised at a stroke, the animal became hemiplegic and soon died with convulsions and hemorrhage." He noted that lesions of the right cerebellar hemisphere affected the right side of the body.

Shortly afterward, more precise cerebellar lesions were made by the French physiologist, Flourens, who concluded, "I have shown that all movements persist following ablation of the cerebellum; all that is missing is that they are not regular and coordinated." He made lesions in pigeons, dogs, and other animals, noting that a slight cerebellar damage produced no impairment of sensory, vital, or intellectual functions, but a lack of motor coordination which he called "drunken"—a drunken swim, a drunken flight, and a drunken gait. These experiments on cerebellar ablations were repeated, but the crude lesions produced inconsistent neurological disturbances. Magendie concluded that the cerebellum controlled equilibrium, but his studies were on acute preparations, many dying before the effects of vascular and neural shock had passed. Other investigators concluded, however, that the cerebellum was a coordinating center for movement. After cerebellectomy in birds, Fedors noted an extensor hypertonus, the significance of which he did not appreciate. It was not until Luigo Luciani, using aseptic techniques, made cerebellar ablations in dogs and apes that the chronic effects of such lesions could be analyzed. Luciani recognized three stages: 1) functional exaltation; 2) deficiency phenomena; and 3) compensatory mechanisms. During the first week or 10 days, the animal had opisthotonoid seizures characterized by head retraction and tonic extensor spasms. These extensor phenomena became apparent within two days of decerebellation in the monkey and after a week or 10 days in the cat and dog, occurring as the animal was beginning to perform voluntary movements. Luciani termed the animal's disturbances asthenia, atonia, and astasia (tremor), later called the "Luciani triad." After a month or so, as the animal began to walk on all fours, these signs became less marked. Luciani concluded that the cerebellum, although exerting a bilateral effect, predominantly involved the ipsilateral extremities, contrary to the contralateral effect of hemispheric lesions. Perhaps Luciani's description of the three stages was oversimplified, but at that time it gave a much clearer insight into the function of the cerebellum than had been possible previously. The compensation for cerebellar defects, Luciani concluded, came primarily from other parts of the cerebellum. David Ferrier reported that stimulation of the anterior part of the middle cerebellar lobe "excites the muscular combinations which would counteract a tendency to fall forward" and that "stimulation of the posterior part of the middle lobe calls into play the muscular adjustments necessary to counteract a backward displacement of the equilibrium." Lesions of the lateral lobes, he believed, caused a disturbance of the equilibrium laterally. Rudolph Magnus, who investigated the tonic labyrinthine and neck reflexes before and after ablation of the cerebellum, found those reflexes little changed and concluded that "the centers responsible for them the [labyrinthine reflexes] lie in a well-defined local arrangement in the brainstem and not in the cerebellum." Thus, the popular idea that the cerebellum was the labyrinthine center was abandoned.

Experimental work on cerebellar functioning emphasized the species differences. As a result, clinical studies of cerebellar function became of great interest. Babinski in 1900 asserted that the disturbances previously considered to be cerebellar dysfunction were due to injury to the vestibular apparatus and that the phenomena attributable to cerebellar affections were "asynergia, adiadochokinesis and cerebellar cataplexy." Sherrington, writing at about the same time, conceived of the cerebellum as the head ganglion of the proprioceptive system. He believed that the organ functioned as a whole and in association with the motor region of the cerebral hemisphere. Subsequent investigations required electrical and physiological techniques that were not developed until the middle of the 20th century.

Localization of Function Within the Cerebellum

Although Luciani thought that there was no localization of function within the cerebellum, Löwenthal in 1895 observed the extensor tonus of decerebrate rigidity, which could be relaxed by stimulation of the superior surface of the cerebellum. With Horsley in 1897 he published a short, preliminary account of stimulation of the cerebellum and cerebrum in cats and dogs. They noted that "when both cerebral hemispheres were removed and, as a result, active extensor tonus of the limbs was obtained, excitation of the upper surface of the cerebellum caused an immediate relaxation of such tonus so long as the current was applied, and that on the latter being shut off the tonus was immediately reestablished." They concluded that when the cerebellum is stimulated with the animal in a decerebrate posture the biceps contracts powerfully and the triceps actively relaxes. They noted that stimulation of both the ipsilateral and contralateral paths of the cerebellum gave rise to this effect although it was more pronounced upon ipsilateral stimulation. Moreover, they reported that stimulation of the cerebellum without decerebrate rigidity would constantly produce a tonic contraction of either the triceps or biceps or both together.

After the turn of the century, extensive investigations of cerebellar function were carried out by Sherrington and others. Evidence for the localization of function within the cerebellum came from the findings of comparative anatomy by Louis Bolk, who stated, "I have reached the following assumptions regarding the localization of cerebellar functions. The anterior lobe contains the coordination center for the group of muscles of the head (eyes, tongue, muscles of mastication, facial muscles) and in addition of the larynx and pharynx; in the lobulus simplex is the coordinating center of the cervical muscles; the upper portion of the lobulus medianus posterior contains the unpaired coordination center for the left and right extremities; in each of the lobuli ansiformis and paramedian is one of the paired centers for the two extremities."

When postmortem examinations became a common procedure, a number of cerebellar abnormalities were recognized and correlated with clinical findings. However, cerebellar dysplasia was noted in some persons who had no clinical manifestations during life.

Congenital Cerebellar Atrophy

Cerebellar dysfunction as the result of atrophy and aplasia has been confused. It seems probable that many cases referred to as "atrophies," especially the so-called "congenital atrophies," are actually aplasias which do not manifest themselves clinically during adolescence or adult life. Accordingly, the congenital cerebellar ataxia described by Batten may be the result of either maldevelopment or atrophy resulting from early disease. Because Batten did not discuss the pathological findings in his cases, it is impossible to determine whether they represent aplasia or atrophy. He noted that the child, typically backward in such developmental phases as walking and talking, was unsteady and ataxic on attempts to stand or walk. Speech was slow and limited to a few jerky words. However, as the child grew older, the disability often lessened. Such patients have one of several pathological lesions. One, assumed to be due to an injury at birth, was characterized by cerebellar atrophy or ulegyria, pronounced in the deeper folia. Spiller in 1896 described a case of cerebellar cortical atrophy with gliosis. In some cases, the granular layer alone was affected, suggesting that the state might have been hereditary. If gliosis of the cerebellar cortex and white matter was present, however, the changes were likely to represent an atrophy rather than an aplasia.

Olivopontocerebellar Atrophy (Dejerine-Thomas)

Dejerine and André Thomas in 1900 described a cerebellar disturbance characterized clinically by an isolated cerebellar syndrome developing in adult life as the result of atrophy of the cerebellar cortex, inferior olives, gray matter of the pons, degeneration of the middle cerebellar peduncle, and partial atrophy of the restiform bodies without evidence of inflammation or sclerosis. Isolated cases not so clearly described had been reported. Although the syndrome reported by André Thomas in 1897 and again with Dejerine in 1900 is a progressive spinocerebellar degeneration, a satisfactory classification of the disorder has not been established.

The designation "olivopontocerebellar atrophy" included many different types of olivopontocerebellar atrophy and accompanying abnormalities of the brain stem, retina, cerebral hemispheres, and neuromuscular systems. That all of these varied neurological disturbances should be included under the umbrella of olivopontocerebellar atrophy is open to question.

Late (Acquired) Cortical Cerebellar Atrophy

Many disorders result in parenchymatous degeneration of the cerebellar cortex: anemia, hypoglycemia, hyperthermia, cerebral lipidosis, Hallervorden-Spatz disease, Wilson's disease, tuberosclerosis, mongolism, Jakob-Creutzfeldt disease, diffuse cerebral degeneration (Alpers), leukodystrophy, and cerebral cholesterinosis. The cerebellar cortex is also involved in infections of the central nervous system such as meningoencephalitis and tuberculous meningitis, which are part of a general affliction. In addition to these disorders, the cerebellum or its cortex is predominantly affected in a number of so-called degenerative diseases: hereditofamilial corticocerebellar degeneration, prolonged alcoholism and malnutrition, remote malignancies, endocrinopathies, intoxications with heavy metals and anticonvulsants, granule cell degeneration, and focal panatrophy sine symptoms.

Crossed Cerebellar Atrophy

When one cerebral hemisphere is damaged in infancy or early childhood, the opposite cerebellar hemisphere does not develop or "becomes atrophic" as the result of trans-synaptic atrophy which may involve cortico-ponto-cerebellar, central tegmental-olivo-cerebellar pathways, or retrograde dentato-thalamic pathways.

Alcoholic Cerebellar Degeneration

In 1897, André Thomas described the clinical manifestations of alcoholic cerebellar ataxia and noted the pathological changes, mainly in the superior vermis. Subsequently, many clinical cases and a few autopsies on verified alcoholic patients were reported. In the 20th century these cases were grouped with neuropathies in alcoholics, many suffering not only from nutritional deficiencies but from deficiencies in essential food elements so that it is probable that the cerebellar (and cerebral) pathological changes resulted from a number of factors in addition to the toxic effects of excessive alcohol.

Hereditary Spinocerebellar Atrophy

In the 19th century, a number of cases diagnosed as hereditary spinocerebellar atrophy were reported, many of which were not confirmed at autopsy. As a result, they probably represented a motley group ranging from muscular atrophies to olivary atrophy occurring in several members of a family. While they might have been variants of a fundamental dysplasia, their classification is unproved. In 1892, Sanger Brown described a familial form of progressive cerebellar ataxia involving the limbs and speech, spasticity, pyramidal tract, and in some cases optic atrophy. One case was autopsied and showed posterior column as well as dorsal spinocerebellar atrophic tracts and some cell loss in Clarke's column and the anterior horn cells. Although a number of other cases were reported, few autopsies were made. As a result, the proper classification of these cases has yet to be determined.

4

The Spinal Cord

In fact, the greater part of all we know of an exact nature concerning this most important organ, the spinal cord, has been accumulated mainly in the last half of the present [19th] century.

—Clevenger

The early Egyptians knew that the spinal column activated the muscles of the body, for the *Edwin Smith papyrus* describes the paralysis, urinary incontinence, and emissio seminalis resulting from a neck injury. It is not clear, however, that the Egyptians understood the role of the various components of the spinal column—bone, membranes, spinal cord, and spinal bone marrow. The Hippocratic writers had a vague concept of the function of the cord that passed through the vertebral bones. Perhaps if the section which Hippocrates stated was being written on the spinal cord had been preserved, their concepts would have been clarified. About a hundred years later, Herophilus described the caudal prolongation of the rhombencephalon, which he termed the "spinal cord" and from which the nerves arose. A more detailed account of its structure and its relationship to the rhombencephalon was given by Galen four centuries later. Galen outlined in detail the vertebral bodies, the intervertebral discs, the anterior spinal ligaments, and the dura mater and pia mater ensheathing the spinal cord, from which a bundle of filaments emerged on each side from the vertebral canal through round lateral foramina. These fibers, he believed, conveyed spirits from the brain to the muscles. In a series of brilliant experiments, Galen defined the topographical arrangement of the nerves supplying the sensory and motor segments of the body, the sympathetic nerves, and the function of the seven cranial nerves identified at that time. Upon his death, Galen's teachings, previously disdained by the sects in Rome, regained favor and within a few centuries were considered the ultimate authority in medicine.

The Structure of the Spinal Cord

More than a thousand years passed before Vesalius in *De humani corporis fabrica* described the spinal cord in greater detail. As had the earlier anatomists, he noted that the spinal cord in its passage through the canal gave off lateral shoots, each of which entered a separate foramen until only a single thread (filum terminale) was attached to the sacrum. Vesalius stated that the number of spinal nerves was not agreed upon, some professors of anatomy noting 30 pairs of nerves and some 29 pairs. This description of the spinal cord and nerve roots was not improved upon for years. Even Willis' sketch of the spinal cord, which depicted cervical and lumbar enlargements, 32 nerve roots, a nerve of the sacral bone, and a fanciful vascular tree on the spinal cord which extended to the sacral sac, was less than accurate. Although the spinal cord was considered a conduit, the origin and termination of the channels were determined centuries later.

The Hippocratic writers knew that damage to one side of the brain would cause spasms and paralysis on the opposite side of the body. Aretaeus reasoned that the channels carrying motor spirits from each side must cross, forming the letter X. The actual crossing was not seen until 1709 when Domenico Mistichelli observed a braiding of fibers in the upper cervical spinal cord. Pourfour du Petit more accurately described the decussation of the fibers of the pyramidal tract; however, his concise description attracted little attention. In 1786, Vicq d'Azyr elaborated upon the arrangement of the fiber bundles of the spinal cord, their varied size and shape at different levels, and their divisions into posterior and two lateral segments (later called columns) and a white anterior commissure.

These descriptions of the gross appearance of the spinal cord were refined some years later when Stilling, using lenses, examined alcohol-fixed preparations. The contrast between the white and gray matter was more apparent, and the longitudinal course of some tracts and the transverse course of others were readily seen. Stilling also noted that fibers radiated from the horns of the central gray to the anterior white matter. Von Kölliker (Fig. 4-1) in 1850, using chromate as a fixative, described the nerve roots in more detail and their passage through the substantia gelatinosa into the substantia grisea, some to turn upward into the posterior column and some to disperse in the lateral column. He noted that some bundles of transverse fibers passed across in the commissure to radiate into the opposite posterior horns.

Early in the 19th century, anatomists interested in the distribution of tracts in the brain and spinal cord devised techniques to trace their course. In 1853, Ludwig Türck demonstrated that injured tracts of the spinal cord degenerated in the direction they normally conducted. By following the degenerated tracts after a transverse myelopathy, he was able to define six pathways on each side of the spinal cord: two anterior, two lateral, and two posterior. One pair "at the decussation of the pyramid [the medullary tract], proceeds to the medulla oblongata . . . of the opposite side where, as the posterior half of the lateral column, it proceeds downward to the vicinity of the termination of the spinal cord." A second and smaller tract left the pyramid uncrossed and ran along the midline sulcus of the spinal cord, but not as far caudally as the lateral tracts. By staining the myelin ensheathing the nerve fibers, Flechsig in 1876 complemented the findings of Türck. Assuming that fibers subserving a specific function would myelinate at earlier or later times than fibers of other tracts, Flechsig was able to define the various bundles of the spinal cord. He supplemented such investi-

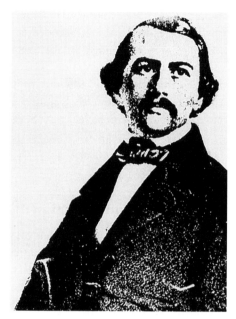

Fig. 4-1. Rudolf Albert von Kölliker (1817-1905). (From the collection of A. Earl Walker)

gations with observations of the secondary degenerations of fiber tracts. Based on these techniques, he was able to analyze the composition of the pyramidal tracts. "Each pyramid contributes about 3.5% to 9% to the direct tract and . . . about 97% to 91% to the lateral (crossed) tract." Flechsig noted that rarely all pyramidal fibers crossed in the lateral tracts so that the direct fibers were absent, and infrequently the fibers crossed only on one side. He presumed that the pyramidal fibers originated in the cerebral cortex and projected to the anterior gray horn of the spinal cord.

Prior to this, the vascular supply of the spinal cord was conceived by anatomists to be a symmetrical arrangement of the vessels along each nerve root. Even Vesalius and Willis illustrated the arterial supply of the cord rather fancifully. It was not until von Haller's exposition that it was realized that only a few nerve roots had accompanying vessels. He noted that there was a regional variation of the vascular supply of the spinal cord. In the cervical segments, the spinal cord on both sides received serial arterial branches along the C2-7 anterior roots. The thoracic segments of the anterior spinal artery had few inputs other than a large artery accompanying the ninth or 10th thoracic roots on one side; occasionally, it entered the spinal canal as high as the T4-5 foramen. Anastomosing arteries passed from the anterior spinal artery around the spinal cord to the posterior roots, especially at the C6-7, T4-5, and T9-10 segments and the lumbosacral enlargement. Von Haller's figures were not only artistic but quite accurate. Somewhat later, Mayer published sketches which were neither as well drawn nor as true to life as von Haller's, although Mayer's descriptions were quite precise. Many subsequent anatomists confirmed this arrangement but a few adhered to the old concepts. In the early 1880s, Adamkiewicz presented his beautiful illustrations of the blood vessels of the spinal cord along with a clear text. Seven years later, Kadyi confirmed the findings. These accounts of the vascular supply of the spinal cord were generally accepted in the 20th century.

The Function of the Spinal Tracts

Galen's remarkable observations on the effects of sectioning the spinal cord at various levels clarified the clinical manifestations of paraplegia. He observed that when oxen were stabbed just behind the first vertebra, the feet of the animal and its respirations were paralyzed. In living, unanesthetized monkeys, Galen noted that transecting the spinal cord more caudally produced the loss of "the capacity of sensation and the capacity of movement" below the cut. These observations led Galen to consider the spinal cord as a tract transmitting spirits between the brain and the body and limbs. Had he observed his animals longer, he might have realized that the cord subserved other functions. As it was, more than a thousand years passed before even cursory investigations were made of isolated spinal cord activity. Leonardo da Vinci concluded that as a decapitated frog twitched when the spinal cord was pricked, it must contain the basis of life and motion.

Legallois in 1812 decapitated frogs and concluded "that decapitation does nothing more than arrest inspiratory motions, and that consequently the source of these motions is in the brain; but the source of the life of the trunk is in the trunk itself." He noted that each part of the body was not animated by the entire cord, but only by the segment innervating it. Hence, destruction of a portion of the cord caused only the related part of the body to "die." Legallois repeated Galen's experiments, making transverse sections of the cord at various levels, and demonstrated that the part of the body corresponding to each segment of the cord had sensation and voluntary movement, although the activity was not as "harmonious" as that of a normal animal. He concluded that there are as many centers of sensation as there are segments of the spinal cord.

It was Whytt, however, who in the 18th century rediscovered the conducting function of the spinal cord and, in addition, its modulating influence on muscular activity. Whytt discarded the old concepts of spirits and concluded that involuntary and voluntary motor activity depended upon the action of the nerves which have not only powers of feeling and motion but sympathy (reflex activity). He recognized that between the afferent and efferent fibers there must be a "sentient principle" which might be located in the brain or spinal cord. After discussing the various possible locations of this principle, Whytt concluded that the spinal cord was essential for such activity. Other writers placed the control locus or *sensorium commune* in places other than the spinal cord—"as widely as the origin of the nerves extend."

In 1832, Haechel developed the concept that the segmented vertebral column was a series of unitary components or metameres, and the whole organism a chain creature. In this frame of reference, the skull was thought of as a modified vertebra and the other parts of the central nervous system as segmented structures. This concept led to the assumption that each unit of the spinal cord must have an input (sensory) from the skin and an output (motor) to an effector organ such as a muscle.

When Alexander Monro secundus, in 1783, described the ganglionated posterior root and the smooth anterior root entering the spinal cord, it seemed that they must be subserving different functions. In 1809, Alexander Walker deduced that the anterior roots were sensory and the posterior roots motor. Charles Bell, after some experimentation, extended this concept. He thought that the cerebrum was the center for movement and sensation, and that these faculties traversed the anterior part of the spinal cord, exiting in the anterior spinal roots. He considered involuntary or reflex activities to be mediated by the cerebellum, the posterior columns, and the posterior roots of the spinal cord. Bell wrote of his findings on a stunned rabbit in a letter to his brother. "I opened the spine and pricked or injured the posterior filaments of the nerves—no motion of the muscles followed. I then touched the anterior division—immediately the parts were convulsed." In a small pamphlet entitled "Idea of a New Anatomy of the Brain" published privately in 1811, Bell further stated, "I found that injury done to the anterior portion of the spinal marrow, convulsed the animal more certainly than injury done to the posterior portion . . . I could cut across the posterior fasciculus of nerves, which took its origin from the posterior portion of the spinal marrow, without convulsing the muscles of the back; but that on touching the anterior fasciculus with the point of the knife, the muscles of the back were immediately convulsed." Although Bell had demonstrated the motor function of the anterior roots, he had not shown the function of the posterior roots; in fact, he thought that "the secret operations of the vital organs were controlled by the posterior roots," which he referred to as autonomic nerves.

Unaware of this work, François Magendie (Fig. 4-2) in 1822 demonstrated that the posterior roots or the sensory conducting spinal nerves subserved a function quite different from that of the anterior roots. Upon reporting his results, Magendie received a letter from Bell's brother-in-law informing him that Bell had performed similar experiments 13 years previously. Magendie

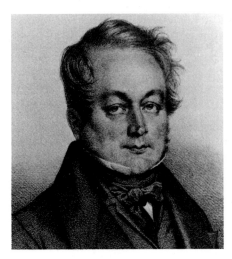

Fig. 4-2. François Magendie (1783–1855). (From A History of Neurosurgery. *Green-blatt SH, Dagi TF, Epstein M, editors. Park Ridge, Ill: American Association of Neurological Surgeons, 1997, p 131)*

acknowledged that Bell had shown that the anterior roots subserved motor function but maintained that the sensory function of the posterior roots had not been demonstrated. Accordingly, Magendie asserted that he had established "that fact in a positive manner." The priority of the concept, however, was argued; that the principle was called "the Bell-Magendie law" is probably an indication of the compromise. Later investigators tried to repeat Magendie's experiments but had equivocal results. Similar tests on frogs led Benedikt Stilling to assert that "the posterior spinal roots are sensory and not motor. The anterior roots are motor and not sensory."

Once the function of the roots was established, the question arose as to whether there was a topical overlap in the innervation. Eckhard, on the basis of experiments, concluded that the same spinal nerve does not always supply the same muscle in the same species of animal. To test sensation, he used an isolation technique by sectioning sensory roots adjacent to the one to be examined. He was able to map out the sensory supply of the lower extremity and concluded "the sensory fibers do not go precisely to the parts of the skin below which lie the muscles supplied by the corresponding motor fibers." Eckhard introduced the terms "myotomes" and "dermotomes" to designate the motor and sensory projections of the nerve roots. His results suggested a fairly specific pattern for the individual posterior spinal roots. Türck's experiments sectioning individual roots seemed to confirm Eckhard's results, but it was Sherrington's nerve root isolation studies in 1906 on apes that provided the most conclusive results, namely, "each sensory spinal skin-field extends to a certain extent across the neighbor's skin fields. . . . The fore and aft overlaps are throughout the body very great and it appears that each point of skin throughout the body is supplied by at least two sensory spinal roots, in certain regions by three." In addition, Sherrington examined the distribution of the motor roots and defined their cells of origin in the anterior horns of the spinal cord.

The Spinal Reflex Arc

Reflex activity, although probably inherent in Galen's description of natural movements and the Elizabethan scientists' theories of sympathy of parts, was not clearly formulated. Even the basis of the many involuntary responses—pupillary contraction and dilatation, wild movements after decapitation, and the contraction of a stretched muscle—was not definitely attributable to a specific part of the nervous system. Although Legallois had demonstrated by sectioning the neural axis that such processes were located in the sensory-motor segment of the spinal cord, quite a few advances in the understanding of neural activity (e.g., the function of the anterior and posterior roots, the localization of function in the cerebral hemispheres, and the concept of a sensorium commune transforming sensory into motor impressions in a zone including the spinal cord) had given new insight into the functioning of the nervous system. It required an analytical mind to bring these ideas into order. Such a singular scientist was Marshall Hall. In 1832, Hall demonstrated in the frog and turtle that the sensory nerves are functional in parts such as the torso even when separated from the rest of the body. The induced movements upon stimulation of sentient nerves do not occur if the spinal cord is destroyed. There may be some doubt as to Hall's priority, but no doubt at all that his research established the concept of a reflex. He asserted that some activity, not requiring perception, was independent of conscious sensory or motor input, that sensory impulses coming into the spinal cord affected other segmental reactions, and that the segmental activity might be influenced by the higher centers of the nervous system. He suggested that in "walking, in man, I imagine the reflex function to play a very considerable part—the contact of the sole with the ground is not unattended by a certain influence upon the action of certain muscles." He introduced the word "arc" to describe the reflex pathway. The implication of reflex activity occasioned considerable discussion as to whether the spinal animal had some sentience and conscience. Hall noted the absent or decreased spinal cord excitability immediately after transection, a condition he called "spinal shock." Bastian believed that such shock was permanent if the spinal cord of man was completely transected, but in 1906 Sherrington and others showed that the reflexes might return upon faradization of the legs unless sepsis or extensive damage to the spinal cord was present.

The conductive capacity of the spinal cord was established by Galen and the segmental activity was demonstrated by Hall, but the function of the specific tracts defined by anatomists was poorly understood. In the middle of the 19th century, Charles-Eduard Brown-Séquard conducted his famous experiments on hemisection of the spinal cord in which he demonstrated that pain sensibility was carried in the lateral part of the cord by fibers that had crossed from the opposite side. Based upon these experiments, he recognized the loss of the contralateral appreciation of noxious stimuli below the lesion and a hyperesthesia on the same side below the lesion. He was apparently aware, however, of the retained ipsilateral proprioceptive appreciation below the lesion.

The clinical significance of the spinal reflexes was appreciated at about the same time by two German neurologists. Wilhelm H. Erb in 1875 described the patellar tendon reflex, which he stated could be easily elicited by tapping the quadriceps tendon either above or below the patella. Karl Westphal, editor of the *Archiv für Psychiatrie und Nervenkrankheiten*, stated that he had used the test but considered it to be a muscle reaction to the blow. He noted that in cases "in which the sign is especially obvious" rhythmic reflex, extension movements (clonus) may develop.

After spinal cord section or injuries, a number of reflex patterns may be modified. Plantar stimulation, instead of inducing the normal flexor pattern, may cause an extensor response of the great toe, a reaction first noted by Remak in 1893, but named after Babinski who, three years later, recognized its significance as a means of distinguishing hysterical from organic hemiplegia. The plantar reflex may be accompanied by fanning of the toes (described by Babinski in 1903) and/or withdrawal of the leg. Occasionally, a crossed extensor thrust may occur (Phillipson's reflex). Clonus at the ankle, knee, or hip may develop after the period of spinal shock has passed. The bladder function reflex may vary, depending upon the presence of sepsis, but is usually passed through three stages—an initial paralysis with retention, then automatic voiding, and finally reflex micturition. The reflex bowel functions may also vary, with an initial fecal retention and decreased peristalsis, then automatic evacuation as peristalsis returns, bowel sounds increase, and the anal reflex returns. When reflex defecation develops, reconditioned regular bowel habits return.

In 1895, Hill showed that splanchnic control of blood pressure remained in the spinal dog placed in an upright position. In spinal man, however, there was poor vascular control with postural changes. Animals with a high transection were poikilothermic, and tetraplegic patients had difficulty controlling their body temperature. With high transections, sweating may be limited to cephalic segments, but in partial sections, the body temperature was usually normal.

In 1917, Riddoch stated that sexual function in males went through stages after spinal shock, with erection, a tactile reflex mediated through S2-4, returning eventually. In partial lesions of the spinal cord, orgasm may or may not be possible, but in transections, it is absent. In females, after the period of shock, menstruation usually recurs but orgasm cannot be achieved, although if erogenous zones in other parts of the body are manipulated, there may be some arousal. Pregnancy may occur even in tetraplegic women and a normal delivery can result.

Inhibition of Spinal Activity

In the early part of the 19th century, the nature and role of inhibition in reflex activity were discussed by Charles Bell, West, and Hering; several hypotheses were suggested to explain the phenomenon. Sherrington's observations clarified not only the central site of the inhibitory mechanism related to skeletal muscle, but also many of the other phenomena associated with inhibition (i.e., postural tone, decerebrate rigidity, stepping reflexes, and crossed extensor reflexes). At the end of the 19th century, Sherrington's classic book entitled *The Integrative Action of the Nervous System* clarified the concepts regarding the final common path, synaptic connections, central inhibition, central excitation, and reciprocal innervation.

The application of the knowledge of the function of the spinal nerve roots to clinical problems was slow to develop. Considering that the studies of Bell and Magendie in the early part of the 19th century had demonstrated the sensory and motor activity of the nerve roots, it seemed probable that the tracts subserving such functions were parcellated within the spinal cord. To determine the location of such tracts, Schiff partially sectioned the spinal cords of innumerable dogs and cats. Based upon these experiments, in 1854, he demonstrated to a commission of the Académie Française that the fibers carrying pain and temperature senses decussated soon after their entry into the spinal cord and that the fibers in the posterior columns, carrying kinesthetic sensation, did not cross. He published his results in 1858. Brown-Séquard's later experiments confirmed the concept of specific sensory paths in the spinal cord and, although his conclusions were only a little more advanced than Schiff's, his name is usually prefixed to the syndrome of hemisection of the spinal cord.

Clinicians supplied the proof of these concepts. Two cases of partial spinal cord injury, one studied by Müller and one by Gowers, confirmed the dissociated sensory loss. That certain afferent fiber bundles crossed to the opposite side of the human spinal cord before proceeding cephalad was demonstrated by Bechterew, although he was uncertain of the sensory modality carried by these fibers. The question was settled by the clinicopathological studies of Spiller in 1905 and Petrén five years later.

Spiller diagnosed involvement of the anterolateral tracts in a tubercular patient by reason of the predominant loss of pain and temperature sensibilities below the lesions. Although the patient had developed a paraplegia, at autopsy the main lesions were found to be tuberculomas of the anterolateral segments of the thoracic spinal cord. This localization within the spinal cord was not generally accepted, and some time later Cushing sectioned the entire spinal cord for the relief of intractable pain. Encouraged by Petrén's clinical confirmation of the anatomical organization of the spinal tracts, Spiller guided Martin as he performed the first cordotomy in man that resulted in satisfactory relief of pain.

Afflictions of the Spinal Cord

As with the brain, the common disorders of the spinal cord were the result of trauma and infections. Other disturbances of spinal cord function (neoplasm, degenerative disorders, deficiency states, and congenital anomalies) were rare. In the 18th and 19th centuries, the treatment of these conditions was simple and usually ineffective.

Spinal Cord Trauma

The earliest medical treatise, the *Edwin Smith papyrus,* written about a thousand years before Christ, describes six cases of spinal injury. The writer obviously knew the results of a broken back—paraplegia, urinary incontenence, and emisso seminis. Little was added regarding such injuries during the Greek and Roman eras, although Aretaeus did observe that paralysis resulting from a unilateral spinal cord lesion was on the side of the injury. Galen's brilliant experiments on the spinal cord revealed its topical organization. His treatment of such crippling injury, however, was little better than the manipulative therapy advocated by Hippocrates. Some centuries later, Paul of Aegina suggested that a broken spine might be operated upon and bony fragments removed. Medieval surgeons with fatalistic views, however, did not attempt such interventions. Later, a few surgeons such as Petrus d'Argelata tried to reduce the angulation by manual pressure. Paré stated that if the patient were paralyzed in the hands and arms, felt no pinpricks, and was incontinent of urine and feces, one might predict death. He added, however, that after informing parents, friends, and assistants of the prognosis, one might make an incision to remove indriven bony spicules compromising the spinal cord and nerves!

A few Renaissance surgeons, aware of the mechanical effects of spinal injuries, were more hopeful. Fabricius Hildanus devised a clasp to grasp the ligamentum flavum so that a pin could be inserted through holes in the jaws of the clasp and the tough ligament (Fig. 4-3). Using the clamp to exert manual traction, it was vainly hoped to separate and realign the displaced spinal fragments. Bolder surgeons of the 18th century operated upon fractures of the spine even if there was cord damage, although Heister commented "death will be generally an inevitable consequence." Yet, there is an early account of complete recovery of function from a spinal lesion.

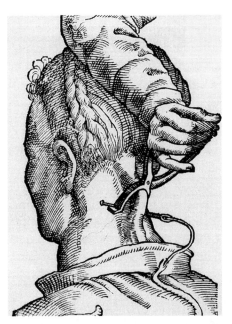

Fig. 4-3. Illustration of the method of Fabricius Hildanus for alignment of a fractured cervical spine. (From the collection of A. Earl Walker)

Louis in 1762 operated upon a paraplegic captain of the French Army, removing bone and metallic fragments from the lumbar spine (probably a cauda equina lesion), and effected a recovery. In 1796, Chopart and Desault advocated operation for spinal cord injury even if there was no evidence of fracture. Surgical intervention in such cases usually failed to improve the paralysis and so operation was vehemently opposed by most surgeons of the 19th century, even after anesthesia and antiseptic techniques were introduced.

Spinal Infections

Probably even more common than traumatic lesions of the spinal cord were destructive processes wrought by infections, particularly tuberculous. Such disease of the vertebral column has been identified by paleopathologists. The peculiar bent posture of the spondylitic patient has been depicted in paintings and sculpture from early times. The majority of such victims were suffering from tuberculous spondylitis, a disease found in Egyptian mummies and referred to in the Hippocratic writings. Oribasius probably was referring to tuberculous spondylitis when he advised curetting and draining abscesses of the vertebral bodies. Paraplegia as the result of such lesions was not noted until Dalechampius in 1610 wrote of its association with spinal caries. Morgagni attributed paralysis of the lower extremities to such lesions and not to neoplasia. At about the same time, Percival Pott discussed spinal deformity and parapareses; also in 1779, J.P. David of France described the condition in greater detail and reported on autopsy findings. It was 1816, however, before Delpech established the etiology; thereafter, these infections were differentiated from spinal neoplasms. Pott's aggressive therapy led to his name being attached to the condition, although David's conservative treatment eventually was adopted by most physicians.

Spinal Cord Tumors

Although thought by some to be a granuloma, perhaps the first documented spinal cord tumor was that treated by Salzmann, to which Morgagni had referred. Other early cases of myelopathy considered to be neoplastic were probably inflammatory or metastatic. The earliest undoubted primary spinal cord neoplasms were described by Velpeau in 1825, Duplay in 1834, and Ollivier in 1837. Velpeau's case involved a cauda equina tumor, Duplay's patient had three "tumors of the arachnoid" (neurofibromatosis), and Ollivier reported four extramedullary tumors. Probably, Phillips' description in 1792 was the earliest account of an intramedullary spinal cord tumor. A fusiform enlargement of the filum terminale was described by Cruveilhier in 1835. None of these tumors was studied histologically. Some years later, Charcot and Marie reported an extramedullary growth which on the basis of microscopic sections was probably a psammomatous meningioma. In 1874, von Leyden described and illustrated an intradural encapsulated neurofibroma. In spite of the discrete nature of these tumors, all surgical attempts at their removal resulted in fatality. Some surgeons expressed the desire to excise well-encapsulated neoplasms of the spinal cord; however, physicians considered the possibility of successfully operating upon such lesions not within the range of practical surgery. The spinal cord tumor diagnosed by Gowers and excised by Horsley in 1888 changed the bleak surgical picture.

The patient was a middle-aged army captain who for three years had suffered severe pain in the back and who over a period of four months had gradually lost all power in his legs. William Gowers, the leading English neurologist, had made a diagnosis of an extramedullary spinal cord tumor and Sir William Jenner had concurred. Victor Horsley, a young surgeon appointed the previous year as neurosurgeon to The National Hospital, Queen Square, was called in consultation. Through his mind must have passed the medical reports of some 57 patients with spinal cord tumors treated by various methods but all dead. He knew the general opinion that the risks preponderated the chances of finding a tumor. Probably unknown to Horsley was a Scotsman by the name of William Macewen who several years previously had successfully removed fibrous neoplasms of the spinal theca. Within a few hours of seeing the patient, Horsley removed the lamina indicated by Gowers without finding a tumor. A lamina above and one below were excised without finding a tumor. Horsley was about to close the wound when his assistant Charles Ballance suggested that he explore still higher, whereupon a tumor was uncovered and removed. After a long convalescence, the patient made a full recovery.

This has been hailed as the first successful extirpation of a spinal cord tumor. Irrespective of the real priority, it was the case that stimulated surgeons in all parts of the world to operate upon the spinal canal for lesions causing paraplegia. The majority of lesions were infectious (tuberculous, parasitic, or pyogenic), and only about a third were neoplastic. Moreover, the surgical technique for laminectomy and tumor removal was still crude and, as a result, successful outcomes were uncommon.

Angiomas of the Spinal Cord

In the 19th century, blood vessel tumors of the spinal cord, usually found at autopsy, were considered to be venous angiomas. A report by Gaupp in 1888 described hemorrhoids of the lumbar pia mater (perhaps secondary to a disc protrusion). In the 20th century, surgeons exposed such lesions at operation when looking for a spinal cord tumor. The earliest angioma successfully extirpated was by Perthes in 1920. In addition to these malformations, true blood vessel tumors, possibly a manifestation of Lindau's disease, were reported. Schubach was the first to name the condition Lindau's disease, although Berklinger credited Berenbruch with describing the condition in a dissertation at Tübingen in 1890.

Intraspinal Cysts

By the end of the 19th century, it was common procedure to explore for a lesion causing progressive paraplegia, especially if a sensory level could be demonstrated; however, a number of conditions other than an expected tumor were exposed. Many were cystic, the nature of which could be determined only by examination of the cyst wall or its contents. Some cysts, lined with epithelial elements and containing epidermal or dermoid matter, might be of developmental or iatrogenic origin. The former were named pearly tumors by Cruveilhier by reason of their shimmering appearance. They were sometimes associated with other anomalies such as syringomyelia or diastematomyelia. When spinal puncture became commonly used to diagnose and treat such conditions as meningitis, cholesteatomas were reported at the level of the needle insertion. Presumably, the tumor resulted from the displacement of a plug of cutaneous epidermal tissue into the subarachnoid space. The less common dermoids and teratomas have been found in the midline of the spinal cord.

Arachnoidal cysts lying anterior or lateral to the spinal cord were described in 1898 by Schlesinger. Such cysts were presumed to arise from faults in the arachnoidal trabeculae and to cause root irritation or spinal cord compression. Hydatid cysts involved the vertebral bodies or the foramina but were usually extradural; cysticercotic cysts were commonly found enmeshed in the subarachnoid or extradural spaces.

When operations upon the spinal cord became common in the 20th century, patients with segmental spinal disorders causing pain and paresis underwent a surgical exploration which often disclosed a thickened and cystic arachnoid. Usually, no specific cause could be identified. Operative excision of these cystic lesions rarely improved the patient's complaints.

Metastatic Neoplasms

Tumors originating in various organs of the body, especially in the abdomen, frequently involve the extradural spinal space, compressing or less commonly invading the spinal cord. In the 19th century, such tumors were rarely operated upon because of the bleak outlook. In 1832, Hodgkin described "swelling of lymph glands, splenic enlargement, fever and severe cachexia which rapidly caused death." Although spinal cord involvement had been noted clinically earlier, Murchison and Sanderson in 1870 first described lymphomas involving the spinal cord.

Spinal Motor Neuron Disease

"Wasting palsy" apparently has been known for centuries, but has such varied manifestations that it is difficult to classify the disorders. Consequently, only a few common conditions of the spinal motor neuron disease such as leprosy and beri-beri were recognized in the early 19th century. Even when the microscope became available to examine the tissues, prominent changes were observed only in the atrophic muscles. Occasionally, other abnormalities were reported. In 1830, Charles Bell referred to two cases, one a lady with her senses but "total want of all motion of the bodily frame" except for respiration, and another, described by Thomas Ingle, of a lady approximately 50 years old who over a period of two years developed complete paralysis of the limbs and eventually of the muscles of the neck and mouth, causing dysphagia. She had no loss of sensibility. At postmortem, the brain showed insignificant abnormalities but the membranes forming the sheath of the spinal cord were thickened and "the anterior half of the cord . . . [was] in a semi-fluid state while the posterior portion possessed its usual firmness." Darwell described a similar case the following year.

Aran-Duchenne Disease

On the wards of the Hôpital St. Antoine in Paris, F.A. Aran in the middle of the 19th century was studying patients with muscular atrophy. His first report appeared in 1848 and two years later in a lengthy paper. Aran described 11 cases, four of which might be considered by current standards as amyotrophic lateral sclerosis. When Cruveilhier examined the spinal cords much later, no lesions were found in the nervous system of one patient; in another, with varying degrees of muscular atrophy, he found shrunken cervical anterior roots and attenuated hypoglossal nerves. Cruveilhier was uncertain whether the atrophy was primary or, more likely, secondary to spinal cord disease. Not until better clinical and neuropathological techniques were available could the issue be resolved. In subsequent papers, Aran described the clinical course of these patients—a slow progressive weakness, wasting, and fine twitching of the hand muscles. As the weakness and muscular atrophy extended to the arm muscles, it eventually involved the trunk and legs. Duchenne studied some of these patients using his electric stimulator and reported upon them in his text of 1861. Because the muscle wasting was not associated with evidence of spinal cord involvement, such as sensory loss or urinary or bowel disturbance, Aran and Duchenne each thought that the condition was primarily an affliction of the muscles.

Later, when Clarke and Luys reported microscopic changes in the anterior horn cells of the spinal cord, a neurogenic origin seemed probable, but some neurologists, such as Friedreich, defended a muscular basis of the condition.

Amyotrophic Lateral Sclerosis (Charcot's Disease)

Shortly after Aran and Duchenne had described the muscle-wasting disorder, Jean M. Charcot (Fig. 4-4), in 1865, wrote an anatomical-pathological account of similar disorders which he classified as protopathic (intrinsic spinal disorders (e.g., Aran-Duchenne disease)) and chronic deuteropathic (secondary spinal disorders (e.g., amyotrophic lateral sclerosis)) myelopathies. In patients with amyotrophic lateral sclerosis, Charcot noted the spinal cord changes associated with the muscle wasting of the upper limbs and the spastic paresis of the lower extremities. The involved muscles showed progressive atrophy and fibrillary contractions but retained responses to faradic stimulation. Early in the disease progression, the small hand and forearm muscles were involved, producing deformities of the fingers and hand. Weakness of the muscles usually preceded obvious atrophy but the disability and wasting could occur at the same time. All modalities of sensation remained intact. The weakness and atrophy spread to involve the proximal mus-

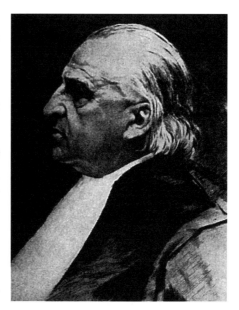

Fig. 4-4. Jean Martin Charcot (1825-1893). (From The Founders of Neurology, *2nd ed. Haymaker W, Schiller F, editors. Springfield, Ill: Charles C Thomas, 1970, p 421)*

cles of the upper extremities. After a few months, the muscles of the lower extremities became weak (especially the extensors) and spastic, but with little atrophy. The bladder and rectum were not affected. In the later stages, the tongue became atrophic and paretic, the palate moved little, the voice was nasal, the facial muscles drooped and, eventually, respiration and deglutition became labored. The entire course lasted only two to three years.

Charcot realized that the clinical cases of spinal myelopathy were a complex group—poliomyelitis, syringomyelia, syphilitic pachymeningitis, Landry's paralysis, Friedreich's ataxia, and hereditary muscular atrophy—and all had to be considered.

Progressive Bulbar Palsy

The muscles of the face, upper alimentary canal, and respiratory tract, innervated by the bulbar brainstem, were noted to become paralyzed in association with local disease such as diphtheria or as the result of a morbid process of the brain stem. This latter condition—labio-glosso-pharyngeal paralysis—was described by Dumeril in 1859 and in greater detail by Duchenne the following year. Duchenne de Boulogne described a condition characterized by "paralysie musculaire progressive de la langue, du voile du palais et des lèvres." The unwieldy title given by Duchenne was changed by Wachsmuth a few years later to "chronic progressive bulbar paralysis." Duchenne's original description of the clinical features was quite complete and few details were subsequently added. Speech disturbances, characterized by indistinct articulation and a nasal intonation, were usually the first indications of the disease. Later, the patient was aware of difficulty drinking and swallowing solid foods, which might cause choking. The facial and masticatory muscles became so weakened that the jaw drooped, although the eyes and forehead remained quite mobile.

This pure syndrome was rare; usually it was accompanied by supranuclear palsies, such as increased masseter reflexes, pathological laughter or crying, and progressive muscular atrophy of the limbs and trunk suggestive of amyotrophic lateral sclerosis. The neural involvement, however, might consist only of spastic limbs with minimal wasting of the muscles. The disease was progressive, but remissions occurred, prolonging the course from one or two years to a number of years.

At postmortem, the involved muscles showed granular and fatty degeneration with varying degrees of atrophy. The motor nerves were usually demyelinated and had fragmented nerve fibers and increased interstitial tissue. Although the brain might appear normal or slightly small to the naked eye, on microscopic examination, the neurons of the motor cranial nerves were small, shrunken, or absent, being replaced by compound granular cells and glial proliferation. The pyramidal tracts were demyelinated, with few nerve fibers and accompanying glial proliferation. The association of bulbar and progressive spinal muscular atrophy, and the frequent combined degenerative changes in the cranial nerve nuclei and spinal anterior horn cells, led Kussmaul to associate the two conditions. Later writers have combined all three clinical disorders as a unit—the motor neuron diseases.

Progressive Nuclear Ophthalmoplegia

In 1856, von Graefe pointed out the similarity between certain cases of progressive ophthalmoplegia and bulbar paralysis. Other writers confirmed this resemblance; Brissaud even affirmed that they were the same disorder.

The initial manifestations—bilateral ptosis—preceded ocular palsies by months or years. After a few years, the paralysis becomes complete except for the preservation of pupillary reactions and some movement of the levator palpebrae superioris. Many of the early cases were attributed to syphilis, multiple sclerosis, or other cerebral lesions. The remaining pure cases had onset of symptoms in early adult life and were rarely examined pathologically, so that the etiology was not established.

Gowers envisioned the motor neuron diseases to be a unit, and if not identical, very similar. The pathological changes were similar in the motor cortex; only small, shrunken, or shadowy ghosts remained. The degeneration of the pyramidal tracts varied, not necessarily corresponding to that of the motor cortex. Usually, the motor projection systems in the brain stem, the motor nuclei, and the projection tracts were severely degenerated. The neurons of the anterior cell columns were most frequently degenerated, although some cells remained. Nerve root fibers from the anterior horn cells were demyelinated, at times only to the margin of the spinal cord. With Marchi stains, patchy degeneration was seen in the anterior roots and the peripheral nerves. The muscles involved showed secondary degenerative changes.

Hereditary Neurogenic Muscular Atrophy (Charcot-Marie-Tooth Disease)

In the 1850s, Virchow and Eulenburg reported on a series of patients who had progressive muscular atrophy with some members of their families similarly afflicted. In 1873, Friedreich concluded that such familial cases were a variant of the muscular atrophy described earlier by Duchenne. Thirteen years later, however, Charcot and Marie published a 40-page paper describing a unique progressive muscular atrophy, often familial, which began in the legs and later involved the hands. In the same year, Tooth wrote a thesis on a progressive type of familial muscular atrophy beginning in the peroneal muscles and later involving other muscles of the leg. Before his short account of the disorder appeared in *Brain* two years later, Hoffmann published a 53-page paper on progressive neuritic muscular atrophy. Although it was obvious that these were the same condition, French writers called it the Charcot-Marie disease, and English authors the Charcot-Marie-Tooth disease. In all three reports, the disorder was clearly defined and differentiated from progressive muscular atrophy.

The disease began with slow but progressive weakness and atrophy of the anterolateral muscles of the legs, so that the afflicted young person had difficulty standing on tip-toes and walked with a high steppage gait. As the result of weak extensors of the toes, the foot developed a high arch. The involved muscles, at first of the leg and later of the thigh, atrophied. When the afflicted person was chilled, fasciculations might be seen. Sensory disturbances were rarely present. Some time later, the legs became paretic and the fingers had difficulty in carrying out fine movements as atrophy of the thenar and interossei muscles became apparent; however, sensory impairment was unusual. In spite of the high steppage gait and the pes cavus, the afflicted person could walk on a wide base. As the leg muscles atrophied, the tendon reflexes diminished and eventually were lost; less commonly, the reflexes of the arms were impaired. The plantar reflexes were flexor or, if the atrophy was profound, no response could be obtained. The skin over the shrunken muscles became cyanotic, thickened, and at times, ulcerated. A number of other neurological disturbances such as cranial nerve paresis, optic atrophy, and visceral disorders might develop as the disorder slowly progressed over the years. In spite of the disability, some patients lived a normal life span.

Although Virchow and Friedreich had noted the fascicular atrophy and myopathic fibers in the muscles, later writers described more extensive abnormalities—endoneurial proliferation, demyelination of the larger fibers of the peripheral nerves, chromatolysis of the lumbar anterior horn cells, demyelination of the tract of Goll and to a lesser extent of the tract of Burdach, and atrophic changes in many of the brain stem nuclei—in the central nervous system.

Charcot-Marie-Tooth disease may be confused with the myopathies, scapulohumeral atrophy, hypertrophic neuritis of Dejerine and Sottas, spinocerebellar degeneration and, in the early stages, a number of local neuritides. Although there is no effective therapy, various palliative orthopedic procedures considerably relieve some contractures.

Scapuloperoneal Syndrome

In the same year that the Charcot-Marie-Tooth syndrome was described, another muscular affliction was reported by Brossard under the title of "syndrome scapulo-distal." It consisted of atrophy of the muscles below the knees, particularly the peroneal muscles, and of the shoulder girdle muscles. Subsequent reports have indicated that in some patients the disorder was myopathic and in others neurogenic.

Werdnig-Hoffmann Disease

Within two years of each other, Werdnig and Hoffmann wrote of infants who in the first year of life developed progressive weakness of the legs and later of the arms, so that they died within a few years. Examination of the brain and spinal cord showed only severe atrophy of the anterior horn cells of the cervical and lumbar regions of the spinal cord as well as atrophy of the muscles they supplied. Subsequently, reports indicated that the clinical course of such cases was quite varied. The most severe forms began in the first three months of life with a sudden loss of movement of previously active limbs, which assumed a hypotonic "frog posture" when the child was on its back. The lower extremities were more severely affected than the upper, and only the ankles and toes could be moved. The rest of the body was less affected, and the heart not at all. Within a year, respiratory infections usually caused death. In the less severe forms, the child might develop normally for six months or so and be able to sit up before muscle impairment incapacitated the infant. Eventually death resulted from respiratory infection. Children who attained the first year of life without serious difficulties developed a waddling gait as the result of weak girdle muscles. After the initial incapacity, some victims compensated and lived for years with slight disability.

Friedreich's Ataxia

Friedreich's papers in the 1860s on hereditary spinal ataxia were classics and "laid the groundwork for all subsequent knowledge of hereditary degenerations of the spinal cord, brain stem and cerebellum . . . the main clinical and pathological observations and ideas are sound and enduring." Friedreich studied nine members of three families who suffered from ataxia, especially of gait. He noted the early onset before or during puberty, affecting predominantly females, and the long course of the disorder with no sensory impairment until the late stages of the disease. The ataxia of both arms and legs was aggravated by voluntary movement. Nystagmus and speech impairment developed. After years of progressive motor and sensory impairment, the tendon reflexes of the legs were lost although the muscles were not atrophied; however, kyphoscoliosis and various deformities of the feet occurred.

In four patients studied at autopsy, Friedreich noted degeneration of the posterior columns, particularly in the lumbar regions, atrophy and demyelination of the nerve fibers, and thinned posterior nerve roots most marked in the lower lumbar and sacral roots. The condition was not considered a distinct entity until Brousse in 1882 proposed that it be called "maladie de Friedreich."

The early prepubertal appearance of the disease limited the chances of inheritance, so that familial cases were the rule. The condition is generally considered to be recessive although sporadic cases may occur. However, each affected family has its own characteristic so various combinations with other degenerative conditions and transitional forms are commonly found.

Fazio-Londe Disease

Bulbar paralysis in adults was recognized in the middle of the 19th century, but it was another quarter of a century before Berger in 1896 reported on a 12-year-old child with progressive bulbar paralysis involving the lower motor nerves and the pyramidal tract. Some years later, Fazio saw a 22-year-old woman and her son who both had lower facial paralysis and paresis of the upper facial muscles, tongue, vocal cords, and dyspnea. Although other cases were reported, only one has had anatomical verification.

Deficiency Neuropathies: Pernicious Anemia

Addison's anemia was described long before the neuropathy was recognized. In 1884, Lichtenstern wrote a paper entitled "Progressive pernicious anaemia in tabetic patients." Three years later, Lichtheim noted the association of pernicious anemia and demyelinizing lesions in the posterior columns, to a lesser extent in the lateral columns, and in other parts of the spinal cord. Several other authors attempted to clarify the situation before Russell, Batten, and Collier gave a complete description of the peripheral nerve and spinal cord involvement. Their report noted the stocking and glove paresthesias, muscle wasting, autonomic disturbances, and absent tendon reflexes.

Hereditary Spinocerebellar Atrophies

The hereditary spinocerebellar atrophies comprise a few familial conditions varying from peripheral muscular atrophy to cerebellopontine disturbances. The families described by Sanger Brown in 1892 had a progressive cerebellar ataxia involving the limbs, and pyramidal tracts causing spasticity and in some cases optic atrophy. At autopsy, the posterior columns as well as the dorsal spinocerebellar tracts were degenerated, with some cell loss in Clarke's column and the anterior horns. Later cases with severe ataxia of all limbs have had degeneration of the entire posterior spinal columns. A suitable classification of these rare dysplasias has not yet been determined.

Carotid Sinus Syndrome

"Stoppage of the pulse" must have been noted by ancient physicians who compressed the neck to produce coma and who relied heavily upon examination of the pulse, but Parry is credited with the first reported observation in 1825 of a slowed heart rate upon compressing the upper part of the neck. Czermak, a physiologist, was the first to recognize cardiac slowing in man upon stimulation of what was thought to be the vagus nerve but later shown to be the carotid sinus.

The following year, de Cyon and Ludwig stimulated the cranial end of a nerve adjacent to the vagosympathetic cervical trunk of animals, producing marked slowing of the heart rate and arterial hypotension. It was not clear, however, as to what structure was stimulated until Hering in 1924 identified the carotid sinus as the receptor and origin of the reflex arc which traversed the glossopharyngeal nerve to the medulla oblongata to activate the efferent arc carried by the autonomic outflow.

5

The Peripheral Nerves

T he early Greek anatomists considered that all of the white "cords" in the body were the same and called them "neurons." Even some blood vessels were included in this term, for Praxagorus thought that the fibrous bands were the endings of arteries, a concept ridiculed by Galen. Although Herophilus supposed that the brain and spinal cord gave rise to motor and sensory nerves, Erasistratus believed that they came from the meninges. The role of these fibrous cords was not clarified by Galen, who referred to three kinds of nerves: 1) voluntary nerves, originating from the brain and spinal cord; 2) ligaments from the bones; and 3) tendons from the muscles. He conceived that the soft nerves, subserving motion, arose from the cerebellum, but he thought that "the source of all the hard nerves is the spinal cord, and its lower extremity is the source of the extremely hard ones." Although Galen had dissected many different species of animals and made exquisite studies of the effects of sectioning the spinal cord at different levels and of cutting certain nerves, such as the phrenic and recurrent laryngeal in the neck, he was perplexed by the plexuses and peripheral nerves. The dissectors during the Middle Ages were also confused by these cords.

The earliest anatomist to clearly describe the nerves and depict their course was Vesalius (Fig. 5-1). His artistic illustrations of nerves of the limbs and trunk show fairly accurately the major plexuses formed by the spinal roots after their emergence from the vertebral canal in both the cervical and lumbosacral regions. The more distal disposition of the nerves, however, is somewhat fanciful.

Although Vesalius accurately portrayed the structures of the nervous system, correcting some Galenic errors, he still wrote of animal spirits flowing from the brain through hollow "nerves" to the muscles.

After the publication of Vesalius' masterpiece, several anatomists described and illustrated the nervous system in figures of varying artistic quality. The cop-

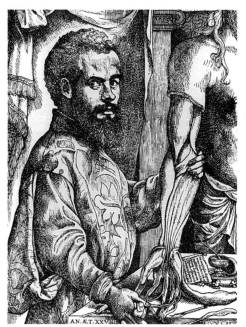

Fig. 5-1. Andreas Vesalius (1514-1564). (From A History of Neurosurgery. *Greenblatt SH, Dagi TF, Epstein M, editors. Park Ridge, Ill: American Association of Neurological Surgeons, 1997, p 102)*

perplate engravings of Eustachius, although not published until 1714, were excellent; the earlier plates had been both less accurate and less pleasing to the eye.

Renaissance Concepts

Descartes was probably the first to suggest a new concept, namely, that "The nerves are not just hollow tubes with valves to regulate the flow of the animal spirits outward from the brain to the muscles but they contain a . . . marrow composed of a large number of exceedingly delicate threads . . . which terminate on the one hand on the internal surface of the brain looking towards the ventricles and on the other hand in the skin or other tissue." He conceived of the human body as a machine controlled by the pineal body, which activated all organs. Descartes believed that the walls of the ventricles received sensitive impulses that determined the outflow of the (motor) animal spirits. As the animal spirits were agitated by the fire continually burning in the heart, there was no need of a soul. Although fantastic, this concept stimulated interest in the workings of the body.

To clarify the earlier mechanical explanation of nerve-muscle activity, Glisson, Regius Professor of Physics at Cambridge in the middle of the 17th century, introduced the concept of irritability—a propensity to react to a stimulus as the fundamental property of nerve and muscle activity. In essence, irritability required perception to initiate a series of factors which eventuated in a voluntary or involuntary reaction.

In a history of physiology, Michael Foster wrote that we owe Glisson not only the concept of "irritability" but also the proof that when a muscle contracts, it does not increase in bulk. In *Tractatus de ventriculo*, Glisson states: "Fit into the top of an oblong glass tube a second tube like a funnel. Let a strong muscular man insert into the mouth of the larger tube the whole of his bared arm, and secure the mouth of the tube all around to the humerus with bandages so that no water can escape from the tube. Then pour water through the funnel until the whole of the larger tube is completely filled and some water rises up into the funnel. This being done, now tell the man to alternately contract powerfully and to relax the muscles of his arm. It will be seen that when the muscles are contracted the water in the tube of the funnel sinks, rising again when relaxation takes place."

Nerve Excitation

Glisson's rather obscure concepts, published *in extenso* after his death, lay dormant for half a century. Then, in the mid-1700s, Albrecht von Haller (Fig. 5-2), a Swiss physiologist, in his famous book *Elementa physiologicae* defined a part of the body as irritable if, upon a slight touch, it contracted independent of the will.

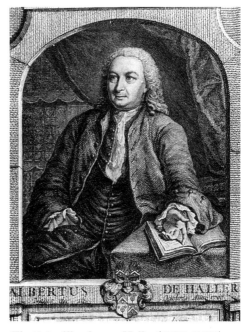

Fig. 5-2. Albrecht von Haller (1708-1777). (From A History of Neurosurgery. Greenblatt SH, Dagi TF, Epstein M, editors. Park Ridge, Ill: American Association of Neurological Surgeons, 1997, p 124)

Von Haller assumed that there must be fluid within nerves which conducted the impulse; he rejected other conducting media (vibrations and electrical transmission). At about the same time, Whytt wrote that "the contraction of an irritated muscle cannot be owing to any effervescence, explosion, ethereal oscillations or electrical energy excited in its fibers or membranes by the mechanical action of stimuli upon them." Several years later, Alexander Monro secundus reiterated that conclusion when he wrote "that the matter on which the energy depends is a secreted fluid, we are, far from being able to prove." But a few years earlier, Stephen Hales, a country clergyman, had asked if the force activating the nerves may not "act along their surfaces like electrical powers?"

Nerve Structure

With only the naked eye to appraise neural and muscular activity, the Elizabethan investigators conjured up many bizarre theories which were acrimoniously debated in almshouses and in print. Some, such as Glisson, had consid-

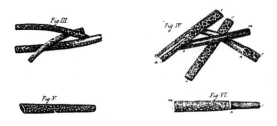

Fig. 5-3. Fontana's illustrations of nerve fiber cylinders. (From the collection of A. Earl Walker)

ered nerve fibers, animal spirits, and muscle juices to be invisible and hypothetical. It was a hundred years later that Fontana clearly defined the nerve fiber as a small, transparent cylinder (Fig. 5-3). Remak, in 1836, first differentiated myelinated and nonmyelinated nerve fibers. He termed the primitive band as the central core of the myelinated fiber, and the entire insulated fiber the primitive tube. The nonmyelinated fibers, which he called organic or primitive, were not enclosed in a sheath but were naked, gelatinous, and much smaller than the primitive tube. That the myelin sheath of the peripheral nerve was interrupted at regular intervals was considered artifactual until Ranvier in 1871, with silver impregnations, defined "small black, transverse lines of remarkable clarity like rungs of a ladder . . . I shall call this ring the constriction ring of the nerve tube." Ranvier noted that the constrictions were equally spaced along the same nerve tube, but somewhat closer together in thin rather than thick tubes. Since each segment of the nerve tube had a single nucleus in the membrane of Schwann, he concluded that the segment was a cellular unit joined to its neighbor at the constrictions.

That the nerve fiber had at its end a sensitive terminal seemed probable. Accordingly, in the middle of the 19th century, a number of investigators searched for such terminals on the afferent fibers and described, in addition to free endings, various specialized cutaneous structures named after their discoverers—Meissner's corpuscles and Krause's end bulbs.

The terminals of the motor nerves were investigated by Willy Kühne of Heidelberg. He noted that some nerves ended beneath the sarcolemma as a large plate or a cluster of fibers. In most cases, "the plate ends in the substrate of nuclei and finely granular protoplasm, but in other cases this residue is absent and the nerve plates, then, have so-called nerve end bulbs."

Electrical Excitability

When electroscopes and the Leyden jar, a powerful source of electricity, became available in the mid 1700s, many experiments on nerves were carried out. Galvani demonstrated that limbs of frogs could be convulsed by both mechanical and electrical stimulation. He noted that a nerve-muscle preparation of a frog would twitch when touched by an observer, that atmospheric electricity induced by a long wire could be used to stimulate a frog's leg, and that it twitched when hung up by brass hooks to an iron railing. This latter response was due to the flow of current between dissimilar metals, although Galvani did not understand that principle. Just before the end of the 18th century, an unknown investigator reported that muscles might twitch in the absence of any metal or external source of electricity if the cut end of a frog's spine lay over a muscle or if a limb was drawn up to touch an exposed sciatic nerve. This, although unrecognized at that time, was due to the current of injury. Von Humboldt, using a galvanometer, demonstrated the flow of current between the cut surface of a muscle and its undamaged surface.

Through the efforts of DuBois-Reymond, a pupil of Johannes Müller, the most renowned physiologist of that time, the middle of the 18th century saw a marked swing away from the metaphysiological concepts of philosophers. Using more precise instrumentation to measure physiological phenomena, DuBois-Reymond confirmed Matteucci's demonstration that nerve-muscle preparations and muscles themselves could produce electricity, which he named muscular current. Consequently, DuBois-Reymond concluded that the activating principle was electricity. This proposal led to acrimonious arguments that the electrical flow was entirely an injury current and not present in normal resting muscle.

Although Müller had said that the time required for a sensation to pass from an extremity to the brain and/or spinal cord and back to the muscle to produce a contraction was infinitely small and immeasurable, his pupil Bernstein hypothesized that the membrane of the inactive nerve or muscle fiber was normally polarized and that the action potential was a self-propagating depolarization of the membrane. These studies carried out in Germany stimulated the English schools of physiology, particularly. At Cambridge University, Michael Foster and his pupils explored the subject with improved instrumentation so that precise and accurate measurements could be made of many of the parameters of nerve and muscle excitation.

Fontana had shown that heart muscle might be activated by a weak stimulus, but once stimulated, developed power which was much greater than that of the initial excitation. He also recognized a refractory period. That skeletal muscle shared these properties was shown by Keith Lucas in 1917 using elaborate electrical techniques for stimulating and recording. The all-or-nothing property of nerve was demonstrated by Gotch. About that time, the earlier concept that the nervous fluid passed uninterrupted from the nerve to muscle was questioned. Kühne, noting the histological differences between muscle and nerve endings, suggested that the action current of the nerve invaded the muscle, causing it to contract (Fig. 5-4). As there was a time delay at the neuromuscular junction, however, the possibility of a chemical mediator was suggested. Elliott, observing that smooth muscle responded to adrenalin when

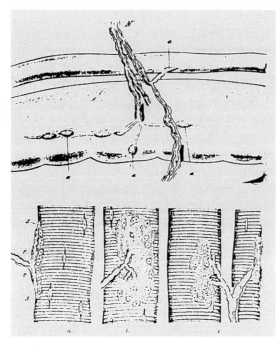

Fig. 5-4. Kühne's illustration of the neuromuscular junction. (From the collection of A. Earl Walker)

deprived of its sympathetic nerve supply, suggested in 1904 that adrenalin was the chemical stimulant liberated when an impulse arrived at the neuromuscular junction. Langley, noting that smooth muscle might either contract or relax when stimulated, postulated two types of receptor substances—one excitatory and one inhibitory. Finally, the potent effect of acetylcholine on arterial pressure and other parasympathetic activities led Dale to consider that it might be the stimulating substance. The proof came from Loewi's demonstration in 1921 that fluid bathing a frog's heart which had been stimulated by its vagus nerve had an inhibitory action upon the beat of another heart—thus proving the existence of a chemical mediator.

The Repair of Nerve Wounds

The confused concept regarding the structures included in the term "nerve" rendered the Hippocratic teachings obscure. Not until the Alexandrian scientists differentiated nerves from similar appearing strands—tendons—was their surgical repair considered. Although Galen defined the function of the spinal nerves and sutured cut tendons of wounded gladiators, he offered no suggestion that severed nerves might be surgically repaired. Later surgeons referring to nerve injuries only closed the wound. Rhazes in a 1511 translation was the first to tell of the approximation of the ends of cut nerves. Surgeons of the 12th to 15th centuries mention wounded nerves but most were ambivalent regarding the treatment of injured nerves; some sutured the nerve with the muscle and skin and others only approximated the wound edges. Ambroise Paré wrote of the painful effect of partially cut nerves and described the misery of King Charles IX of France, who suffered from causalgia. His advice was to section the wounded nerve to relieve the pain and prevent convulsions.

The earliest attempt at suturing a severed nerve was probably made by Gabriele Ferrara in 1608. He used a split tortoise tendon soaked in hot red wine to suture the ends of the nerve. Such repairs were not expedient on the battlefields of Europe, however, where even in the 17th century, a completely severed nerve was left untreated as the wound was closed. A painful or spasmic partially sectioned nerve might be treated by having the scarred nerve excised, or in the case of an extremity nerve, an amputation performed.

Even during the American Civil War, Mitchell (Fig. 5-5) did not recommend direct nerve sutures but instead applied electrical stimulation to the denervated muscle.

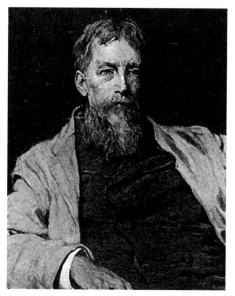

Fig. 5-5. S. Weir Mitchell (1829-1914). (From The Founders of Neurology, *2nd ed. Haymaker W, Schiller F, editors. Springfield, Ill: Charles C Thomas, 1970, p. 480)*

The Return of Nerve Function

Experimental and clinical studies were each demonstrating that the function of a denervated muscle might return if the ends of the severed nerve were approximated by sutures. Cruikshank in 1795 showed that the severed peripheral nerves of dogs reunited if opposed. Some observers saw only a bridging scar at the site of the section, but Fontana reported nerve fibers crossing the gap. Michaels in 1785 cut the nerves of dogs and later noted the return of a response to painful stimuli. The interpretation of these early experiments is open to question; better controlled studies were carried out in the next century. Clinical experiences of Swan, Wood, and others confirmed such functional regeneration of interrupted nerves. Some surgeons reported recovery even after resection of long segments of major nerves of the limbs.

The reason for the functional recovery was not clear, for Langier and others reported return of function within a few days of suturing the nerve. Weir Mitchell et al in their 1864 manual on gunshot wounds and injuries to the nerves maintained that such rapid recovery was due to the overlap of adjacent nerves and not to regeneration of the severed nerve.

As it became evident that an end-to-end anastomosis was not feasible for coapting nerve ends in many cases, attention was given to means of bridging the gap, the most suitable suturing material, and the best means of handling the neuromas at the site of the wounded nerve. As most of these factors were resolved after World Wars I and II and are admirably discussed by Browne, they are omitted here.

Clinicians in the early part of the 19th century considered that the sensori-motor centers were located in the spinal cord and brainstem. As a result, neurological treatises of that time emphasized the role of the peripheral nerves and the spinal cord in disease but paid scant attention to the cerebral hemispheres. Thus, in the first edition of Romberg's 1853 textbook, of the 13 sections on the sensory neuroses, only two related to the brain; in the 26 sections on motor neuroses, only five concerned cerebral dysfunction. Many disorders were termed neuropathies, although later careful and detailed neuropathological examinations with modern techniques have revealed a wider distribution of the lesions.

Clinical Disorders of the Nerves: Neuropathies

In the 16th and 17th centuries, most disorders of the nervous system were considered to be diseases of the peripheral nerves rather than of the spinal cord or brain. It is evident that the neurologists of that time were better acquainted with afflictions of the peripheral nerves than those of the central nervous system. In a modern textbook of neurology, one would expect that two thirds of the subject matter would be devoted to telencephalic disorders.

Leprosy

From ancient times, the leper was considered to have a contagious and fatal disease with myriad manifestations. Only in the last century has it been shown to be essentially a disorder of the peripheral nerves; other manifestations were secondary phenomena. The causative agent, *Mycobacterium leprae,* was discovered by Hansen in 1874. Based upon pathological studies, Virchow established that the peripheral nerves were the seat of the infection. Subsequent investigators have shown that "all leprosy is neural leprosy" and that the principal tissue to react is the Schwann cell.

Diabetic Neuropathy

Although Rollo in 1797 described the sensory and motor manifestations of diabetic neuropathy, it was not generally appreciated until Charles-Jacob Marchal published a small monograph on the subject in 1864. A few years later, Ogle wrote that the cranial nerves, especially the sixth, may be affected in diabetes. In 1884, Bouchard showed that the muscle stretch reflexes were absent in diabetic patients. Althaus noted the resemblance of diabetic neuropathy to tabes dorsalis; in 1890, Leval-Picquechef referred to diabetic neuropathy as pseudotabes diabetica. Gowers also recognized the similarity between diabetic neuritis and alcoholic neuropathy. It required neuropathological techniques developed in the latter part of the 19th century to show the different changes in the spinal cord and peripheral nerves in these conditions.

Hyperthyroid Neuropathy

In severe thyrotoxicosis, a motor neuropathy was initially described by Charcot and somewhat later by Joffroy as "Basedow's paraplegia."

Hypertrophic Neuropathy

In 1893, Dejerine and Sottas described two siblings with weakness of the extensors of the toes and of the dorsiflexors and evertors of the ankles, kyphoscoliosis, distal wasting and sensory loss, incoordination of the arms, areflexia, miosis, and nystagmus. At autopsy, in one case, the peripheral nerves were found to be thickened. The condition was considered to be a variant of Charcot-Marie-Tooth disease, although Dejerine and Sottas maintained that it was a separate condition. Other clinical syndromes characterized by hypertrophic nerves were subsequently reported, so that hypertrophic neuropathy came to be considered a nonspecific syndrome with varied pathogenesis.

The enlargement of the nerves may be of any degree, even sufficient to cause a partial spinal block. The thickened nerves have myelinated fibers interspersed with many onion-skin cellular proliferations. The clinical course is variable—some cases being progressive, some intermittent or relapsing, and some stationary.

Beri-Beri

In China, the swelling of legs and an unsteady gait were recognized as a "leg and air" disease, described in the 1st century AD. In 1642, Bontius, a Dutch physician who suffered from burning feet, gave a clear description of what is now called beri-beri and which the natives of the east attributed to "land winds." In other parts of the world, the condition has been apparent in times of war and famine when food was restricted. It was generally considered to be an infectious disorder until Eijkman in 1896 showed that, in chickens, dehusked rice was responsible. Clinically, it was apparent that the deficiency, frequently complicated by chronic alcoholism, caused a complex disturbance consisting of gastrointestinal disorders and systemic infections. The typical neurological finding was a severe polyneuropathy. Funk, a Polish chemist, demonstrated that the disorder could be remedied by the administration of a pyrimidine base which he called a vitamine—a vital amine; when it was shown that the compound was not an amine, the "e" was dropped from the name.

Pellagra

This deficiency disease, probably present although not recognized in ancient times, characterized by erythema of the skin, "mal de la rosa," bowel disorders, and severe mental disturbances, was described posthumously by Gaspar Casal y Julian in 1762. He considered it to be a form of leprosy which could be cured by a diet of milk, cheese, eggs, and fresh meat. In 1897, Henry Strachan wrote of a multiple neuritis occurring in the Indians of Jamaica.

Pellagra was characterized by painful, burning paresthesias and muscular cramps in the legs. The appreciation of pain and temperature, and later, position and vibratory sense, was impaired in the lower extremities. As the muscles wasted, the tendon reflexes diminished. When walking, the ataxic feet felt as if they were stepping on cotton. The skin mucous membranes became fissured and lacerated. A few years later, Stannes, noting the dermal condition, called the state "pellagra" (rough skin), but Frapolli earlier had given it the same name. This condition occurs in countries or situations in which the people have an inadequate food intake and a diet deficient in niacin.

Nerve Compression Syndromes

Pain as the result of nerve compression has probably plagued mankind for ages, although the cause has only recently been established. Sciatica, described by the Hippocratic writers from early times, has been attributed to both physical and ethereal factors. Just after the beginning of the 20th century, it was shown to be due most often to degenerative changes in the intervertebral disc. Other compressive lesions had been recognized somewhat earlier. In 1896, Pierre Marie noted in a case of acromegaly that the patient had complained of tingling and weakness of the left hand. Three years later, Stern described nocturnal acroparesthesias as the result of compression of the median nerve. The carpal tunnel syndrome was not generally recognized, however, until Woltman's report in 1941. Since that time, a number of other nerve compression syndromes have been described (e.g., thoracic outlet, peroneal, and tic douloureux).

Hereditary Sensory Radicular Neuropathy

In 1852, an unsigned report, probably by Nélaton, described a cabinet maker with indolent ulcers of his feet requiring repeated amputations. His two brothers and three children were similarly afflicted. Somewhat similar cases were reported in the next 50 years; one case had degeneration of the dorsal root ganglia (hereditary sensory radicular neuropathy). A number of other disorders— pes cavus, syringomyelia, spina bifida occulta, and various disorders resulting from muscular wasting, malnutrition, diabetes, and alcohol—must be considered in isolated cases which probably have a different basic pathogenesis.

Hereditary Recurring Neuropathy

Although hereditary progressive polyneuropathy has been known since it was described by Charcot and Marie and Tooth, cases with a relapsing course are rarer and less well understood. In 1886, Dreschfeld described two sisters who had acute attacks of pain and weakness in the shoulders and arms which slowly subsided. Similar familial palsies, usually involving the upper extremities, have been reported, but recurrent familial peripheral nerve palsies are less common.

Neuropathy Secondary to Cancer

It was probably Oppenheim in 1888 who was the first to report the association of cancer and peripheral neuropathy. Reports by Auché and others soon followed. The sensory and/or sensorimotor manifestations often antedated the discovery of the primary cancer by months or even years. Although pure sensory neuropathy was described by Weber and Hill in association with a carcinoma in 1893, they considered it only a coincidence; the association of carcinoma and encephalopathy, myelopathy, and neuropathy was described later. These neuropathies may be associated with many different types of malignancy but the most common are bronchogenic carcinoma, lymphoma, leukemia, and myeloma.

"Restless Legs"

Although Thomas Willis may have referred to "restless legs" as is averred by Critchley, it was more than a century and a half before the complaint was again mentioned in medical literature. In 1849, Magnus Huss wrote of three alcoholics who complained, while lying down, of creeping sensations in both legs and an irrepressible desire to move them. At night, the afflicted had to get up and walk about to obtain relief. In 1861, Wittmark referred to a condition he called "anxietas tibiarum" which suggests restless legs. Although later writers mentioned a similar condition, K.A. Ekbom gave the first detailed description of the disturbance. He noted that the principal complaint was a peculiar, creeping sensation beneath the skin in the muscles, even in the bones, involving one or both legs and, rarely, the arms. The annoying creeping sensation might be associated with a weak or heavy feeling in the involved members. It only occurred when the person was at rest, usually in the evening, when tired or in bed. The feeling might persist for hours, keeping the patient awake. Walking about or massaging the legs might give relief; cold applications, even cold air, seemed to help. Both sexes were afflicted, at times for years. In a few cases, an iron deficiency was responsible, but usually no cause or cure could be found.

6

Clinical and Pathological Examination of Patients with Neurological Disorders

For thousands of years, the status of the human body was assessed by a few simple maneuvers—inspection, palpation, and auscultation—that assured the examiner of the functional state of the human body. Such examinations, however, were not appropriate for determining the activity of the brain and spinal cord, which were encased in bone. For defining the activity of that system, a means of stimulating a part and noting a reaction had to be devised. When Hall demonstrated certain reflex activities in 1836, a principle was disclosed whereby the responsivity of a tissue could be tested. The clinical neurologists in Europe recognized the significance of such examinations. It was obvious that each segment of the nervous system would have specific responses that could be elicited if the reflex arc was functional. Based upon the many reflex arcs of the body, in a short time neurologists were able to formulate series of tests that would assess the reactivity of the nervous system from head to foot, and combined them to produce a formal neurological examination.

The Clinical Neurological Examination

During the Middle Ages, the physician's examination of a patient consisted of inspection, palpation of the pulse, and urinoscopy. Some healers based their therapy solely upon the inspection of the urine bottle; depending upon the appearance of the fluid—its color, consistency, suspended matter, and presence of particulate matter—the patient's disorder would be diagnosed and therapy could be prescribed.

157

During the Renaissance Period, physicians became more interested in the patient's history. The complaint was considered to be the disease and was treated as such rather than as a symptom of an underlying condition. In the 16th century, physicians began to abandon humoral concepts as postmortem examinations became common, and sought a somatic basis for most complaints. Accordingly, a weak arm was recognized not only as a local affliction of the limb, but as a disturbance of the brain or spinal cord. As these structures were encased in bone, little information regarding their function could be obtained from a superficial examination. Not until scientists had disclosed the neural basis of sensory, motor, and reflex activity could an objective assessment be made of their activity.

The scientific basis of the examination of the nervous system developed during the 19th century. In 1836, Marshall Hall elucidated the excitomotor system, later termed the reflex arc. He emphasized that an appropriate stimulus was followed by a contraction of certain muscles independent of voluntary control. Thus, the comatose patient breathed normally; the tone of the muscles distal to a spinal cord section after a period of shock remained normal or might be augmented. Much of the neurological examination was developed upon such principles, but it was some time before clinicians who were exploring the nervous system utilized those guides. In the first manual of neurology written by Romberg in 1844, the sensory and motor neuroses (afflictions of the peripheral nerves) were presented in detail, but the means for determining their dysfunction was not discussed. A few isolated tests for sensory impairment (the "Romberg test") and motor loss were mentioned, but of the reflexes only the cremasteric was described. The pupillary reactions, although recognized by Avicenna centuries earlier, were not listed. A short while later, Duchenne expounded on the normal and pathological electrical reactions of muscles and nerves, but gave few clinical correlations. Hammond in 1871 listed such technical aids as the ophthalmoscope, cephalohemometer (used to measure intracranial pressure), esthesiometer, thermometer, dynamometer, biopsy trocar, and electrical stimulators; however, no instruments used to examine the reflexes were mentioned.

It was not until the French clinicians became interested in neurological disorders that a systematic routine for examining the functions of the nervous system was formulated in the latter part of the 19th century. In 1877, Charcot described a "methodical examination of a patient." After a brief discussion of the history, Charcot observed for his attentive audience any obvious motor disturbances such as tremor or abnormal posturing. He tested the strength of the limbs, the presence of spinal epilepsy (clonus), muscle contractures, circulatory disturbances, and the skin temperature. Based on these observations, Charcot would discuss the differential diagnosis of the patient's presenting complaint.

Some physicians made a more detailed examination of as many neurological functions as possible. In 1882, Bramwell outlined the examination of a patient with a spinal cord disorder. After eliciting the history, he evaluated the general appearance of the patient—his facial expression, attitude, gait, and nutrition— made from observations as the history was being taken. The muscular strength was assessed with a dynamometer. The irritability of the muscles was tested using faradic, galvanic, and mechanical stimulation. The tone of the muscles was assessed by their resistance to passive movement. The reflexes—superficial (plantar, gluteal, cremasteric, abdominal, epigastric, and interscapular), deep (knee jerk and ankle clonus), and the organic (vesical and rectal)—were examined. Muscular coordination was tested. The sensory functions were appraised by responses to questions regarding pain, numbness, tingling, formication, and thermal paresthesias. The appreciation of touch, pain, and temperature was assayed. Vasomotor responses and trophic changes in the skin were noted. The spinal column was palpated to assess its mobility and discomfort on movement. It is apparent that this examination would give a satisfactory appraisal of the state of the spine and spinal cord.

In 1888, Gowers published a book on diseases of the nervous system, in which he outlined a clinical neurological examination under the headings of motor symptoms, sensory symptoms, reflexes, changes in nutrition, and electrical irritability. In another section of the book, Gowers described the examination of the cranial nerves. In 1890, Oppenheim gave a similarly detailed account of the neurological examination. Table 1 outlines the clinical examinations used by Wernicke in 1881 and Mills in 1898.

Some physicians not thoroughly indoctrinated in basic neurology relied upon the demonstration of certain signs and symptoms for the diagnosis. If the patient's neurological status matched such a constellation, often in the form of an algorithm, the nature of the disorder would be considered established.

The Cranial Nerves

The early anatomists divided the nerves into two groups—those that took origin from the brain and those that arose from the spinal cord. The cranial nerves that came from the base of the brain and passed out the bony orifices of the skull must have been recognized by the Alexandrian anatomists, although they gave little attention to their distribution. Their methods of dissecting the brain in situ precluded a satisfactory examination of the nerves at the base. As a result, the cranial nerves were not codified until Galen, studying the brains of oxen, enumerated seven pairs of cranial nerves based upon the rostral-caudal location of their sites of exit from the cranium. Galen recognized that some nerves passing out of a foramen consisted of several disparate bundles of fibers. Centuries later, von Soemmerring, aware that such variations implied functional differences, proposed an anatomicophysiological division into 12 nerves, a classification still in use.

The clinical or bedside examination of the cranial nerves has changed little

TABLE 1

NEUROLOGICAL EXAMINATION CIRCA LATE 19TH CENTURY

Wernicke (1881)	Mills (1898)
Subjective Data	
–headache, dizziness, vomiting	–impaired mentation, pain, headache, visual and auditory disturbances
Objective Findings	
–sensorium and mental status	–mental examination noting mood and memory
–vegetative functions (temperature, pulse, appetite, urine)	–vasomotor, trophic and secretory status, pulse, thermometry
–cranial nerves (optic fundi)	–smell, fundus examination, visual and occular status, pupillary reactions, facial sensation and movement, taste and hearing
–motor disturbances (paralysis, reflexes, abnormal movements)	–motor status – power, coordination, muscle status, fibrillations, electrical reactions
	–reflexes, cutaneous (abdominal, plantar, cremasteric, anal)), deep (tibial, radial, patellar, toe jerk, ankle clonus, biceps, triceps and radial)
–sensory disturbances (hemianesthesia, hypesthesia)	–sensory status (esthesiometry, 2-point discrimination, temperature, pressure, muscle, position)
–station and gait	–Romberg test
–speech (stuttering, cadence, etc.)	

in the past century. The tests of cranial nerve function which Gowers outlined in his textbook of 1888 differ only slightly from those employed at the present time. The cranial nerves were examined as follows.

The Olfactory Nerve

Although the appreciation of odors was recognized by the early Grecian philosophers as arising from the nose, the neural pathways were not identified until Galen described the conduits (olfactory tracts) carrying odors from the nose to the brain. This concept was accepted until 800 AD, when a monograph by an unknown writer suggested that the cords from the nasal cavity were not conduits, carrying odors to the brain, but nerves conveying spirits from the nose. Another 800 years passed before this concept was further elaborated upon by the Renaissance anatomists. Observing that the white tracts coming from the nose varied in size depending upon the phylogenetic importance of the olfactory organ, Willis concluded that they conveyed information regarding smell to the ventricles. This interpretation was not accepted by all philosophers; some thought that an odor was carried by the blood to be appreciated.

Both anatomical and clinical evidence was accumulating to indicate that the first cranial nerve of Willis subserved olfaction. Although the loss of smell was infrequently mentioned in the earlier literature, occasional observations were made. Lower described anosmia as the result of a "scirrhous pituitary tumor" which might have been an olfactory groove meningioma compressing the olfactory bulbs. Longet reported a case in which the olfactory tracts were absent and the subject had a congenital absence of olfaction but preservation of the sense of touch in the nose. The anatomists of the 19th century were tracing the fibers of the olfactory tract to the base of the brain and thalamus. Yet the issue was not settled, for Magendie thought that the sensory (trigeminal) nerve of the face subserved olfaction.

When clinicians began to study the functions of the nervous system in sequence, anosmia was noted. Hughlings Jackson examined a man who, as the result of being kicked in the head by a horse, lost "the sense of smell forever." Six years later, in 1870, Notta wrote of a man who lost his sense of smell but recovered it in 8 weeks. Ogle in the same year queried whether the sense of smell was not lost in these cases as the result of tearing the olfactory nerve at the cribriform plate. He distinguished the loss of smell from that of taste, for the latter might be preserved when the former was lost. In 1876 Ferrier confirmed this differentiation for he noted that the sense of smell might be permanently lost, although taste might recover, after a head injury. These clinical observations confirmed the role of the first cranial nerve in olfaction.

The Optic Nerves

Blindness has been noted to follow injury to the eyeballs from time immemorial. The earliest account appears to be that of Hippocrates, who wrote "dimness of vision occurs in injuries to the brow." Galen was somewhat more specific in stating that injury to the optic nerves caused blindness. Although the Arab physicians contributed to the understanding of vision, they added little to the knowledge of the central visual pathways. Willis recognized the "seeing nerves" as carriers of the animal spirits from the orbital globes to the chambers of the optic nerves or thalami at the base of the brain. From these bodies, the image or "sensible species" was assumed to pass to the common sensory center. The introduction of postmortem examinations made it possible to verify the nature and extent of visual disturbances. In a report dated 1780,

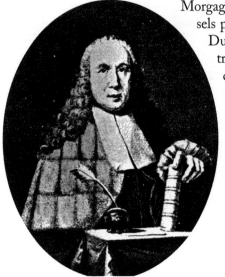

Fig. 6-1. Giovanni Battista Morgagni (1682-1771). (From Classics of Neurology. *Huntington, NY: Krieger, 1971)*

Morgagni ascribed blindness to swollen vessels pressing on the optic nerves. In 1822, Duponchel described the effects of trauma to the optic nerves; a more detailed account was given by Chassaignac of blindness resulting from a basal skull fracture involving the sphenoid bone.

A few years later, Nuhn described the damage resulting from a fracture passing through the optic canal. When the ophthalmoscope was invented, the fundal and optic disc changes secondary to basal skull fractures could be seen.

Trauma to the optic chiasm was not reported until 1883 by Nieden. The resulting defects in the visual fields were described the next year by Tuffier and Shöler and Uhthoff. Although the central visual pathways were not known in 1719, Morgagni described a homonymous hemianopsia in a person who had an occipital lobe lesion (Fig. 6-1). The visual field disturbances after head injuries were shown by Gowers. Because of their position, the optic tract and lateral geniculate bodies were rarely affected by trauma alone. Steffen was most likely the first to describe an optic tract lesion and which was confirmed at autopsy reported by Willbrand et al in 1885.

Gowers used charts that tested the visual acuity and color appreciation. The visual fields were plotted, giving the characteristic defects indicative of optic nerve, chiasm, tract, and radiation lesions.

The Oculomotor, Trochlear, and Abducens Nerves

Eye movements were examined by asking the patient to follow the examiner's finger as it was moved about the visual field. The extent and smoothness of the movements and the presence of nystagmus were observed. The status of the pupils—their size, shape, reactions to light, and accommodation—was noted. The palpebral fissures were observed as well as sweating on the face.

The Trigeminal Nerve

The appreciation of touch and pain over the three branches of the trigeminal nerve was ascertained. The strength and contraction of the masseter muscles were appraised.

The Facial Nerve

Although Galen grouped the facial and auditory nerves, Willis separated them; thereafter, they were considered to be individual nerves. To test the strength of the upper and lower facial muscles, various grimaces were observed. At the same time, tremors, fibrillations, and spasms of the face could be noted. The loss of taste was assessed by having the patient identify salt, sour, sweet, and bitter objects applied to the tongue. Following head injuries, taste was often absent, although the precise nerve involved was not clear. Ferrier noted that smell and taste could be individually involved; however, the locale for the appreciation of taste and the neural pathways were not clarified until neurosurgeons observed the effects of cutting various peripheral nerves related to the face.

The Auditory and Vestibular Nerves

The auditory and vestibular nerves were identified by the early anatomists and the Roman physicians. Tests for their function were crude in those days but after the Renaissance period, auditory acuity was assessed using a tuning fork and vestibular function was assessed by injecting warm and cold water into the external auditory canals. Aural vertigo was described by P. Ménière in 1861; Charcot in 1874 termed it "vertigo ab aure loesa." In the early part of the 19th century, Purkinje and Flourens, on the basis of their experiments, concluded that nystagmus resulted from cerebellar or vestibular disorders.

The Glossopharyngeal Nerve

Gowers admitted that the testing of the glossopharyngeal nerve was uncertain, although he observed the patient for weakness of the upper pharynx.

The Vagus Nerve

To assess vagus nerve function, the quality of the voice was noted and the ease of swallowing was tested. Spasms of the throat, esophagus, and stomach were assessed. Palatal movements and reflexes were tested, although Gowers admitted that they might not be a vagus nerve function.

The Spinal Accessory Nerve

Gowers included laryngeal movements as well as sternocleidomastoid and trapezius muscle movements as activities of the spinal accessory nerve.

The Hypoglossal Nerve

The hypoglossal nerve was tested by noting the movements of the tongue, both voluntary and involuntary.

Gowers discussed cutaneous and muscle or tendon reflexes under reflex action. Cutaneous reflexes included the plantar, gluteal, cremasteric, and abdominal reflexes, and of the cranial nerves, the conjunctival, iris (pupillary), and neck reflexes. The tendon reflexes included the knee jerk and the ankle jerk which, if exaggerated, becomes ankle clonus.

Thus, by the end of the 19th century, the neurological examination had quite a modern garb, although a number of tests—those for higher mental function, cranial nerve activity, muscle tone, astereognosis, and pathological plantar reflexes—were not yet routinely incorporated in the battery of tests.

Electrical Activity of the Brain

Another technique used to determine cortical function was the study of the brain's electrical activity. Stimulated by DuBois-Reymond's report of action potentials when muscles contracted, Richard Caton, a Liverpool physician, wondered if there might be the same potentials in the brain. To test that possibility, Caton exposed the brains of rabbits and monkeys and placed galvanometer electrodes on the gray matter. He noted varying fluctuating potentials recorded from electrodes on the surface of the animal's brain. These potentials changed on one side when the opposite eye was illuminated. The oscillations of the baseline, he demonstrated, were not related to respiratory or cardiac rhythms. By changing the depth of anoxia or anesthesia, and by killing the animal, Caton showed that they were of biological cerebral origin. Moreover, with his electrodes on the external surface of the skull, Caton could detect a feeble flow of current producing electrical waves. He presented his findings in 1887 at the Ninth International Medical Congress held in Washington, D.C.

Caton's discovery in 1875 of the electrical potentials generated in the brain received little notice, as his report appeared in the *British Medical Journal*, which was seldom read by physiologists. Brain waves were rediscovered by Adolph Beck about 15 years later. Beck reported that in the brains of frogs, rabbits, and dogs, "there was a continuous waxing and waning variation." Like Caton, Beck noted augmented electrical activity in the occipital cortex which was superimposed upon the slow wave pattern of the resting brain when a burning magnesium ribbon was flashed before an animal's eye.

When Beck's claim was published, a physiology professor in Vienna named Fleischl von Marxow wrote to the journal claiming that he had shown that sensory stimulation induced electrical activity in the brain detectable by a sensitive galvanometer. His experiments were reported in a sealed letter dated 1883 held in the vault of the Imperial Academy of Sciences at Vienna. Although he had registered the electrical activity from the skull, he wrote, "perhaps it will be possible to observe, by recording from the scalp, currents evoked by various psychological acts of one's own brain."

The question of priority seemed to be settled when Caton referred to his publication in the *British Medical Journal*. However, a year later, a Russian, Vasili Yakovlevich Danilevsky, wrote to the editor of the *Zentralblatt für Physiologie*, stating that in his doctoral thesis of 1876 he had "revealed spontaneous electrical activity" in the brain. In fact, several other Russian investigators had demonstrated such electrical activity earlier than Beck.

When the thermionic tube was developed for amplication of the electrical potentials, brain recording was revived by Hans Berger (Fig. 6-2), a psychiatrist in Jena who confirmed the findings of Caton and extended the work to man. Berger named the process "electroencephalography" and demonstrated the abnormalities of such potentials in disease, thus opening a new approach for clinicians and physiologists to explore the brain.

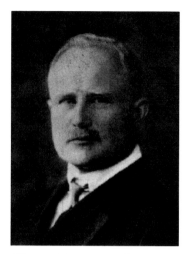

Fig. 6-2. Hans Berger (1873-1941). (From A History of Neurosurgery. *Greenblatt SH, Dagi TF, Epstein M, editors. Park Ridge, Ill: American Association of Neurological Surgeons, 1997, p 241)*

Medical Illustrations

In the early neurological literature, the pathological state was rarely illustrated, although it was usually described in vivid language. Photography had been introduced in the first half of the 19th century, but most books were illustrated with line drawings; artistic sketches such as those of Charles Bell were rare. Hammond's book of 1871 had fewer than three illustrations per hundred pages of text. Charcot in his lectures on diseases of the nervous system used eight prints per 100 pages of text. Gower's manual contained 28 figures and Oppenheim's *Lehrbuch*, 30 figures per 100 pages. Macewen's book on brain infections had 17 figures per 100 pages. Duret in 1905 used 36 figures per 100 pages; Cushing in 1908 had 56 figures per 100 pages—the majority of pages contained photographs. The medical artist was just appearing on the horizon.

The Chemical Products of Neural Activity

Cerebrospinal Fluid

A watery fluid in the meninges was mentioned in the *Edwin Smith papyrus*, but it was forgotten as the early philosophers focused attention upon the cavities within the brain. Although the Greeks and Romans knew of these cavities, they apparently were not aware that they contained fluid. Berengario da Carpi did mention a watery excrement of the brain which usually could be seen in the ventricles when the head was dissected; however, the first explicit account of ventricular fluid was given by the Italian anatomist Massa, who practiced in Venice in the early part of the 16th century. He states, in referring to the ventricles, "observe the watery superfluity in these cavities, sent there from other parts of the brain and expurgated through a foramen from the cavities of the ventricles. It is particularly noteworthy that I have always found these cavities full or half full of the aforementioned watery superfluity of the rational brain."

In the following centuries, the presence of ventricular fluid was mentioned by various anatomists. Thomas Willis speculated about the function of these humors in the ventricles.

> The moderns consider these places as vile and assert them to be merely sewers for the carrying away of excreted matter. . . . Some substance has been added to this belief because in the dead these ventricles are often observed to be filled with water; furthermore, ways seem to lie open from the ventricles for excretion through the infundibulum and to the cribriform plate.

This reference to drainage from the cribriform plate, which had been earlier noted by Schneider and elaborated upon by Lower and Willis as nasal catarrhs, may have been cerebrospinal fluid rhinorrhea; if so, Willis did not understand its significance.

Until this time, however, attention had been directed almost entirely to the liquid within the ventricular system. In 1692, Valsalva made a passing reference to a collection of humor around the brainstem similar to that found in joints. In the next century, Swedenborg, in a treatise on the brain published from 1741 to 1744, described the lymph of "the cerebellum and choroid plexus of the fourth ventricle," a fluid which he stated was present about the medulla oblongata and spinal cord. Undoubtedly, Swedenborg was referring to cerebrospinal fluid, but as his work was not published until 1882-1887, he received little credit for his observations. Later, both von Haller and Morgagni referred casually to fluid surrounding the base of the brain.

It remained for Domenico Cotugno (Fig. 6-3) in his famous book *De ischiade nervosa commentarius* to point out that extracerebral and spinal fluid had not been seen in the past because of the method of dissecting the head. Cotugno stated:

> Hitherto anatomists have not observed this large collection of water in the spine and around the brain because of the ridiculous method usually employed for the dissection of bodies. When they are about to examine the brain they usually cut off the head with the neck, and when this had been done, and the tube of dura mater descending through the spine of the neck has been cut through, all of the fluid collected around the brain and the spinal marrow is at once lost.

Cotugno was aware that the fluid in the ventricles could pass through the aqueduct of Sylvius and fourth ventricle to mix with the water about the spinal cord. Although historians have given him great credit for his discovery, in actuality, his observations, published in a small book on sciatica, were little read or appreciated.

It was not until Magendie reported his investigations of what he designated "le liquide cephalo-spinal" (cerebrospinal fluid) that the true nature and distribution of the water in and about the brain and spinal cord were appreciated. In a paper presented on January 10, 1825, Magendie pointed out that cerebrospinal fluid was a nor-

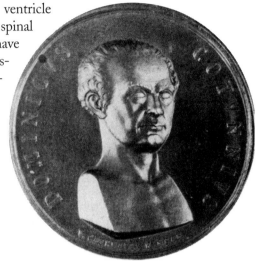

Fig. 6-3. Domenico Cotugno (1736-1822). (From the collection of A. Earl Walker)

mal watery constituent located between the pia mater and arachnoid membranes of man and animals. The ventricles, he stated, were constantly full of fluid which might measure as much as two ounces without producing a defect of intellectual function, but if more than that quantity were present, a paralysis of movement and dementia might result. Magendie noted that the fluid produced in the spinal canal could pass into the cavities of the brain or, vice versa, that the fluid produced in the ventricles could pass into the posterior ventricle and through a midline opening into the spinal fluid system at the base of the brain and then down along the spinal cord as far as the sacral sac. In a paper presented to the Academie des Science of Paris, Magendie described and depicted in a wax model the posterior midline foramen, subsequently named after him, between the fourth ventricle and the cisterna magna. He believed that the fluid within these cavities was continuously agitated by the respiratory excursions, so that "[w]hen we draw air into our chest to breath the liquid partly passes out from the cerebral cavities into the spinal canal; on the contrary, at the moment in which we breathe out from the lungs by expiration, the liquid returns into these cavities passing across the conduits mentioned above and particularly running through the aqueduct which thus carries the liquid in one direction and again in the opposite direction." A clever observation indeed!

The lateral recesses of the fourth ventricle were subsequently described by Luschka in a beautifully illustrated monograph on the choroid plexuses of the brain (Fig. 6-4). Luschka expressed doubt that the cerebrospinal fluid was a simple capillary transudate from the vessels to the pia mater or from the ependyma. He states, "it cannot escape unbiased observation that the most

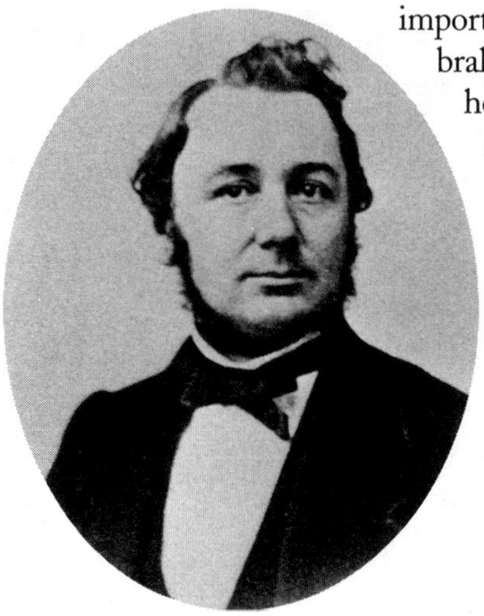

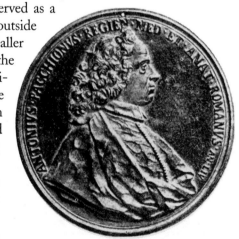

Fig. 6-4. Luschka, who described the lateral recesses of the fourth ventricle. (From the collection of A. Earl Walker)

important sources for the formation of the cerebral spinal fluid are the choroid plexuses; however, as may be concluded from the metamorphosis of its epithelium, the ependyma, and outer vascular membrane (pia mater) also participate in it."

In the early part of the 19th century, Munro and Kellie collaborated in establishing that the skull, being a closed box, maintained a constant fluid content. Roy and Sherrington in 1890 challenged this assumption, however, and reasoned that the cerebral circulation had to respond to arterial pressure and to the requirements of the cerebral parts being irrigated. It was a half century later that Cobb and his associates showed that there was intrinsic control of the cerebral circulation.

Function of the Cerebrospinal Fluid

Although several physicians knew of water within and at the base of the brain, none had suggested a valid reason for its presence. Willis had deduced that it served as a sewer to carry away excretions to outside sites. In the next century, von Haller wrote that a thin humor from the arteries was excreted into the ventricles and drawn back through the veins. A half century previously, in 1705, Antonio Pacchioni had described the arachnoidal tufting along the vascular sinuses (Fig. 6-5). Their function remained obscure until Faivre in 1853 suggested that they might be involved in the elimination of non-organic substances in the spinal fluid. This concept was further developed by the experimental studies of Key and Retzius, who demonstrated that dye injected

Fig. 6-5. Antonio Pacchioni, who described arachnoidal tufting along the vascular sinuses. (From the collection of A. Earl Walker)

into the subarachnoid space passed through the tufts into the blood sinuses. Little additional research was done on this subject until Dandy and Blackfan produced experimental hydrocephalus early in the 20th century (Fig. 6-6). Dandy and Blackfan occluded the foramen of Munro after removing the choroid plexus and found that hydrocephalus did not develop; it was on the basis of their studies that they concluded that cerebrospinal fluid was formed from the choroid plexus and absorbed diffusely from the subarachnoid space.

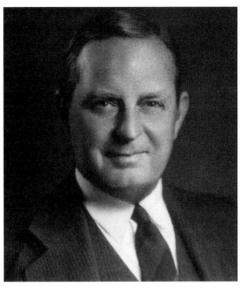

Fig. 6-6. Walter E. Dandy made fundamental discoveries in the pathogenesis of hydrocephalus. (From the collection of A. Earl Walker)

Dilated cerebral ventricles had been tapped for the relief of hydrocephalus by early physicians, but it was 60 years after Magendie's demonstration of the cerebrospinal fluid that, in 1885, Corning introduced a needle into the subarachnoid space to inject cocaine as an anesthesetic. No attempt was made to remove or examine the fluid. Approximately six years later, neurologists in Russia and England independently needled the lumbar subarachnoid space for the purpose of relieving intracranial pressure. Quincke reported on this procedure before an international congress and has been given the credit for introducing lumbar puncture, although Morton and Wynter in England used the procedure to relieve intracranial pressure at about the same time. The possibility that examination of the spinal fluid might be of diagnostic value was explored by Fürbringer and Netter in patients suffering from meningitis, brain tumor, and meningeal hemorrhage. Shortly thereafter, in 1901, Widal, Sicard, and Ravaut reported on the cytological changes found in various diseases of the nervous system. Two years later, Froin described xanthochromia and spontaneous clotting in loculated spinal fluid from inflammatory or neoplastic involvement of the meninges (spinal block); the syndrome was named after him. In those days, practically any patient having a neurological disorder was suspected to be suffering from syphilis. The Wassermann test, introduced in 1906, and the colloidal gold reaction of the spinal fluid perfected somewhat later were important diagnostic aids. It was somewhat later that Mestrezat systematically described the constituents of the spinal fluid in health and disease.

Cerebrospinal Fluid Fistula

It is surprising that the Greek and Roman physicians who dissected the brain and spinal cord did not refer to the water surrounding and within these structures. The Renaissance anatomists were aware of the ventricular fluid; Willis referred to its secretion from the cribriform plate. Earlier, Schneider had described the nasal discharge as a catarrh, a concept which was accepted for centuries. The presence of fluid about the brainstem and spinal cord, although briefly mentioned earlier, was clearly described by Cotugno in 1762.

Morgagni reported a case of clear nasal discharge but was unaware of its genesis. King concluded that in the 18th century such a flow of fluid from the intracranial cavity was "a protective mechanism of animal economy to ward off an already general anasarca." That fluid might drip spontaneously from the nose was asserted by Charles Miller in 1826. He probed an opening "above and to the right of the crista galia" to verify that the fluid came from the nasal cavity.

Watery fluid dripping from the ear of a person after a head injury was reported in 1780 by Stalpart Van der Weil; Berengario da Carpi had also written of another case. Langier in 1778 concluded that this fluid, which he assumed was serum from a blood clot, was evidence of a skull fracture. Rarely the otorrhea arose spontaneously from a fistula in the external auditory canal.

Robert in 1847 and Tillaux in 1877 determined that the chemical constituency of the fluid was the same as that of the spinal fluid. The appellation "cerebrospinal fluid rhinorrhea" was introduced by Thompson in 1899; otorrhea was a natural sequence.

Abnormal Intracranial Gaseous Material

The presence of gas within the scalp was described by Werner in 1873 as "subcutaneous emphysema" or "pneumatocele." In 1914, Wolff termed intracranial gas "pneumozephalus." Most cases were the result of gas-forming organisms which were responsible for the chronic mastoiditis, but some were due to coughing or sneezing foreign air into the subgaleal space. The presence of air in the extradural, subdural, subarachnoid, ventricular, or intracerebral spaces, usually due to basal skull fractures, was described much later.

The Examination of the Pathological Nervous System—
The Evolution of Neuropathology

An examination of the human brain was rarely made in early times because of tribal taboos or religious tenets. Some knowledge of the gross structure of the intracranial contents was obtained by treating head wounds of warfare; however, there is no evidence that a systematic examination for abnormalities of the brain was made. The Alexandrian physicians and surgeons were primarily interested in the anatomy and physiology of the brain. Since their subjects most frequently died of trauma by the age of 20 or 30, they would rarely encounter other pathological lesions in the nervous system. For this reason, it is understandable that the medical writings of that early period make little reference to diseased states of the brain.

Occasionally, bony lesions other than traumatic ones bore mute evidence of a pathological condition. Erosion of the skull base by tumors, or of the vertex by neoplasm, infections, or hyperostoses give an indication of some conditions which afflicted ancient people.

After the Greek and Roman periods, autopsies were banned and for a thousand years knowledge of the morbid effects of disease on the human brain was not advanced. During the plague epidemic in the 13th century, the authorities permitted a few autopsies to determine possible causes and treatment for the affliction. Although anatomical dissections were performed at a number of medical schools in the 14th century, it was not until 1562 that Paré conducted the first legal autopsy.

In the 16th century, some physicians and surgeons requested permission to examine the bodies of their patients. One of the earliest was Berengario da Carpi, who is more renowned for his anatomical observations than his pathological findings. A number of Paduan physicians of that time dissected the human body to examine its tissue morphology rather than to determine the cause of death. Two Italian scientists, Bernard Tornini in 1485 and Antonio Beniviene in 1507, published accounts of clinical data and autopsy findings in considerable detail. Beniviene's 54-page book on postmortem examinations gave a nearly modern account of the gross pathology.

In 1554, Fernel of the Paris faculty wrote an unillustrated section on postmortem examinations which Long called the first pathology textbook. At about the same time, Paré was performing legal autopsies. His most famous case involved the postmortem examination on Henry II, who died in 1559 of a head wound received in a joust. Henry II's brain revealed a large subdural hematoma on the side opposite the wound. In the next century, Bartholin, Professor of Anatomy at Copenhagen, encouraged the verification of disease by autopsy. In Geneva, Theophile Bonet reported on all the autopsies performed since ancient times—some 3,000 cases, many described so fragmentarily that later writers criticized the work. It was, however, the stimulus for scientific investigation of disease in the 17th century.

These early treatises often neglected to mention the brain, so that neurological disorders were little advanced. Moreover, the custom of cutting off the head at the neck and examining it some time after the general autopsy led to an isolation of the cephalic findings. This was particularly noteworthy in the fascinating reports of Thomas Willis. His clinical accounts with limited autopsy findings, at times, are difficult to reconcile with modern disease. Yet, some of his histories are sufficiently detailed to identify the pathological state.

An example is the account of a woman about 30 years of age who, after suffering from a severe pain in the head for 6 months, developed weakness of her limbs and fell into a deep sleep. She regained consciousness, continued to suffer headaches, again lapsed into a sleepy distemper, and died. When her skull was opened, a scirrhous tumor was found between the dura and pia mater. Does this not suggest a meningeal tumor which any modern neurosurgeon could resect?

The more detailed accounts by Morgagni in the next century, many reported previously, were the basis of modern pathology, especially of the nervous system. Without the aid of the microscope or stains, he described the gross abnormalities of the brain so precisely that most cases can be diagnosed; however, for more detailed examination, physicians sought a means of preserving the organ. Boyle had found that wine hardened tissues and Willis subsequently immersed brains in that fluid. A century later, Vicq d'Azyr and Reil used alcohol for organ preservation. With such fixatives to harden the brain, Meynert, Burdach, and Stilling described much of the gross anatomical structure of the central nervous system. The introduction by Hannover of chromic acid and its salts as fixatives was the next great advance. At the end of the 19th century, Blum, while studying the antiseptic properties of formaldehyde, noted its effect upon his own fingers and suggested its use as a hardening agent. Within a few years, formaldehyde was universally recognized as an ideal fixative for pathological work.

When the brain was fixed in situ, its structural configuration remained, so that distortions of the tissues were retained. Consequently, displacements of cerebral or cerebellar tissue into normal spinal fluid cisterns were observed by Pagenstecher in 1871. Twenty years later, Chiari described the distortions and caudal displacement of the cerebellum by traction due to spinal dysraphism. In 1894, Arnold referred to the caudal transposition of the cerebellar tonsils by myeloceles. Two years later, Hill demonstrated that increasing the intracranial volume with a balloon raised the pressure, greatest in the supratentorial space, less in the subtentorial space, and least in the spinal subarachnoidal space, which he attributed to a tamponade at the tentorial notch and foramen magnum. In 1900, Marie described the downward displacement of the cerebellar tonsils resulting from intracranial space-occupying lesions. Cushing a few years later used the term "cerebellar pressure cone" to define this state. These displacements were elaborated upon later by Meyer, Kernohan, and Cairns.

Although thin sections of the brain and spinal cord had been made previously, Benedict Stilling was the first to cut serial sections by hand to study the minute structure of the spinal cord and brainstem (Fig. 6-7). Shortly thereafter, a microtome was invented which allowed thinner and more uniform sectioning. At first, the tissue blocks were frozen, but later various embedding methods were utilized. In 1869, Edwin Klebs described paraffin embedding, and a decade later, Duval introduced collodion, from which celloidin was later compounded.

In the early unstained sections, the fine structure of the central nervous system was not seen. Cochineal was first used to stain the tissue but the elements were not differentiated. Although Boehmer had differentially stained cells and myelin by mordanting in alum before

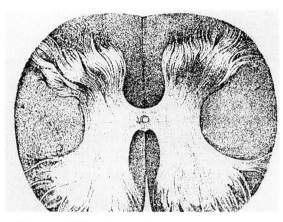

Fig. 6-7. Stilling's illustration of a cross-section of the spinal cord. (From the collection of A. Earl Walker)

dyeing in hematoxylin, the technique was perfected by Weigert in 1882. Using these neurohistological techniques, the normal and pathological elements of the nervous system could be studied. Another method to stain myelinated tracts was subsequently developed. Although Nasse in 1839 and Waller in 1850 had noted the breakdown of myelin in nerve fibers whose axons were damaged centrally, it

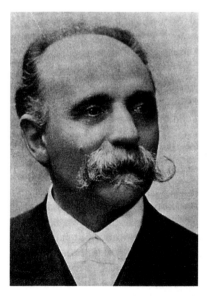

Fig. 6-8. Camillo Golgi (1843-1926). (From The Founders of Neurology, 2nd ed. Haymaker W, Schiller F, editors. Springfield, Ill: Charles C Thomas, 1970, p 36)

was Marchi in 1886 who demonstrated that products of myelin degeneration could be specifically stained by osmic acid after mordanting with chromic salt. Thus, it was possible to follow a sectioned myelinated fiber tract from the transection almost to its termination, a technique by which Marchi traced many fiber pathways within the central nervous system.

The minute histology of the neuron was described by both Golgi and Nissl. In 1881, Camillo Golgi (Fig. 6-8) showed that the fine structure of the neuron could be revealed by encrustating the nerve cell, its contents, and its ramifications with silver and gold salts. Using this technique, Spanish anatomists led by Golgi and Ramon y Cajal investigated all parts of the central nervous system. Nissl found that toluidine blue, an aniline dye, had a particular affinity for certain chromatophilic substances within the cell cytoplasm and nucleus. In 1892, he demonstrated the intracellular changes which take place after axon injury. With these histological techniques, it was possible to demonstrate pathological changes in neurons, fiber tracts, and blood vessels of the brain.

Neuropathology as a specialized branch of pathology did not exist until well into the 19th century. It was born as a bastard offspring of neuropsychiatrists, who sought the morphological cerebral changes underlying mental disease. Previously, pathologists with little interest in psychiatric disorders had ignored the special techniques necessary for studying the nervous system. Kraepelin and others like him took to the microtome and used aniline dyes to find an anatomical basis for the psychoses. As a result, they discovered the fundamental neuronal and glial reactions to disease, which they described with a novel nomenclature that remained a barrier to communication between neuropathologists and general pathologists for almost a century. In Paris, the mecca of neurology in the 19th century, Charcot founded a neuropathology laboratory in which, using the new staining techniques, he established the histological basis of a number of diseases such as poliomyelitis, amyotrophic lateral sclerosis, multiple sclerosis, tabes dorsalis, and muscular dystrophy. His pupils, including Pierre Marie, Jules Dejerine, and Joseph Babinski, studied the neuropathological changes in the superb clinical material which came from the French hospitals. They were the pioneer explorers of the disorders of the brain.

In the 20th century, new technical methods for the study of neuropathology changed its face almost completely. The Spanish school studied the characteristics of brain tumors as revealed by silver and gold impregnations. Electron microscopy solved many problems of nervous system structure in health and disease. Chemical studies of the brain initiated in the 19th century with the work of Thudichum developed into neurochemistry, histochemistry, and enzyme chemistry. And so the neuropathologist has become part of the total effort to explore the mysteries of the nervous system.

7

Manifestations of Cerebral Disorders: Headache, Epilepsy, Sleep Disorders, and Cerebrovascular Disease

Headache

Pain in the head was known as "cephalea" in Roman and Greek times and was a common affliction. When associated with fever, it was termed "cephalalgia." Roman physicians (e.g., Themison, Thessalus, and Soranus) discussed pain in the head in detail, thinking that it was due to physical stress such as chills or sunstroke. They recognized that the pain may be in a portion of or in the entire head; if confined to one side, it was called hemicrania. The attack was said to begin in the depth of the eyes or back of the head and extend over the entire head or down the spine. These writers referred to a dimming of vision, nausea and vomiting with tearing, and photophobia. Lying down in a darkened room with astringent plasters applied to the forehead was the usual treatment and afforded some relief. After fasting for three days, the patient was usually well enough to be given food and drink. If the pain persisted, the patient's hair was clipped down to the skin and plasters, cupping, and in desperate cases even scarification, were tried. Other therapies might be prescribed such as warm applications locally, clysters to relieve the bowels, and simple foods. As the pain eased, the patient was gotten up into a chair, walked about, and given passive exercises. Baths, rest, and a liquid diet were augmented by leavened bread, eggs, vegetables, and tender fish or birds. The physical and dietetic regimen after some time might be terminated by a sea voyage.

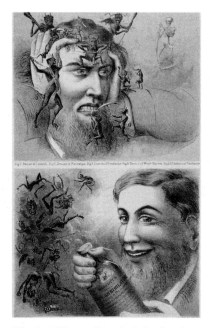

Fig. 7-1. Illustrations depicting head-ache and other painful conditions. (From Medicine: A Treasury of Art and Lit-erature. *A Carmichael and R Rotzan, editors. New York: Harkavy, 1991)*

Obviously, this treatment recommended by the Greek and Roman Methodists included considerable physiotherapy and psychotherapy. Later writers such as Are-taeus of Cappadocia did refer to hetercra-nia, but not even Galen's discussion of the effect of black bile was a satisfactory remedy. The Arabs and the later physi-cians of the Middle Ages added little to the understanding of headache; however, with the Renaissance, interest was revived (Fig. 7-1).

In his rather long discourse on head-ache, Thomas Willis (1621-1675) noted that the pain may be due to structures either without or within the skull but that the former is more rare and more gentle because the skull is not as sensitive as the interior meninges. Yet Willis maintained that the brain, cerebellum, and their med-ullary dependencies "are free from pains because they want sensible fibers."

Migrainous headaches were well known to Willis. "The pain may be uni-versal, affecting the entire head, or it may be remitted in some private region, sometimes producing a meagrim on the side, sometimes in the forepart and sometimes in the hinder part of the head." As an example, Willis cited the case of a noblewoman who had a typical migraine headache. Headache due to intracranial pressure was described. "Yea, I have known Inflammations, Imposthumes, Whelks, Scirrhous tumors growing to the Meninges with the Skull, and other Diseases of an evil conformation, excited in the Membranes of the Brain; by which, at first, for a long time, fre-quent headaches, and most cruel, and then afterwards a sleepy and deadly dis-temper hath been induced; the cause of the Disease not detected, but after death by Anatomy."

Willis related the case of a woman about 50 years of age who, after suffering from grievous pain in the head for six months, fell into a lethargy with a partial resolution of her limbs; she came to but continued to suffer headaches, relapsed into a sleepy distemper and died. When her skull was opened, a scirrhous tumor was found, occupying the space between the dura mater and the pia mater.

Two of Willis' cases might well have been subdural hematomas. One, a young man of the university, had had for a fortnight most grievous pain in the head, later aggravated by fever and afterward making convulsive movements and idle talking. Various remedies did not help, and he ultimately died. "His skull being opened, the Vessels leading the Meninges were full of blood and very much distended, as if the whole Mass of Blood had flowed thither, so that the bosoms being dissected and opened, the Blood presently rushing forth, flowed to the weight of several ounces above half a pint; further, the membranes themselves being distempered throughout the whole, with a fiery Tumor, appeared discolored: These coverings being taken away, all the infoldings of the Brain and of its Ventricles, were full of a clear water, and its substance being too much watered was wet, and not firm." In a second case, the collection of blood was described as being under the temporal suture.

Willis' treatment of the headache (i.e., abstention from eating, rest, and evacuation of the bowels by an enema) was not particularly imaginative, the aim being that the "matter be suffered to evaporate from the membranes of the head." Sometimes he applied blisters to the back of the head. Willis apparently had little use for surgical intervention, for he stated that, in some cases, trephination had been advised, but none that he knew of were willing to submit to it. In fact, he thought that there could be "anything of certainty expected from the opening of the Skull where it pained; if an imposthum lay hid there, this had been the only way of Cure, but that would rather have caused sleepy distempers or deadly convulsions than Headache."

The concepts of headache and the principles of treatment changed little over the next few centuries. Robert Whytt (1714-1766) wrote of periodic headaches in much the same terms as the Elizabethan physicians and his best remedy ("vomits, laxatives and bitters") was about the same as that advocated by the earlier physicians. It is of interest that in all violent headaches, the primary treatment was bleeding in one form or another.

Various causes of headache were suggested. Wepfer attributed the headache to the stasis of blood in dilated vessels. Later, Fothergill described "sick headaches" but did not suggest their pathogenesis. In a lengthy analysis of the factors producing headache, Tissot in 1788 concluded that migraine was the result of disturbances of the gastrointestinal tract producing cerebral vasomotor upsets. In his first textbook of neurology written in 1842, Romberg discussed "neuralgie cerebralis or hemicrania (la migrene)" as a miserable headache coming on with or without warning by pain on one side of the head, usually the left, gradually increasing in intensity and aggravated by light, noise, or activity. The eye on the involved side watered and the hair on that side was sensitive. Scotomata and tinnitus developed as the headache reached its acme. When the patient became nauseated and vomited, the pain usually abated and the patient slept. Romberg pointed out that there was a familial incidence.

The treatment, however, was little different from that of the 16th century— rest in a darkened room, drinking tepid tea to induce vomiting, and a mild clyster at the end of the attack to open the bowels. If the patient was dyspeptic, mineral water was prescribed; if anemic, arsenic in the form of Fowler's solution was usually given.

In 1860, DuBois-Reymond suggested that the headaches were the result of vasomotor neurosis irritating the sympathetic nerves and causing constriction of the blood vessels. At about the same time, Liveing likened a migrainous attack to an epileptic seizure. At the end of the 19th century, Gowers discussed the subject in his textbook. He recognized the hereditary disposition and that certain conditions such as trauma and infection of the nervous system might initiate the disorder. Gowers gave a detailed account of the symptomatology— the neurological disturbances, sensory concomitants, motor and speech alterations, mental confusion, varied head pains with the accompanying nausea and vomiting, as well as the associated manifestations or equivalents. Gowers attempted to explain the mechanisms involved in the production of the headache, which he attributed to toxic and metabolic states. Although he advised mainly symptomatic remedies, the general discussion has a modern approach.

Complicated Migraine

It was recognized early that headache might be associated with other disturbances, which were referred to as "complicated migraine" or "migraine accompagnée or associé." These various states might accompany or be quite independent of the headache. Such so-called migraine equivalents might take the form of scintillating scotomata, auras, recurrent vertigo, visceral or abdominal disorders, and mental disturbances such as agnosias, mood changes, transient mania, and amnesic episodes. Occasionally, the migraine equivalent might be a paralytic episode involving the extraocular or limb musculature. Probably the most common and best known were the scotomata, which had been described in colorful terms throughout the ages from the time of the Roman writers.

Ophthalmoplegic Migraine

In 1883, Feré described a rare familial migraine which is accompanied by a paralysis of one or more ocular muscles. The palsy lasts for some time after the headache, only gradually clearing.

Hemiplegic Migraine

It was noted early that headache might be associated with motor disturbances such as transitory weakness of an extremity of one side of the body or of an eye muscle or muscles. Although the weakness usually cleared, the paresis was not always benign. Oppenheim described a woman who suffered migraine with a visual or dysphasic aura and who four months postpartum had a migrainous attack with dysphasia, which developed into a right hemiplegia and progressed to coma. At postmortem examination, the left middle cerebral artery had a recent extensive thrombosis. Liveing described hemiplegic migraine and noted its familial occurrence; Charcot also reported a familial case.

As physicians became aware of the vascular factors in many migraines, an attempt was made to classify them on an anatomical basis. The headaches associated with visual disturbances were attributed to posterior cerebral artery alterations, hemiplegic manifestations to middle cerebral artery spasms, and generalized "sick headaches" to more diffuse vascular changes. Even basilar vessels were thought to produce a specific cephalalgia. In his discussion of borderline epilepsy, Gowers cites the case of an 18-year-old girl who suffered a right-sided migraine. After 10 years of such episodes, she had an attack in which it seemed that a black curtain dropped and she saw stars—"brilliant with thousands of golden points." The girl became dizzy and her arms, legs, and jaw experienced dysesthesias for 10 minutes, whereupon she lost consciousness. When she recovered after 15 minutes, she suffered a severe occipital headache that lasted two hours. Bickerstaff and Adams suggested that such attacks represented a basilar artery migraine.

Migraine Variants

It is not surprising that a common complaint such as headache should have aberrant manifestations. Although such well-defined headaches were probably known throughout the ages, the most typical, often called "facial migraine," appears to have been first described in recent literature by Mollendorf in 1867. This severe headache occurring in middle-aged men is an agonizing, unilateral facial pain beginning in the cheek and spreading to the adjacent head and neck. It is characterized by flushing of the face and injection of the ipsilateral conjunctiva. As the pain becomes worse, thin mucus runs from the nostril. The discomfort reaches an acme in a half hour or so, lasts for several hours, and is usually accompanied by nausea and vomiting. In 1883, Eulenburg gave an excellent clinical description of what he called "hemicrania angioparalytica sine neuroparalytica." Subsequent writers have given various names—ciliary neuralgia, periodic migrainous neuralgia, erythromelalgia of the head, histamine cephalalgia, greater superficial petrosal neuralgia, and Horton's headache; however, the descriptive term "cluster headache" is commonly used. Because small injections of histamine precipitated the headache and desensitization relieved the discomfort, the state has been assumed to be a hypersensitivity disorder; however, the etiological factor is not yet established.

In 1890, Hutchinson described a syndrome of a swollen, tender temporal artery associated with fever and localized headache. Forty years later, Horton emphasized the fact that the condition may involve other vessels (such as the retinal arteries) and cause blindness. The affliction occurred in older people and was characterized by fever, anorexia, malaise, and weight loss. The temporal artery was swollen, tender, and often nonpulsatile. If the ophthalmic artery were involved, blindness might result. The pathological changes, usually confined to one side but occasionally involving the cerebral vessels, consisted of endarteritis with giant cells.

Many factors have been suggested to account for specific types of headache. At one time or another, all of the following have been held responsible for headache: psychiatric causes, muscle tension, coughing, exercise, sexual intercourse, head traumas, dental disturbances, barometric changes, cervical spine abnormalities, and temporomandibular arthritis, as well as various metabolic factors. A common factor has not been found to cause all cephalalgias.

An understanding of the basic causes and treatment of migraine was not forthcoming until the studies of Graham and Wolff showed that the pathogenesis was complicated but related to the excessive pulsations of the cerebral vessels, which could be minimized by ergotamine tartate.

Epilepsy

The episodic disturbances of unawareness, at times amounting to unconsciousness and often associated with convulsive movements, were recognized as epileptic attacks in the 17th and 18th centuries; persons subject to such episodes were often confined to mental hospitals. If the manifestations were a generalized seizure, the person was labeled an epileptic; if the disturbance was of a psychic nature, the subject was considered to be a lunatic and confined to the madhouse. It was the unruly epileptics that led to the use of the first effective drug for the treatment of seizures. In the latter half of the 19th century, many medications (e.g., sodium nitrite, borax, belladonna, digitalis, arsenic, zinc, picrotoxin, antipyrine, and various nerve tonics) had been prescribed for seizures with little success. The only effective medication—bromide of potassium—was introduced by Sir Charles Locock in 1857. He had noted that epileptic patients given the drug for various other disorders had a marked decrease in their attacks. In spite of side effects (e.g., skin rash, drowsiness, and sluggish behavior), the drug was the sole effective agent for the treatment of epilepsy for more than a half century.

It is said that Locock had prescribed bromide of potassium for epilepsy occurring in women during menstrual periods based upon the report of a German who became impotent when taking excessive bromides; Locock thought that the drug would only be of value in cases of menstrual seizures. Another version of the original use of the drug stated that unruly epileptic patients were not only quieted by the drug but that their seizures were alleviated.

At the beginning of the 19th century, the convulsing epileptic was considered to be suffering from a predisposing factor related to heredity or to have one or more of some 28 exciting causes ranging from joy or terror to, more commonly, an organic brain lesion disclosed by postmortem examination. The pathological anatomy usually found in the brains of these patients was assumed to be responsible for the epileptic state, although van Sweeten stressed that the cerebral abnormalities might be only a secondary factor or unrelated to the seizures.

From early times, the impairment of cerebral circulation has been considered a factor in the production of a seizure. Cooper in 1836 produced convulsions in rabbits by temporary cerebral anemia. At about the same time, Marshall Hall was inducing neurological paroxysms by modifying the blood supply to the brain. He considered an induced laryngismus to cause venous congestion. Noting the facial pallor which, at times, preceded a convulsion, Brown-Séquard concluded that a generalized cerebral vasoconstriction was responsible for the convulsions. John Hughlings Jackson (Fig. 7-2) admitted that "contraction of the blood vessels in epilepsy was the established theory of the day." Based upon the premise that the attacks were initiated by cerebral vasoconstriction, to dilate the cerebral ventricles, Alexander in 1899 carried out a cervical sympathectomy. Horsley, however, denied a vascular etiology; he considered the attacks to be related to a general excitation of the nervous system.

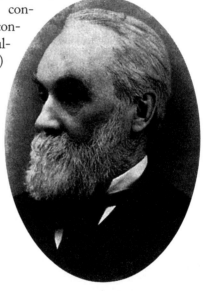

Based upon the assumption that the seizures were caused by a gross disturbance of the brain, surgeons sought means of repairing a defect or eliminating a responsible lesion. In the 19th century, operating upon the brain carried significant risk from both the procedure itself and from complications,

Fig. 7-2. John Hughlings Jackson (1835-1911). (From The Founders of Neurology, 2nd ed. Haymaker W, Schiller F, editors. Springfield, Ill: Charles C Thomas, 1970, p 457)

especially infection. Although the introduction of anesthesia and aseptic techniques had lowered the operative mortality to 7% in the best hospitals in the 1890s, the outlook was poor for the person having any but the simplest brain operation.

To relieve seizures, a number of surgeons devised ingenious accoutrements

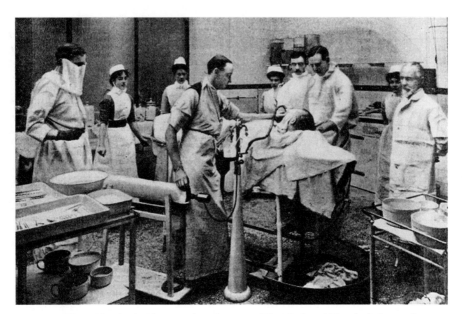

Fig. 7-3. Victor Horsley in his operating theatre at The National Hospital, Queen Square. (From A History of Neurosurgery. *Greenblatt SH, Dagi TF, Epstein M, editors. Park Ridge, Ill: American Association of Neurological Surgeons, 1997, p 377)*

based upon the presumed causative factor. Kocher, noting the increased fluid in the subarachnoid space of epileptic brains, concluded that sudden changes in pressure caused a convulsion. To prevent such rapid fluctuations in pressure, he devised a "moveable valve"—essentially a decompressive mechanism made by removing a large piece of calvarium, incising the underlying dura mater, and suturing the three adjoining scalp flaps, thus providing a means of compensating for a sudden increase in intracranial pressure which was thought to initiate a seizure. Although this device was used by several European surgeons, it was abandoned within a few years.

Cortical resection for the relief of epilepsy was initiated shortly after Fritsch and Hitzig demonstrated the electrical excitability of the cerebral cortex of animals. Victor Horsley, who had stimulated the cortex of apes and induced generalized seizures by the injection of absinthe, was appointed surgeon to The National Hospital for the Paralysed and Epileptics in 1881 (Fig. 7-3). His first operation was a surgical exploration for the firing focus of a young man suffering intractable seizures. Horsley recounted his exploration for the excitable focus at the margin of the scar and his resection of the cortical focus with relief of seizures. His second case required electrical stimulation to locate the thumb area of the cerebral cortex. As the patient's spontaneous attacks began with twitching of the thumb, Horsley excised that zone by a subpial resection. He considered that point in the cerebral cortex as the "primary spasmic center." Although Horsley's success stimulated European surgeons to operate for the relief of epilepsy, their results after a time were less encouraging, so that at the end of the 19th century, surgery for epilepsy fell off until new diagnostic methods (electroencephalography) and improved surgical techniques were introduced in the next century.

A number of other surgical procedures to relieve seizures were attempted. Unverricht in 1883 sectioned the corpus callosum to prevent a focal seizure from becoming generalized. For the relief of posttraumatic seizures, a transventricular choroid plexectomy was carried out, but without success. Based upon Hall's theory of reflex epilepsy, a number of peripheral nerve procedures were propounded. Romberg suggested tying strings about the arm of a patient whose fits began in the hand. Lente removed cutaneous scars from which attacks seem to be generated; Hammond (Fig. 7-4) excised scars in which a peripheral nerve seemed to be entangled and initiated an aura. Krause even excised the gasserian ganglion to denervate a trigger zone in a facial scar.

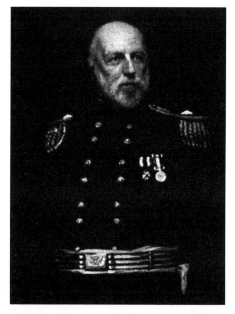

Based upon the Hippocratic comment that excessive venery caused convulsions, a number of operations upon the genitalia were performed. Masturbation, often noted in the mentally retarded, was considered by Tissot and Romberg as a significant etiological agent. Consequently, castration, clitoridectomy, and ovariectomy were frequently performed, although some neurologists such as Gowers deprecated such procedures.

Fig. 7-4. William Alexander Hammond (1828-1900). (From The Founders of Neurology, *2nd ed. Haymaker W, Schiller F, editors. Springfield, Ill: Charles C Thomas, 1970, p 445)*

Based upon the observation that epileptic patients were frequently constipated, Axtell in 1910 repaired colonic angulations which he assumed were causing autointoxications. Although Reed later reported on a series of bowel resections, the procedure did not gain general acceptance when cerebral resections were being perfected.

Disorders of Sleep

From the beginning of time, both sensory and motor activities have disturbed the rest of mankind. Such parasomniac activity occurs more frequently in young children and adolescents than in adults. Sleep disorders were often considered as psychotic abnormalities rather than neurological afflictions. Dreams (often vivid and colorful), sleep walking, sleep talking, nightmares, and head-banging have all been attributed to psychotic aberrations. Some nocturnal disturbances, such as enuresis, snoring, sleep apnea, and insomnia, have been shown to have a neurological basis. In the 19th century, however, few sleep disturbances were defined. The most prominent was narcolepsy, a state with many ramifications.

In his discussion of "continued sleepiness" published in 1685, Thomas Willis wrote "many authors call this not a disease, but a drowsy disposition; for the affected as to other things are well enough, they eat and drink well, they walk abroad, they take care indifferently of their household affairs, but in speaking, or walking, or eating, nay their mouths being full of meat, they now and then nod, and unless they are stirred by others, they are presently overwhelmed with sleep." Later medical writers in the 19th century called this condition by various names—Caffe makes reference to "sleeping sickness," Fischer to "epileptic sleep," and Westphal to "episodic sleep." However, it was Gélineau's designation of that sudden, short lasting, and overwhelming desire to sleep as "narcolepsy" which gained general acceptance. In 1926, Adie gave a detailed description of the varied manifestations of the disorder and declared it to be a disease "sui generis." Somewhat akin to narcolepsy is sleep paralysis, a state of inertness, usually on awakening or falling asleep, lasting a few minutes, and clearing immediately when the subject is stimulated.

In 1902, Lowenfeldt called attention to the frequent association of episodic somnolence and transient attacks of powerlessness or ataxia of the limbs, which he noted to be frequently induced by emotional outbursts. This state, which Henneburg in 1916 termed "catalepsy," consisted of a sudden loss of muscular tone and strength brought on by such intense emotions as laughter, anger, and joy, caused a person to fall or the head to nod usually without losing consciousness.

A trance is a sleep-like state that has been recognized for ages; in ancient times, a trance was probably assumed to be due to the soul temporarily leaving the body. As the concepts of the soul changed, however, the term was applied to a variety of sleep-like states not implicating such a metaphysical structure. Thus, a trance is considered referred to sleep-walking, lethargy, and hypnotic states, all having the common condition of unawareness of the normal milieu of the individual or of the unconscious state associated with anesthetic drugs, cerebral ischemia, or traumatic impairment of the brain. The term may be more specifically applied to ecstatic or hypnotic trance.

These states have been described in the 19th-century literature in different ways. Gowers, under the heading of induced hypnotism, following Charcot, lists three conditions—catalepsy, lethargy, and somnambulism. Catalepsy, a rare occurrence, may present in persons of either sex, although it most frequently occurs in young women. It is characterized by a sudden loss of consciousness or contact with the environment associated with a peculiar rigidity of the limbs such that the stiff member may be moved, as if made of softened wax, into any position which can be maintained indefinitely. The state may last from a few minutes to hours, passing off without residua. Lethargy, or trance, is a sleep state which may occur quickly or gradually and last from hours to days. It is associated with no neurological abnormalities except the unresponsive state, which in extreme cases has been called the "death trance." The termination is usually gradual and may be associated with nervous manifestations such as anxiety, sweating, and sluggish mentation. Somnambulism, or walking in one's sleep, is more common in children but more complex in adults who often perform complicated acts such as dressing or walking about a room without bumping into objects. Upon awakening, the subject has no recollection of the activities.

Most 19th-century writers classified these activities as hysterical manifestations. Gowers included narcolepsy in this category, although he distinguished it from trance by its brevity, its recurrence, and the ability to arouse the subject. However, considering the various manifestations of narcolepsy—sleep episodes, cataplexy, sleep paralysis, and hallucinatory phenomena—it may not be a pure disorder. Certainly, a number of conditions, such as tumors of the third ventricle, head injuries, and various afflictions of the diencephalon, are known to have narcoleptic manifestations. The sudden, intense desire to sleep, the dozing off, and awakening refreshed, even when the lapse was accompanied by a vivid dream, the content of which cannot be remembered, are difficult to distinguish from normal sleep. Associated with narcolepsy may be attacks of cataplexy, sleep paralysis, hallucinations, or somnambulism.

The Kleine-Levin syndrome is characterized by recurrent periods of prolonged sleep (up to 18 hours) and hyperphagia, with normal interludes but in which episodic sexual exhibitionism, delusions, hallucinations, amnesias, and other mental disturbances may occur. It is likely to develop in young girls at the beginning of the menses and to be associated with bizarre behavior.

Although from the beginning of time, trances, sleep walking, and nightmares have disturbed the sleep of the weary, relatively little of its neural control was understood at the end of the 19th century.

Cerebrovascular Disease (Apoplexy)

Although both Galen (129-210 AD) and Vesalius (1514-1564) believed that the brain received "a substantial portion of the vital spirits" from both the carotid and vertebral arteries so that "it is not surprising that the brain performs its functions . . . for a long time"; after all, vessels to it are cut off except those passing through the transverse processes of the vertebrae. That the anastomoses between arteries at the base of the brain provided a channel for irrigating it if a feeding vessel were obstructed, however, was affirmed by Willis, who commented that a patient with the lumen of the right carotid artery almost occluded by plaque "had not died of apoplexy." At that time, the term "apoplexy" was used to describe any sudden loss of consciousness and motion, except respiration. It included a number of bodily disorders as well as neurological infirmities which caused "a breach of the unity within the brain." The disclosure of the nature of this disturbance is generally credited to Wepfer, who reported in 1658 a patient who died of apoplexy within two hours. A postmortem examination disclosed an intracerebral hemorrhage which had ruptured through the floor of the lateral ventricle into the subarachnoid space. Based upon this observation, Wepfer concluded that rupture of a diseased cerebral artery might be the cause of apoplexy. It was another 35 years before Morgagni suggested that such hemorrhages were due to a ruptured cerebral aneurysm. He wrote:

> . . . nothing is more natural, when we see these caverns in the brain, and blood semiconcreted therein, or effus'd in great quantity into the neighboring parts, than to call to mind the rupture of aneurisms in the belly or thorax, and even to imagine, that something similar to this might sometimes happen within the cavity of the cranium.

Morgagni recognized two types of apoplexy: sanguinous (cerebral hemorrhage) and serous (infarction). Of the latter, he gave several examples. In the brain of a palsied man "the corpus striatum was entirely separated from the remainder of the cerebrum by reason of an erosion." He noted in a senile patient "multiple softenings looking like three little caverns covered by a scar with yellowish discoloration of the adjacent hemisphere."

Later, Abercrombie on the basis of clinicopathological studies pointed out that local disease might obliterate the lumen of the vessel or breaches in the vessel wall might allow an extravasation of blood. These occlusive changes, later termed "arteriosclerosis," were considered precursors of outpouchings of the vessel wall and the basis of spurious aneurysms. Some apoplexies were found to be the result of yellow softening caused by a thrombus obstructing a feeding artery; occasionally, the lesion was not associated with an occluded vessel and so the concept of cerebral arterial spasm or obliterative vascular disease without thrombosis was introduced. In 1914, Hunt suggested that narrowing or occlusion of the carotid arteries in the neck might cause a cerebral infarction.

The multiple periarterial bloody discharges often found in the brain of persons suffering cerebral hemorrhages led Charcot and Bouchard to reject an arteriosclerotic etiology and to suggest that rupture of periarterial miliary aneurysms was responsible for the extravasation of blood. In the early 20th century, Pick showed that the miliary lesions were not aneurysms but mural hematomas; several perivascular alterations (i.e., softening, disintegration, and vasospasm) were postulated as factors weakening the vessel wall and leaving it vulnerable to intravascular pressure changes.

Although Hasse had suggested as early as 1866 that increased "tension of the blood column" and Kirkes in 1855 that chronic renal disease were both associated with apoplexy, another quarter-century elapsed before Westphal demonstrated that elevated arterial tension was a decisive factor in cerebral hemorrhage. This denouement clarified the roles of systemic arterial disease and cerebrovascular disorders in the pathogenesis of the apoplexies. Thus, strokes were thought to be either the result of vascular occlusion or vessel disruption with resultant hemorrhage. Shortly, however, other factors were recognized as responsible for some forms of apoplexy (e.g., cardiac disorders and systemic disturbances) so that the term in the classical sense was discarded.

Cerebrovascular Anomalies

Although it is suggested that the demise of some ancient Greeks and Romans was the result of the rupture of an intracranial vessel, the first verified vascular anomalies were found by pathologists at postmortem examinations. Morgagni noted dilatation of the vertebral vessels. Biumi of Milan in 1765 described the clinical features and postmortem appearance of a ruptured aneurysm. Early in the 19th century, Blackall related the clinical history of a 20-year-old woman who died of a ruptured aneurysm at the bifurcation of the basilar artery. By the middle of the 19th century, reports of intracranial aneurysms were common. Gull in 1859 reviewed 62 cases of aneurysm of the cerebral vessels and concluded that, although one might suspect the presence of an aneurysm in young persons dying of apoplexy, there were no symptoms or signs upon which a certain diagnosis could be based. Ten years later, Adams pointed out the combination of paralysis of the third, fourth, fifth, and sixth cranial nerves as the result of a cavernous sinus aneurysm of the internal carotid artery. At that time such aneurysms were considered to be syphilitic in origin. Not until Fernsides in 1916 reviewed the clinical and pathological findings in 44 cases, none of which had evidence of syphilis, was congenital weakness of the arterial wall at a junctional point considered to be a causative factor.

Based upon the clinical history and findings, a nontraumatic saccular aneurysm was diagnosed by Hutchinson, who advised a carotid ligation, which the patient refused; 11 years later, at autopsy, a solid aneurysm the size of a bantam's egg was found in the middle fossa. In 1872, Bartholow of Cincinnati wrote a paper on the symptomatology, diagnosis, and treatment of aneurysms at the base of the brain. He suggested that the earlier writers of the 19th century had probably classified such lesions as apoplexy.

Gowers calculated the frequency of the occurrence of aneurysms on the cere-

TABLE 1

INCIDENCE OF CEREBRAL ANEURYSMS REPORTED BEFORE 1872*

Artery	No. of Cases
Middle cerebral	44
Basilar	41
Internal carotid	23
Anterior cerebral	14
Posterior communicating	8
Anterior communicating	8
Vertebral	7
Posterior cerebral	6
Inferior cerebellar	3
Total	154

*Modified from Gowers (1881).

bral vessels in 154 cases taken from the literature prior to 1872 (Table 1).

Although the clinical manifestations of subarachnoid hemorrhage—sudden, throbbing headache often referred to the eye or side of the head and associated with ocular paresis—suggested the diagnosis, the introduction of lumbar puncture by Heinrich Quincke in 1891 made its verification relatively simple. In his textbook published in 1888, Gowers discussed the diagnosis of aneurysms of the different intracranial arteries, concluding that an aneurysm of each cerebral artery produced a distinct set of symptoms. He noted, however, that some aneurysms did not rupture, and that a few healed spontaneously after rupture. Gowers referred to one internal carotid aneurysm for which the common carotid artery was ligated successfully, and thought that if a basilar aneurysm was suspected, the vertebral arteries could be tied! Other physicians were aware of the entity, for Steinheil in 1895 had diagnosed a bleeding aneurysm on clinical grounds.

The early aneurysms were operated upon as mistaken brain tumors; Beadles referred to an aneurysm arising from the right internal carotid artery that Horsley in 1902 unexpectedly found and treated by ligating the common carotid artery in the neck. The patient was well five years later. Probably the first elective cerebrovascular surgical procedure (carotid ligation for a traumatic internal carotid aneurysm (carotid cavernous fistula)) was carried out in October 1924 by Trotter and successfully relieved the bruit. Dandy ligated the internal carotid artery for a saccular intracranial aneurysm, but had to untie the ligature as the patient became hemiplegic. In 1933, Dott treated two cases of saccular aneurysm by ligation of the carotid artery in the neck (Fig. 7-5). The previous year he had wrapped a saccular aneurysm. Following these initial reports, neurosurgeons carried out many more such procedures.

As the diagnosis at that time was based upon the clinical findings, only those aneurysms at the base of the brain producing cranial nerve pareses were amenable to surgery. Thus, Dandy's first successfully treated case was a posterior cerebral artery aneurysm producing periorbital pain and a third nerve palsy. On the basis of these findings, Dandy exposed the lesion subtemporally and successfully placed a clip upon its neck. The subsequent development of cerebral aneurysm surgery was aided by the introduction of angiography, of arterial clips appropriate for any vessel at any angle, of anesthesia which did not increase the intracranial pressure, of techniques for shrinking the brain, and specialized postoperative care to prevent or relieve spasm of the parent vessel.

Arteriovenous Aneurysms of the Cavernous Sinus

The pulsating exophthalmos produced by an arteriovenous aneurysm of the cavernous sinus and the bruit audible to the patient early attracted the attention of physicians and surgeons. In 1809, Travers, in such a case, noted that compression of the carotid artery stopped the bruit; accordingly, he ligated the artery with eventual relief of the complaints

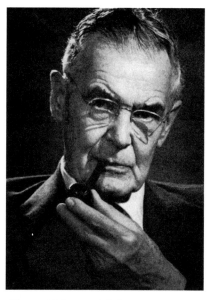

Fig. 7-5. Norman M. Dott successfully treated intracranial aneurysms prior to the development of angiography. (from Clinical Neurosurgery, *vol. 16, 1969)*

(Fig. 7-6). Subsequently, many cases were so treated but with a mortality of 4% to 50% and a morbidity consisting mainly of hemiplegia and recurrence. To avoid these sequelae, various occlusive procedures on the common, internal, and external carotid arteries were tried. Embolization by a muscle fragment to block the fistula was described by Brooks in 1930, and subsequently used with variations. Trapping of the fistulous vessel was first performed in 1931 by Hamby and Gardner after an unsuccessful attempt at embolization. Four years later, Dandy trapped the fistula by clipping the internal carotid artery intracranially and ligating the carotid vessels in the neck.

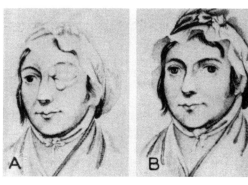

Fig. 7-6. Travers' case of carotid ligation for exophthalmos. (From the collection of A. Earl Walker)

8

Congenital Anomalies
of the Nervous System

Congenital deformities are classified as monstrosities or anomalies depending upon the degree of the abnormality. In the nervous system, monstrous defects such as anencephaly are usually incompatible with life, so that most fetuses with severe maldevelopments are stillborn. Neural anomalies are usually the result of early or delayed fusion in the development of midline structures, resulting in such anomalies as encephaloceles, myeloceles, or hydrocephalus. Many aberrations are presumably a coincidence of hereditary and environmental factors occurring at a time when the antecedents of the brain or spinal cord are developing. Thus, oxycephaly, cyclopia, and other such defects may be produced in susceptible experimental animals; in man, they are caused by agents affecting the spinal or cephalic segments between the 15th and 25th week of development.

"Double monsters," although rare, probably result from the premature splitting of a single fertilized ovum producing two bodies with parts still in continuity, so that various combinations of cephalic or spinal elements of twins may develop. Occasionally, one of the rudimentary twins is so retarded in its development that it becomes a parasite of the other, viable fetus. Paré described and illustrated several such twins with spinal and cranial fusions.

Anencephalic Monsters

Fetuses born with only a membrane over the cranial cavity are usually stillborn, although a few have sufficient brainstem to respire for a few hours. Geoffroy Saint-Hilaire, the founder of modern embryology, has reported such monsters in varying degrees of encephalic aplasia. Such deformed fetuses have been mentioned in Hippocratic and later Roman works. After printing was introduced, anencephalic monsters were described and illustrated, at times rather fancifully. In Paré's book on *Des monstres et prodiges*, first published in 1573, a number of sketches depict the various maldevelopments of the body including several of the head, brain, and spinal cord. One of the illustrations, said to be of an anencephalic, depicts a decapitated child that a reviewer comments "was more of a tribute to the imagination than to the power of observation." Paré attributed such monsters to 13 bizarre causes ranging from the glory of God or devils to the imagination.

In a more serious study, William Harvey in 1651 examined such deformities and concluded that they represented aberrations of normal development. After that time, reports of cephalic deformities were relatively common. Morgagni described two fetuses with no trace of cerebrum, cerebellum, or brainstem; Fontanus reported a similar case in which the cerebrospinal axis contained only limpid water. Geoffroy Saint-Hilaire, in a three-volume classic published in 1832, illustrated and classified cephalic anomalies as anencephalus and pseudoencephalus according to whether there was complete absence or preservation of some rudimentary elements of the brain. Another 50 years passed before the minor congenital defects of the brain received attention. Kundrat in Austria and Cleland in England in the early 1880s described the anomalous development of the brain resulting in anencephaly and lesser defects of the cerebrum. A few years later, Taruffi in a book on teratology introduced the term "holoacrania" to denote the total absence of the brain and "meracrania" to indicate partial developmental defects of the brain.

Developmental Defects of the
Brain and Its Coverings

Abnormalities of the cephalic nervous system may involve any tissue of the head. Congenital foldings of the scalp producing anterior-to-posterior furrows have been known as the washboard scalp. It is not usually associated with intracranial abnormalities. Although defective closure of the skull is a less frequent occurrence than that of the lower spine, it obviously is a defect as the maldevelopment of the frontal and ethmoid bones produces a grotesque countenance. The cranial developmental abnormalities may be divided into those of the cranial vault and those of the base. Anomalies of the vault are much less common, less numerous, and less disfiguring than those of the base.

Anomalies of the Cranial Vault

Vertex skull anomalies are usually related to the premature closure of the cranial sutures causing various distortions of the head. Depending upon the suture involved in early closure, the cranial and facial appearance varies.

Craniosynostosis

Interest in the contour of the head has been evident from the earliest times, when artificial cranial deformation was common. Disfiguration caused by premature molding of the skull was known to many peoples of the world, including the Greeks. Aristophanes referred to oxycephaly, although just what was meant is uncertain. The first systematic study of the relationship of premature sutural closure to cranial deformity was made by von Soemmerring in 1800. Half a century later, Virchow advanced the theory that the deformations were due to fetal meningitis causing edema and fusion of the sutures. The situation regarding synostosis was confused by the primary and secondary sutural closures—the primary craniosynostosis being premature closure and the secondary being normal closure in cases of microcephalus.

The common primary premature closure takes place in the sagittal suture, producing a long narrow head. An early closure of the coronal suture produces an oxycephalic skull. Closure of the metopic suture at an early stage leads to a midline ridge. These cranial anomalies are often associated with other delayed or absent bony developments such as a cleft palate.

Late Sutural Closure

Delayed cranial osteogenesis or sutural fusion may be of any degree. Cranium bifida and cranium bifida occultum are of no clinical significance unless associated with an underlying defect of dura mater or encephalon causing a cranial meningocele or encephalocele, a condition much more common in certain European and Asiatic countries than in the Americas.

The failure of fusion of the occipital squamous centers is the most common type of late sutural closure and may be associated with a meningocele or encephalocele. The defect is frequently complicated by hydrocephalus due to aqueductal stenosis or posterior fossa anomalies such as the Arnold-Chiari malformation or Klippel-Feil deformity. Parietal encephaloceles, less common than the occipital defects, are the result of a midline osseous defect. These malformations usually contain neural tissue as well as meninges. As a rule, frontal encephaloceles, frequent in Southeast Asia, contain neural tissue. The herniation may be into the nasofrontal, ethmoidal, or orbital regions. Basal encephalomeningoceles may present in the inner canthus of the eye or the nasopharyngeal, or oropharyngeal regions.

Craniolacunia

Symmetrical or asymmetrical cranial defects have been recognized for many years. Such craniolacunia, consisting of round depressed areas of the inner table of the skull bordered by denser bone, often disappear in the first year of life but may be associated with severe neurological defects. In 1874, J. Hoffmann described the condition which may have been recognized the following year by West. It has been called "lacunar skull," "Lückenschädel," or "craniolacunia." The term, however, is applied to a number of states characterized by radiologically demonstrable cranial defects, often associated with encephaloceles or meningomyeloceles.

Bilateral oval perforations in the parasagittal regions of the parietal bones through which emissary veins may pass have been termed "foramina parietalis permagna." They may be 1 to 2 cm in diameter and occasionally present only on one side, such as in the cases described by Lancisi and Morgagni in 1701. This defect tends to occur in families—in 16 of 56 members of five generations of the Catlin family—and accordingly has been called "the Catlin mark." Often the defect is associated with other skull abnormalities or disorders of the nervous system.

Anomalies of the Base of the Skull

The developmental defects of the basal structures of the cranium are much more numerous and more complicated than those of the vault. They may involve the bones of the base, symmetrically or asymmetrically. As a result, grotesque distortions of the face and head often occur. The earliest cases recorded were the cyclopian races of mythology. Although Ulysses is said to have fought the one-eyed Polyphemus, medical history records no such monsters surviving infancy (Adelmann).

These anomalies, now termed "holoprosencephaly" or "arrhinencephaly," may have a varied facial dysplasia ranging from a cyclopia to median cleft lip and be associated with various brain malformations. The latter vary from severe holoprosencephaly with failure to cleave into cerebral hemispheres to mild midline dysplasias of the interhemispheric fissure, cingulate gyrus, or corpus callosum. The olfactory system may share in the maldevelopment.

Iniencephaly

Iniencephaly is a rare malformation noted by Geoffroy Saint-Hilaire and described in detail by Ballantyne. It is a deformation of the basal skull at the foramen magnum with some degree of rachischisis and retroflexion of the cervical spine, so that the fetus's face is turned upward with the back of the head adjoining the lower back. The anomaly, which may be associated with an encephalocele protruding from a dilated foramen magnum, is usually incompatible with life. The Klippel-Feil deformity has been considered a mild form of this malformation. A number of other anomalies are often present in the craniospinal axis as well as in other organs.

Hypertelorism

Although the wide spacing of the eyes has been noted by artists as a look of innocence or guilt (demonic) and closely set eyes as an indication of a miserly personality, the association of excessive interocular and cerebral anomalies has only recently been recognized. A sketch by della Porta did depict a face with widely set eyes. The reverse, narrow-set eyes, may be associated with holoprosencephaly and arrhinencephaly as described by Geoffroy Saint-Hilaire and later Kundrat. In 1924, Greig named the condition of widely spaced eyes "hypertelorism." Later, the reverse condition, "hypotelorism," was described.

In rare instances, the sphenoid bone on one side is aplastic; however, more frequently, an aplastic condition of the greater and lesser wings of the sphenoid is associated with a deficiency of the orbital plate of the frontal bone. As a result, the exophthalmic globe pulsates and orbital contents are displaced downward. Dandy in 1929 described this condition and proposed an operation to repair the orbital defect. This anomaly may be associated with von Recklinghausen's neurofibromatosis.

Encephalic Anomalies

In addition to the gross cranial abnormalities accompanying primordial defects of the neural tube, many less severe developmental disturbances affect the neural structures, often without other systemic defects. These anomalies may involve almost any part of the brain, symmetrically or asymmetrically.

Aplasia of the Cranial Nerves

The lack of development of the cranial nerves is more often incomplete than absolute, although clinically the condition is referred to as agenesis or dysgenesis of the nerve. The congenital defects of the cranial nerves are generally symmetrical, but in the case of the eye muscles, the lesion may be predominantly unilateral.

The Olfactory Nerve. Developmental defects of the olfactory nerve are usually associated with more severe abnormalities of the frontal lobes or corpus callosum.

The Optic Nerve. Abnormalities of the optic nerve frequently accompany other developmental defects such as anencephaly or hydrocephalus. True aplasia of the optic nerve is a great rarity. In most reported cases, some elements of the nerve—a hypoplastic optic nerve—have been preserved, thus saving some vision and the central retinal vessels. Seiler, according to Rosenbaum, reported that an eye from a person with congenital hydrocephalus had neither ganglion cells nor optic nerve. Such a person has a true aplasia of the optic nerve. In 1923, Cords reviewed the earlier reports and noted that in many cases the anomaly was bilateral and present in more than one member of a family. The optic foramen on the involved side was small.

Third, Fourth, and Sixth Cranial Nerves. On clinical examination, paresis of one or more of the third, fourth, and sixth nerves is difficult to determine in an infant. An aplasia may be at any point along the nerve or in its supranuclear course. Usually, more than one nerve is involved, although occasionally an isolated nerve is paretic. The manifestation may be an impairment of upward gaze due to muscular or neural factors, at times in the frontal or temporal eye fields.

Congenital ptosis with associated abnormal eye movements was reported by Marcus Gunn in 1883. His original patient was a woman with a left congenital ptosis whose eyelid elevated involuntarily when the jaw was opened or moved to the left. Later, Sinclair identified four types of "jaw winking" depending upon the direction of ocular movement—midline and/or lateral—required to elicit the elevation of the lid. The generally accepted explanation is that in addition to receiving innervation from its usual source, the levator palpebrae muscle gets aberrant fibers from the trigeminal motor nucleus. This hypothesis is corroborated by reports of fibers regenerating after facial nerve lesions to structures not normally innervated by that nerve ("misdirected regeneration").

Duane in 1905 described ocular retraction upon attempting to adduct the eyes. This phenomenon, previously described by both Türk and Stilling, may have a number of etiologies. It occurs in some families as an irregular, dominant factor. The usual explanation is that the paretic lateral rectus muscle receives aberrant nerve supply from the oculomotor nerve; as a result, it contracts with the other oculomotor innervated muscles, causing retraction of the globe.

The Trigeminal Nerve. Congenital abnormalities of the trigeminal nerve are usually of the motor division of the nerve, rarely of the sensory branches. The aplastic trigeminal motor nucleus is commonly associated with concomitant dysplasia of other lower cranial motor nerves, especially the hypoglossal, with sparing of the ninth, 10th, and 11th cranial nerves.

The Facial Nerve. In 1880, von Graefe described congenital facial paralysis and pointed out its frequent association with abducens palsy or total ophthalmoplegia. In 1885 and 1890, Moebius published on the subject, noting that the condition was usually bilateral.

The Acoustic Nerve. Congenital absence of development of the inner ear—a rare condition—was described by Michel in 1863. Eight years later, Mondini-Alexander reported a case in which only the basal cochlea was present.

Ninth, 10th, and 11th Cranial Nerves. It is rare to have defects in the ninth, 10th, and 11th nerves without involvement of other cranial nerves. Such aplasias producing visceral dysfunction seem to be incompatible with life.

The Hypoglossal Nerve. The tongue is often afflicted along with congenital lesions of the facial nerve and other motor cranial nerves.

Anomalies of the Telencephalon

Developmental anomalies of the cerebral hemispheres usually affect symmetrical parts, although not necessarily to the same degree. Accordingly, unilateral afflictions occurring in intrauterine life are assumed to be the result of other factors.

Hydranencephaly

Hydranencephaly, the complete absence of the telencephalon, leaving a calvarium filled with ventricular fluid, was first described by Cruveilhier. He termed the condition "anencéphalie hydrocéphalique"; however, it is probable that Paré referred to the condition. It has been described using many different names.

Lissencephaly

Lissencephaly is the term applied by Owen to describe smooth, unconvoluted cerebral cortex. Earlier, Hildanus, referring to the hydrocephalic brain, noted that in some cases "the circonvolutions and turns . . . were no more seen." Other possible cases were mentioned by Morgagni. This rare developmental defect associated with mental retardation and impaired vision may cause no obvious motor disturbance during the limited life of afflicted infants. The cerebral hemispheres have smooth cortical surfaces with no evidence of lamination but numerous irregular heterotopias. The basal ganglia and thalami consist of sparse, disorganized neuronal constituents with no discernible nuclear structure. The pyramidal tracts are absent. The poorly developed cerebellum may have many heterotopias.

Status Verrucosus or Verrucose Dysplasia

The warty, nodular appearance of the cerebral cortex resembling the cerebral mantle at the fifth month of development was described by Ranke in 1905. Earlier cases, such as that of Meschede in 1864, were associated with marked mental retardation. Most infants with such brains died early, but a few have survived to adult life.

Megaloencephaly

In the early part of the 19th century, when postmortem examinations became commonplace, unusually large brains were reported; the majority were in persons of early adult life and sometimes in infancy. Such hypertrophied brains were found in individuals suffering from impaired intelligence; in some cases, this amounted to idiocy, vertigo or dizziness, disturbed coordination in the limbs, or epilepsy. An early case reported by Scoutetta was a 5½-year-old child with a head of adult size, so heavy that when attempting to run, the child would fall forward. The child died of enteritis. On examination, it was noted that the bones of the skull were much thicker than normal; also, the brain contained little fluid and was symmetrically overdeveloped above the ventricles. Bouillaud, Dance, and Schupman as well as Andral in the 1830s reported other autopsy cases with gross anatomical descriptions of the brain.

Subsequently, large brains have been referred to in such terms as cephaloma, hypertrophy of the brain, megalocephaly, and macrocephaly. Fletcher introduced the term megaloencephaly to designate a symmetrical enlargement of the entire brain. The term, however, has been applied to three different types of large brains: primary, secondary, and unilateral megaloencephaly. The primary class consists of large brains in which there is no apparent etiological factor. The secondary type is associated with some other type of disorder, usually systemic, such as metabolic or toxic. Achondroplastic dwarfs and persons suffering from neurofibromatosis or tuberous sclerosis may fall into this class. The unilateral type consists of persons with hemimegaloencephaly and either normal or asymmetrical body parts. If there is an asymmetry, the megalohemisphere is usually on the same side as the larger limbs. Such individuals are usually mentally retarded and have numerous minor neurological abnormalities. Many are subject to epileptic seizures. Their brains may be grossly normal, except for their size and cytoarchitectural abnormalities.

Microencephaly

This cranial abnormality has been noted for centuries and ascribed to various factors. Individuals with an unusually small head and brain commonly have a skull capacity less than 1350 cc and clinically are mentally retarded. Warkany reviewed the condition beginning with the 17th century.

Porencephaly

The term "porencephaly" was used by Kundrat to describe brain cavitation, usually communicating with the ventricle. The earliest cases were reported by Piorry in 1829 and Smith in 1846 and emphasized the atrophy of the pyramidal tract and the contralateral cerebellar hemisphere in addition to the ventricular enlargement. Somewhat later, Gotard noted the thickening of the skull over the atrophic hemisphere, a finding which was confirmed roentgenographically by Dyke et al.

Schizoencephaly

The term "schizoencephaly" was introduced to describe symmetrical defects in the wall of the cerebral mantle. The earliest report was that of Kundrat in 1882 who considered all such porencephalies to be due to softenings as the result of circulatory disturbances. Schattenberg in 1889 was the first to suggest that symmetrical deformities might be the result of developmental arrest, a conclusion with which Freud agreed. The genesis of the condition, however, was clarified by Yakovlev and Wadsworth in 1946.

Primary Cerebral Hemiatrophy

This term refers to a marked hypoplasia and paucity of cortical neurons without glial scarring of one cerebral hemisphere, presumably a congenital defect. Spielmayer is said to have described the primary type in 1906. It has been confused with the secondary atrophy caused by softening; Jacoby clarified the distinction between the two types. Although it has been said that the primary and secondary forms may be distinguished on the basis of the time the clinical signs become apparent, this criterion does not always hold.

Temporal Agenesis

In the earlier surgical literature, temporal agenesis was described as an arachnoidal cyst or chronic subdural hematoma. Robinson has shown that it is a developmental anomaly of the temporal region occurring about the sixth month of fetal life.

Agenesis of the Corpus Callosum

The failure of the corpus callosum to develop normally was recognized only after postmortem examination of the brain became common. Bianchi in 1748 appears to have been the first to describe this anomaly; 64 years passed before another case was reported by Reil. In 1922, Mingazzini noted that occasional cases had been published in the previous century. But it was not until special radiological examinations were available that the diagnosis could be established during life. With the aid of pneumoencephalography, Davidoff and Dyke confirmed the absence of the corpus callosum in three cases. Unterharnscheidt et al were able to collect 275 cases—the majority diagnosed radiologically—and to analyze the clinical findings. Perhaps as many as 10% were asymptomatic. Mild neurological dysfunctions such as increased muscle tone, seizures, and hydrocephalus, due probably to associated anomalies, were the common complaints. Psychological deficits of a nonspecific nature were present in about half of the cases. Many other abnormalities including trisomy 13-15 and trisomy 18 were noted. The psychological deficits that occur after surgical division of the corpus callosum were uncommon.

Anomalies of the Vascular System

The vessels supplying the brain were well known to the ancient anatomists, but their functional arrangement was confused both by the failure to understand the circulation and the mistaken conception of the rete mirabile.

Aberrations of the major vessels supplying the brain have been noted from the time of the 17th century anatomists. In fact, Casserius missed fame because his drawing of the vessels at the base of the brain failed to show a complete circle, presumably due to the fact that the brain he dissected for his illustration lacked an anterior communicating artery.

The venous system of the cerebral hemispheres, although recognized by the Alexandrian neuroanatomists, received little attention. After Herophilus described the main vascular channels, the cerebral circulation was ignored until the 17th century. In view of their interest in the circulation, it is surprising that Willis and his associates paid little attention to the venous system of the brain.

Bridging veins were described in detail by Rüdinger in 1875. That the longitudinal sinus, when dividing asymmetrically at the torcula, usually passed predominantly to the right lateral sinus was noted by Vicq d'Azyr in 1786 and von Sömmerring in 1800, who attributed the disparity to the fact that most people sleep on the right side.

The vascular malformations (e.g., varices and angiomas) that lie upon the cerebral cortex were seen and described by the early pathologists. They were curiosities, however, until surgeons began to operate upon the brain and exposed such lesions.

Anomalies of the Ventricular System

The cavities of the brain, termed "ventricles," were known to Aristotle in the 4th century BC and to the Alexandrians, Erasistratus, and Herophilus. Galen quoted Erasistratus "when he was an old man" as writing of the brain: "It had a ventricle placed longitudinally on each side and these were [joined to each other] by another ventricle . . . which extended to the cerebellum where there was a smaller ventricle [fourth]." Herophilus called the worm-like processes within the ventricles "choroid meninges" because of their fine transparent nature. Later physicians, especially Galen, thought that choroid "worms" or plexuses were a source of animal spirits—a concept that remained in vogue until the time of Willis. Mondinus wrote of "a bright red substance formed like a long worm which constricts and closes the passage from the anterior to the middle [ventricle]."

In the 15th and 16th centuries, occasional observers noted water in the ventricles after death. Vesalius, after describing the cavities, stated that they drained from the third ventricle to the nasopharnyx (Fig. 8-1). Paré observed that fluid might accumulate in the ventricles in dead persons. He stated that both Albucasis and Vesalius had described patients with enormous heads with intraventricular fluid. Paré stated that the pericranial collections might be drained and cured by incision; however, he had never seen a case of water within the brain cured. Although Berengario da Carpi (Fig. 8-2) referred to water within the ventricles, the consensus at that time maintained that the ventricles contained spirits, not aqueous matter. The first clear account of the ventricular fluid was given by the Italian anatomist Nicholaus Massa (Fig. 8-3) in the early part of the 16th century. He observed "the watery superfluity in these cavities [ventricles] sent there from the other parts of the brain and expurgated through a foramen from the cavities of the ventricles." Massa stated that he had always found the cavities full or half full of water. In the ensuing centuries, the presence of ventricular fluid was noted by many anatomists. Harken to the words of Thomas Willis: "Almost all anatomists of more recent times have given to this more inward chamber of the brain the vile duty of a sewer. Some substance has been added to this belief because in the dead, these ventricles are often observed to be filled with water."

Although attention was being directed to the ventricular collection and expulsion of superfluities, Anton M. Valsalva (Fig. 8-4) in 1692 referred to fluid about the medulla oblongata similar to that in joints. Von Haller also had observed fluid about the inferior brainstem. In 1764, Cotugno in a treatise on sciatica described fluid about the brainstem and spinal cord and explained the failure of previous anatomists to have noted it "because of the ridiculous

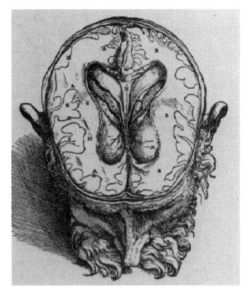

Fig. 8-1. Vesalius' description of the anatomy of the cerebral ventricles. (From A History of Neurosurgery. *Greenblatt SH, Dagi TF, Epstein M, editors. Park Ridge, Ill: American Association of Neurological Surgeons, 1997, p 109)*

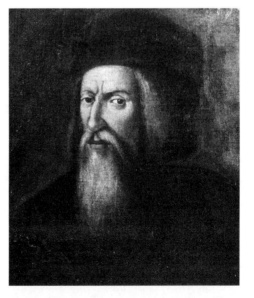

Fig. 8-2. Berengario da Carpi (1470-1530). (From the collection of A. Earl Walker)

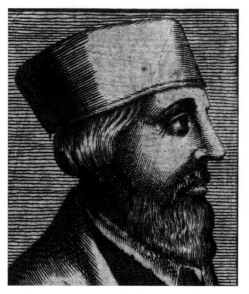

Fig. 8-3. Nicolaus Massa described ventricular fluid. (From the collection of A. Earl Walker)

method usually employed for the dissection of the body... they usually cut off the head with the neck and ... all the fluid collected around the brain and spinal marrow is at once lost." But this publication was little noted, so it remained for Magendie in a series of papers to establish "le liquide cephalospinal." By experiments on animals, he demonstrated that the fluid in the ventricles had free communication from the posterior or fourth ventricle through a midline opening to the spaces around the medulla oblongata and along the spinal cord. This passageway bears his name, although it had been described by both Cotugno and von Haller, neither of whom recognized its significance. Luschka confirmed Magendie's findings and further pointed out that there were lateral openings from the fourth ventricle, a finding which was doubted by some anatomists even after its confirmation by Key and Retzius in 1872.

That the cerebrospinal fluid originated from the choroid plexus was suggested by Faivre in 1853, but this view was not generally accepted until the anatomical studies of Lewis Weed and the surgical observations of choroidal sweating by Cushing in the early part of the 20th century (Fig. 8-5). The subsequent studies of Dandy and Blackfan showed that hydrocephalus developed if the foramen of Monro was obstructed, but not if the choroid plexuses of the lateral ventricles were removed. This observation suggested that the absorption of the spinal fluid took place from the surface of the brain, where Key and Retzius had noted

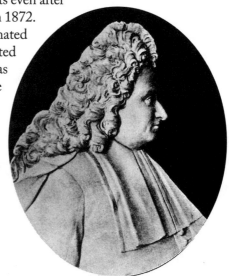

Fig. 8-4. Anton M. Valsalva described fluid surrounding the medulla. (From the collection of A. Earl Walker)

that dyes injected into the ventricular fluid accumulated in the pacchionian granulations. Because these granulations are absent in infancy and in the brain of many species of animals, it seemed that the cerebrospinal fluid must be absorbed diffusely. Although Weed stated, on the basis of experimental work, that the cerebrospinal fluid was produced by the choroidal plexus, Cushing in his Cameron Lectures of 1925 concluded that it had not been conclusively proved.

Ventricular Dilatation and Hydrocephalus

Although the cephalic deformity characteristic of a hydrocephalic baby was known to the Greeks as the Olympian brow, its relationship to enlarged ventricles seems not to have been recognized. Herophilus, who

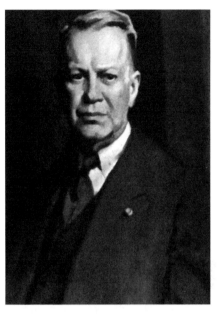

Fig. 8-5. Lewis Weed clarified the structure and function of the choroid plexus. (From the collection of A. Earl Walker)

described the cavities within the brain, makes no reference to their dilatation. Quite probably, the Greek and Roman writers who mention water on the brain were describing extracerebral collections of fluid. Celsus described edema of the scalp as hydrocephalus. Galen refers to four types of hydrocephalus—fluid in the subdural, extradural, pericranial, and subgaleal spaces—but makes no reference to fluid within the ventricular system. Later Roman physicians (Aetius and Paulus Aeginatus) drained water from the scalp or extradural spaces. The Arab surgeons who cauterized the suture lines to remove fluid collections were referring to subgaleal hematomas (Rhazes), although Albucasis described a large head due to intraventricular water.

In the next thousand years, physicians and surgeons rarely mentioned fluid within the head. Da Vinci made a cast of the ventricles but did not refer to their contents. Vesalius described hydrocephalus as water in the cavity of the brain. Paré recognized that hydrocephalus might be due to fluid between the scalp, muscle and pericranium, the pericranium and skull, the skull and dura mater, or in the ventricles. He had never, however, seen a case of water within the brain cured.

Most Renaissance physicians were not acquainted with water in the brain. Mercurialis and Wepfer noted large quantities of water within the brain cavities, a condition which Boerhaave later called hydrocephalus. Some authors reported that they had found the brain and spinal cord abnormal or missing in such cases. Lancisi observed that the contents of the enlarged head communicated with a spinal tumor because pressure over the head was transmitted to the spinal mass. Moreover, the head enlarged as the lower mass grew in size, indicating that they communicated. Morgagni believed that hydrocephalus was of two types—one a rarely seen collection of water between the scalp and cranium, and the other, water within the enlarged cavities of the cerebral hemispheres—as the result of the bones of the skull being pushed asunder, or as seen in adults, by a dropsy of the brain. Morgagni believed that such anomalies could be explained by a dropsy of the head and spine due to a tumor at the lower spine where the bones of the vertebrae gaped (spina bifida). Moreover, he noted that there were nerves entangled in the spinal tumor, which might cause bladder or bowel palsy, if in the sacral region. He stated that "we must not always expect a hydrocephalus to exist in the same patient in whom there is a hydrorachitis but if they do occur together, the patient has convulsions and dies." He admitted that some surgeons thought that the cystic mass was the urinary bladder, but noted that its incision caused the patient's death. Accordingly, Morgagni questioned whether the surgeon should operate on such cases. Paré admitted that he had never seen a patient recover after surgery but that if no operation was undertaken, the patient might live for several years.

Morgagni stated that the entire brain in some hydrocephalic cases might be dissolved into mucus or a limpid bloody water so that all of the ventricular system was a single sac. The cerebral cortex might be so compressed that it was as thin as the dura mater; in such cases, the brainstem and cerebellum might be greatly attenuated.

Apparently unaware of the Italian contributions to hydrocephalus, English writers in the latter part of the 18th century became interested in the subject. Whytt in 1768 wrote that no previous author had presented the "signs by which we may distinguish a dropsy of the ventricles of the brain." He did note Petit's reference to water within the ventricles but commented disparagingly regarding Petit's discussion of the clinical features of the condition. Of Le Dran, who wrote later, Whytt comments that his description was of "such a manner as would make one believe he had never seen the distemper." Whytt noted that considering the frequent occurrence in children (he had about 20 cases) of the condition, it was strange that it "should have been almost unknown to the ancients." He described three stages in considerable detail but admits that he had "never been so lucky to cure one person who had those symptoms, which with certainty denote this disease." He states that "in a dropsy of the ventricles of the brain, any such attempt to draw off the water could have no other effect than to hasten death." As his patients probably had tuberculous meningitis, the outcome is understandable.

The treatment of hydrocephalus has varied greatly throughout the ages.

TABLE 1

TREATMENT OF HYDROCEPHALUS

1. Ancient therapies
   scarification
   trephination

2. Pre-Lister therapies
   bloodletting
   purging
   various drugs (e.g., mercury, salicylates, and bromides)
   physical measures
      compression bandages
      intraventricular caustics such as iodine
      heliotherapy
      compression of carotid arteries
      ventricular puncture through fontanelle, nose, or orbit;
         puncture through trephine hole (usually fatal)
      lumbar puncture

The ancient Greeks incised the scalp and may have punctured the dilated ventricle to allow the fluid to drain. Fabricius Hildanus inserted a trocar to evacuate the fluid. This practice was continued in the 17th and 18th centuries, removing as much as two liters of fluid. These tappings were combined with compression bandages. Various substances (e.g., iodine and astringents) were injected into the dilated ventricles, usually with disastrous results. After lumbar puncture was introduced, spinal fluid was removed to relieve hydrocephalus.

Assuming that the condition was a dropsy of the brain analogous to other dropsies, diuretics were advocated. Even in the early part of the 19th century, the usual treatment was the administration of mercury, a supportive diet, and wine; at that time, Cooke stated that surgery was rarely successful. Such conservative measures, with external compression of the head by bandaging, in some cases seemed to give relief, although the diagnosis may have been erroneous.

The fact that there have been so many medical and surgical approaches to the treatment of hydrocephalus is an indication that a satisfactory method of handling the problem never evolved. Table 1 indicates the ingenious but usually futile procedures that have been used in the past.

Stenosis of the Aqueduct of Sylvius

Although the third circulation was established when Magendie published his research on the cerebrospinal fluid in 1842, it was 20 years before the effect of obstructing the passage of ventricular fluid through the aqueduct of Sylvius was recognized. Hilton in 1863 is said to have been the first to describe such a ventricular block. His patient was a hydrocephalic infant girl who died at five months of age with an imperforate aqueduct. In 1900, Bourneville and Noir reported another such case. Two years later, Spiller described the microscopic pathology of a narrowed aqueduct producing hydrocephalus. Presumably, the size and shape of the aqueduct are genetically determined, so that an idiopathic narrowing represents a hereditary fault. This assumption finds confirmation in the fact that families with several afflicted members have been reported (Bickers and Adams). The defect may be a simple stenosis, an aqueductal forking, or a gliosis surrounding the aqueduct. The latter is considered to be the result of an inflammatory reaction, obstruction by intraluminal debris (blood, blood products, or inflammatory tissue), compression by an adjacent tumor, uncal herniation, or an ependymal proliferation plugging the lumen. Aqueductal maldevelopment is likely to represent a genetic fault; the other obstructions probably result from environmental insults.

The resulting clinical syndrome consists of impaired upward conjugate gaze with downward drift, producing the sunset eye sign, anisocoria, and pupils unresponsive to light, convergence nystagmus, and vertical nystagmus. Various related signs may be present.

Anomalies of the Meninges

Dura Mater Anomalies

The tough membrane covering the brain, the "dura mater," was known to the ancient warriors who frequently saw it exposed in wounds of the head. In the earliest manuscripts extant—the *Edwin Smith papyrus*—the membranes covering the brain are referred to but without comment upon their origin. Even the early anatomists made no reference to the development and anomalies of the membranes of the brain.

Meningeal Anomalies

In association with cranial and encephalic abnormalities, the cranial meninges often have developmental defects. Primitive anomalies of the neural tube are usually manifested by rudimentary meningeal coverings. The tentorium also shares in defects of the encephalon, so that a hemitentorium or absence of the tentorium may accompany a severe encephalic defect.

Congenital Tumors of the Central Nervous System

Intracranial Cysts

Arachnoidal cysts are commonly found around the sella turcica in the supra-, para-, or intrasellar region. In the same basal part of the calvarium, a number of other cysts occur—Rathke's pouch or cleft cyst, craniopharyngiomas, colloidal cysts, and suprasellar cysts. Arachnoidal cysts may be found in the Rolandic area, or the frontal, temporal, or parietal cortex; some are the result of trauma, others are genetic. These arachnoidal cysts are often asymptomatic even though the skull may be deformed by the mass. Pathologically, they may be subdural hygromas, hematomas, or subdural fluid due to arachnoidal tears.

Such arachnoidal cysts of the posterior fossa may be the result of a number of factors. In the cerebellopontine angle, they commonly surround a tumor of the eighth nerve or, less frequently, a neoplasm of other structures. Occasionally, such posterior fossa cysts occur in the absence of a neoplasm. An imperforate foramen of Luschka may cause a pouch lined by ependyma to extend outward from the angle of the fourth ventricle. These glial-lined pouches may even extend into the cisterna magna.

Extradural Spinal Cysts

Cysts lying in the space between the dura mater and the bony spinal canal wall have been long known and long a subject of discussion. Elsberg in 1933 considered that they might arise as the result of trauma—operation or spinal puncture—or as a congenital anomaly. The cyst wall consists of arachnoidal membrane or, in some cases, of dura mater which envelops the diverticulum. The lesion is usually in the thoracolumbar or thoracic region; in the latter case, the condition may be associated with kyphosis dorsalis juvenilis. Occasionally, the cyst lies anterior to the vertebral column, forming an anterior sacral meningocele or an occult intrasacral meningocele with the dilated spinal canal containing a lipoma. The symptoms depend upon the location of the cyst.

Intradural Arachnoid Cysts

Thin-walled (often transparent) cysts lying in the subdural space, sometimes communicating with the subarachnoid space, usually at a root sleeve, have been variously described as diverticuli, adhesive arachnoiditis, circumscribed or chronic arachnoiditis, or meningitis and other states of the arachnoid. Although their true nature is not agreed upon, they have continued to be encountered at myelography, with other spinal imaging studies, and at the operating table. The earliest case seems to have been reported by Spiller et al in 1903. Many subsequent cases so diagnosed have been related to infections— syphilitic, tubercular, parasitic, or traumatic. In some instances, the cyst has extended extradurally.

Perineural Cysts

Somewhat similar cysts are found in the sacral spinal canal. Marburg, who first described cysts surrounding the sacral nerve roots at their exit at the intervertebral foramina, believed that they might be the late result of hemorrhage or be of ependymal origin; however, Tarlov, who rediscovered these cysts, noted that they were common and often multiple. They usually are not accompanied by symptoms.

Anomalies of the Rhombencephalon

Developmental anomalies of the posterior fossa structures are less common than those of the supratentorial region. This is probably due to the fact that rhombencephalic defects are incompatible with life and that only fetuses with lesser anomalies survive.

Cerebellar Developmental Anomalies

Cerebellar agenesis was first described by Combettes in an 11-year-old girl whose cerebellum consisted of a membranous tent connected to aplastic peduncles. Since then, many cases with varying degrees of cerebellar aplasia have been reported in individuals who have survived to childhood or even adult life. Although most of these individuals were mentally defective, they had remarkably few evidences of cerebellar dysfunction.

Agenesis of the cerebellar hemispheres has been reported with varied clinical disturbances and inconstant abnormalities of other posterior fossa structures. Some cases were incidental findings at autopsy. Usually when a hypoplastic cerebellar hemisphere was found, the contralateral olives were atrophic and associated brainstem structures were variously altered. Persons found to have hypoplastic cerebella at autopsy frequently had no history of cerebellar disturbances.

Vermian Aplasia

Abnormalities of the vermis are not uncommon findings at autopsy; many have been found in patients with no clinical history of neurological abnormalities. Some such persons have had psychomotor retardation and some incoordination of gait. The earliest case of total aplasia of the vermis, described by Rossi, was found in a mentally defective woman; the cerebellar hemispheres had an abnormal convolutional pattern. In patients with atresia of the foramina of Luschka and Magendie in whom the vermis is vestigial, no clinical neurological abnormalities may be detectable.

Congenital Atresia of the Foramina of Luschka and Magendie (Dandy-Walker Syndrome)

This developmental anomaly of the posterior fossa structures has been ascribed to the failure of the foramina of Luschka and Magendie to open at the end of the fourth month of fetal life (Fig. 8-6). At that time, the occipital lobes

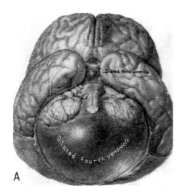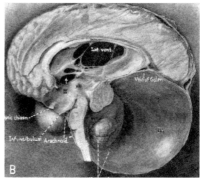

Fig. 8-6. Illustration of hydrocephalus secondary to obstruction of the foramina of Luschka and Magendie. (From Neurosurgical Classics)

have not completed their migration posteriorly and so the lateral sinuses retain their fetal position in the parietal region. Enlargement of the head is the presenting complaint, although there may be no symptoms of intracranial hypertension. Perhaps this is the result of the early occurrence of these lesions when the skull is malleable. In some cases, neurological examination reveals no significant abnormalities except for slight mental retardation and papilledema.

In infants, there is little to distinguish this condition from communicating hydrocephalus except for the prominent occipital region, the roentgenological evidence of the elevated position of the lateral sinuses, and the large posterior fossa. The earliest case was probably described by Sutton in 1887, although Virchow referred to a case of hydrocele of the fourth ventricle but gave no further description.

Dysplasias of the Cervical Spinal Cord and Canal

From the time of Hippocrates, watery cysts on the lower back of newborn babies have been noted; a few cysts with well-defined necks have undergone ligation, alas, with disastrous results. Morgagni was probably the first to observe (but not to understand the relationship) that such anomalies were often accompanied by increased water in the brain. Even when internal hydrocephalus was recognized in the 17th century, the significance of its association with spina bifida was not appreciated. It was an Englishman, John Cleland, who in 1883 pointed out the relationship of lumbosacral meningomyeloceles to the caudal displacement of the cerebellar tonsils and medulla oblongata. This paper, however, received little attention on the continent. Eleven years later, Arnold reported that in a newborn child with a lumbosacral myelocyst, the cerebellar tonsils and medulla oblongata were herniated through the foramen magnum. A year later, Chiari, professor of pathological anatomy in

Prague, in a small monograph, reviewed a series of 24 cases of hydrocephalus. He classified the changes at the foramen magnum into four groups. Type I was a protrusion of the cerebellar tonsils through the foramen magnum, characteristic of long-standing intracranial pressure or hydrocephalus. Type II was the deformity of the cerebellar tonsils, adjacent cerebellar hemispheres, and the caudal medulla oblongata resulting from herniation through the foramen magnum—the malformation commonly termed the "Arnold-Chiari malformation." Type III was an elongated brainstem with ectopic cerebellar tissue in a cervical meningocele. Type IV consisted of a hypoplastic cerebellum and associated anomalies.

The common Type II deformity consisted of a prolongation of the cerebellar vermis and caudal fourth ventricle into the upper cervical canal with a kinking of the medulla oblongata at its junction with the abnormally lowly situated cervical spinal cord. Various other anomalies of the brainstem at the foramen magnum often distorted the medulla oblongata and upper cervical cord. In association with the deformity, congenital anomalies of the spinal cord (e.g., meningomyelocele, hydromyelia, and syringomyelia) are common and some degree of hydrocephalus is a constant. Some years later, Arnold's pupils, Schwalbe and Gredig noted the hypoplastic rhombencephalon, caudal displacement, and dorsal kinking of the medulla oblongata covered by a hypoplastic cerebellar vermis that extended caudally over the upper cervical cord. To describe this condition, they proposed the term "Arnold-Chiari malformation."

The condition was rarely discussed until Russell and Donald emphasized its constant occurrence in meningomyeloceles and associated it with the accompanying hydrocephalus. Various causes of the malformation and the associated abnormalities have been propounded. The two most well-known theories, one the hydrodynamic theory advocated by Chiari and later by Gardner and the other the tethering theory, which indicates that the condition is caused by an associated myelocele, have both failed to explain why these factors are not constantly present. A pronounced maldevelopment of the neuraxis at the pontomedullary junction seems to account for the occurrence of the malformation independent of the neural anomalies.

In 1912, Klippel and Feil described and beautifully illustrated a patient who had such a short neck that the head seemed to be attached to the trunk. Neck movements were limited due to several fused cervical vertebrae. Subsequently, such cases were described with brainstem and cerebellar abnormalities, all of which have been grouped in the Klippel-Feil syndrome. Probably included would be Morgagni's case of anomalous fusion of the lamina of the atlas to the base of the skull, as well as fusion of the bodies of C2 and C3.

Another maldevelopment of the craniospinal junction, "aplasia of the dens," was described by Bevan in the middle of the 19th century. This produced an unstable upper neck due to the absence or rudimentary state of the dens. As a result of unusual mobility of the atlanto-occipital joint, the spinal cord was compromised by sudden movements of the head, resulting in tetraplegia and/ or vertebrobasilar insufficiency.

It was not until roentgenography was commonly used that the frequent occurrence of anomalous craniovertebral dysplasias was recognized. Many such abnormalities—hemivertebrae, unfused or absent dens, hemilaminae sometimes fused to adjacent structures, absent laminae, and defective articular arches—were then described. A few of the earlier described anomalies were designated by eponyms.

Spina Bifida Cystica

Although the Hippocratic physicians are said to have been aware of developmental defects of the lower spine associated with an external mass, they knew naught of its nature. Rhazes was the earliest writer to describe spina bifida. Even Paré does not mention the lumbar cysts. In the 16th and 17th centuries these cystic masses were thought to be related to the urinary bladder, although a few physicians recognized that they originated from dysplastic neural tissue. Tulpius in 1641 described six such cystic masses (Fig. 8-7); he ligated the neck of one, but the child died shortly thereafter. Fifty years later, in a report of 10 cases, Ruysch noted the frequent association of paralysis of the lower limbs. He thought that nothing could be done for the condition. Morgagni assumed that the dysplasia was caused by excessive spinal fluid resulting from scrofula, syphilis, or an inflammatory state. He recognized that it might occur alone or in association with hydrocephalus. Cruveilhier believed that a maldevelopment was responsible for the cystic condition. In 1886, von Recklinghausen in his classical report of the various types of this mal-

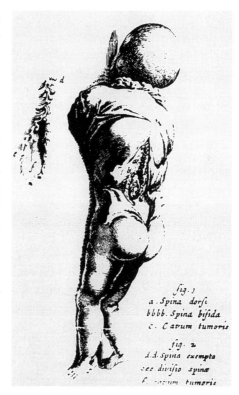

Fig. 8-7. Tulpius' 1641 illustration of spina bifida cystica. (From the collection of A. Earl Walker)

formation described such anomalies as a result of a primary defect in the vertebrae and meninges and considered hydromyelia as a secondary manifestation. If there was an overt sac in the vertebral defect, he called the condition spina bifida cystica; if the malformation was covered with skin, it was named spina bifida occulta—a term Virchow had previously coined. Von Recklinghausen noted that the sac was usually in the lumbar or lumbosacral region and might consist of one of the following: meninges (meningocele), meninges and neural elements (meningomyelocele), or imperfectly developed spinal cord (myelocele).

In 1881, Lebendorff analyzed such defects in birds and man; he concluded that the causative factor was a failure of the neural tube to close in early fetal life. Two years later, Cleland described findings in a case of myelocele in considerable detail. He noted the neural plaque and the dilated spinal canal which extended from the anomaly to within 1.25 cm of the caudally displaced fourth ventricle lying along the cervical spinal cord. Other rhombencephalic anomalies included a deformity of the quadrigeminal plate, now known as "tectal beaking." Cleland attributed these anomalies to either excess production of fluid or abnormal growth of the rhombencephalon. In 1885, Humphrey analyzed the neuroanatomical relationships of meningoceles and pointed out that the spinal cord may be split by a bony spur, a condition known as diastematomyelia. The following year, von Recklinghausen in a discussion of spina bifida concluded that the neural tube was completely closed but was incorporated in the sac wall. To collapse such "tumors," various necrotizing solutions were injected to produce a fibrous scar. This treatment was an advance over the earlier drainage techniques, although not a cure.

Hydromyelia and Syringomyelia

In 1546, Estienne in an anatomy text described a cavity within the spinal cord along the central canal, to which he attached no significance. Eight years later, Fernel in his *Medicina* wrote of a canal within the spinal cord. When autopsies became more commonplace, such anomalies were frequently encountered. Morgagni reported finding an enlarged central canal associated with a meningomyelocele in a hydrocephalic person. Although the patient had no symptoms referable to the spinal cord, he had "a cavity within the beginning of the spinal marrow of so large a size, that I have never seen the like." Later, Portal pointed out that a dilated central canal could cause neurological impairment. Ollivier d'Angers in 1824 described an excessive dilatation of the central canal of the spinal cord which communicated with the caudal end of the fourth ventricle, a condition which he considered to be a developmental anomaly that he termed "syringomyelia." After demonstrating that the central canal was open in all vertebrates and often open in childhood, Stilling in 1856 concluded that the condition should be called "hydromyelia" and the term "syringomyelia" be reserved for other spinal cavities. At about the same time,

Simon proposed that "syringomyelia" should be applied to intraspinal cavities associated with tumors, gliosis, and intrinsic cord lesions and "hydromyelia" used when referring to a dilated central canal. Chiari in 1888 noted that the syringomyelic cavity usually communicated with the central canal. Three years later, he described associated anomalies of the cerebellum which gave rise to hydrocephalus. Such malformations of the posterior fossa structures had been noted by Langhans in 1881, and were described in more detail by Arnold in 1894. As a result, the anomaly was termed the "Arnold-Chiari malformation." Gowers in his text described the clinical and pathological characteristics of this anomaly. He emphasized that the damage to the gray matter caused muscular atrophy and anesthesia of the shoulders and back, extending at times into the arms and hands. Gowers recognized that the condition was progressive, with death in two or three years.

The subject remained quiescent for a third of a century, until 1935 when Russell and Donald reviewed the anomalies of the posterior fossa. They noted the association of spina bifida with defects of the spinal cord and concomitant abnormalities of the posterior fossa structures. Several years later, Gardner in a series of papers (1959-1973) affirmed that the cystic dilatation of the spinal cord was caused by partial or complete obstruction of the foramen of Magendie, shunting the ventricular fluid into the central canal of the spinal cord, causing it to dilate and rupture its walls, thus producing various pathological lesions of the cord—syringomyelia, diastematomyelia, meningomyeloceles, etc. Because this view did not explain all the abnormalities associated with a dilated central canal, other investigators have maintained that the malformation is the result of a primary failure of the neural tube to close.

Aberrant Meningoceles

Instead of presenting in the midline posteriorly, meningoceles may extend anteriorly or laterally from the spinal canal into the pelvic cavity. Probably the earliest such case was reported by an unidentified surgeon who delivered a fetus piecemeal through a birth canal which was obstructed by a pelvic mass. The patient died of puerperal fever; at postmortem examination, the obstruction was seen to be due to a cyst communicating with the spinal canal. The earliest case of a lateral or anterior lumbar meningocele was reported by Robinson in 1903. The patient was an 11-month-old infant with a left talipes equinovarus and a dilated central spinal canal. An abdominal mass was found to communicate with the spinal canal; its neck was ligated, but the infant died of meningitis. Intrathoracic meningoceles usually extend into the retropleural space. Probably the earliest such case reported was that of Pohl; the patient was a 47-year-old woman with cutaneous neurofibromatosis who succumbed from empyema after excision of a retropleural mass.

Sacral Agenesis

The congenital absence of the sacrum or sacral agenesis was first reported and illustrated in 1852 by Hohl in a stillborn fetus with multiple anomalies of the spine, spinal cord, and abdominal organs. Thereafter, isolated cases of rumpless infants—some stillborn—have been described in the medical literature.

9

Infections and Inflammatory Involvement of the Central Nervous System

B rain fevers of ancient times were a motley group of cerebral disorders characterized by fever and "phrenitis"—a generic term encompassing all mental derangements. Not until postmortem examinations became common in the 18th century were some associated pathological lesions defined by the naked eye. Such inspections were inadequate to identify many pathological afflictions. Recall that Whytt, who so clearly described the dilated, water-filled ventricles of hydrocephalic brains, did not notice the arachnoidal infiltrations at the base of the brain. Therefore, a French clinician later described tuberculous meningitis. Even if the pathological state was known, its pathogenesis might be misunderstood. Recall that prior to Morgagni's investigations, intracranial suppuration was considered to be the cause of a draining ear and not the reverse. Because the phrenetic disorders of the nervous system were examined only at late stages, it was difficult to determine the early and subtle pathology of the disorders. Purulent exudates were so compounded by debris and vascular changes that the primary alterations were unrecognizable on naked eye examination. For that reason, the early postmortem descriptions of meningeal suppuration are difficult to interpret and accordingly are of limited value in defining extradural, subdural, meningeal and, in some cases, even cerebral involvement.

Cranial Infections

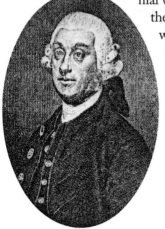

Although fluid draining from the ear and exuding cranial wounds were well known to Medieval physicians, their pathogenesis was poorly understood. Trauma was generally considered to be responsible for the exudates, which were essential for the healing process. Morgagni noted, without explanation, that carious cranial bones were found in association with a draining sinus, but Percivall Pott (Fig. 9-1) pointed out the relationship of a pericranial abscess and the presence of extradural pus. Lannelongue in 1879 demonstrated that the suppurative changes in cranial bone were analogous to those sustained in septic long bones, changes previously thought to be caused by cold, trauma, overwork, or scrofula. When pathological changes due to infection were understood, a rational explanation of the process was introduced. To describe the state of the bone, Lannelongue proposed the term "osteomyelitis." The extradural abscesses described by Paré and later by Pott were purulent extensions from infected sinuses or from osteolytic bone.

Fig. 9-1. Percivall Pott (1713-1788). (From the collection of A. Earl Walker)

Treatment of the diseased cranium varied. Gay in 1797 successfully drained pus from the dura mater. In the latter part of the 18th century, Percivall Pott advised incising a fluctuating scalp abscess and trephining bone to allow purulent material to drain. The inflammatory reaction was attributed to the underlying dura mater and diploic vessels, which were often thrombosed. To evacuate the pus, extensive scalp incisions were advised, but frequently failed as a fatal meningitis developed. Obviously, the cranial infection had spread to the underlying tissues.

Subdural Abscesses

In the 17th and 18th centuries, it was difficult to determine the origin of an intracranial abscess because at the patient's death the lesion had spread widely from the subdural into the subarachnoid space, the adjacent cortex, white matter, and even into the ventricle. As the result of this diffusion, before the time of Morgagni, it was thought that an intracranial empyema arose in the brain and that its extension into the meningeal spaces was secondary. Morgagni wrote of a 60-year-old man who fell on his head, sustaining a scalp wound at the lambdoidal suture. Within a week, he had developed paralysis of the left arm and became stuporous; he died three weeks after the injury. The wound was purulent and, at the separated lambdoidal suture, pus drained from an abscess between the discolored dura and pia mater. In 1834, Abercrombie described another case and referred to the difficulty defining the confines of the infarction. Twenty years later, von Bruns reported a collection of pus in the arachnoid of a patient. Thereafter, sporadic cases secondary to middle ear or mastoid infections occurred in the literature, usually treated by draining through an open wound. Jansen in 1895, Witzel in 1897, and Delstanche in 1898 used iodoform gauze to tamponade the margins of the exposure in order to prevent subdural extension of the infection. Little was added to improve the technique until the chemotherapeutic and antibiotic eras.

Brain Abscesses

Recovery from chronic abscesses of the brain never takes place.
—Hammond

In ancient times, abscesses of the brain were not recognized as such but included in the general term "phrenitis." Although pus-containing cavities within the brain have been known for centuries, their precise situation (e.g., extradural, subdural, or intracerebral) has been difficult to determine from the available descriptions. Renowned surgeons such as Paré referred to nondescript pus pockets. Morand in the 18th century trephined carious bone over a draining mastoid sinus and inserted catgut tents to keep the wound margins open for drainage. Two weeks later, he opened the dura mater with a cruciate incision and explored a purulent cavity with his fingertip. To maintain the escape of pus, he inserted a slender silver tube into the opening; the tube was shortened as the cavity shrunk. The wound eventually healed and the patient survived. In 1821 Roux trephined the skull, allowing an arachnoidal abscess to ulcerate the dura mater and drain. After these successful cases, others were reported. Dupuytren in 1823 treated a patient with a knife wound of the scalp and cranium; he re-explored the old wound and cut into the underlying cortex to open and drain an abscess cavity. Unfortunately, the patient succumbed. Detmold also reported death in a patient after a second operation to drain a subcortical abscess. However, treatment was occasionally successful. The introduction of anesthesia and asepsis in the middle of the 19th century encouraged bold surgeons to explore a weeping wound of a stuporous or comatose patient and even incise the brain in the hope of encountering and draining an abscess. In 1872, Weeds recorded his exploration of an old wound of the scalp; he found the dura mater slightly lacer-

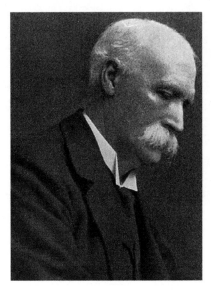

Fig. 9-2. Sir William Macewen (1848-1924). (From A History of Neurosurgery. Greenblatt SH, Dagi TF, Epstein M, editors. Park Ridge, Ill: American Association of Neurological Surgeons, 1997, p 148)

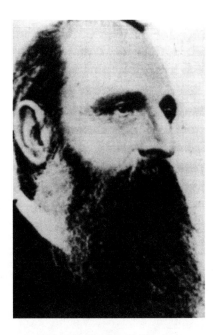

ated and, after plunging his scalpel into the brain, dark green pus escaped. His patient was ambulating in a fortnight. Using aseptic techniques, others also tapped the brain. For this exploration, the use of a cannula or needle and syringe inserted through a small drill hole (Maas) or larger trephine opening (Hulke), to puncture the brain, greatly enhanced the chance of encountering an abscess. When located, the abscess might be aspirated or incised and evacuated.

Henrici attributed the use of a drainage tube to ensure a continued flow of pus to Esmarch, who in 1880 placed a decalcified bone drain into the cavity of a brain abscess. However, Thomas maintained that he had used this same principle in 1875. The method was popularized in 1882 by Wernicke and Hahn's report in the German literature. In his book on brain abscesses, Macewen (Fig. 9-2) referred to this drainage technique using hollow chicken bones. Various antiseptic solutions (e.g., carbolic acid, iodine, and hydrogen peroxide) were used to irrigate and to wash out debris from the abscess cavity.

In the early 1900s, Antony Chipault in a review of brain surgery noted that abscesses were more common than other intracranial lesions, even tumors. Durante (Fig. 9-3) in Rome had operated

Fig. 9-3. Francesco Durante (1844-1934). (From A History of Neurosurgery. Greenblatt SH, Dagi TF, Epstein M, editors. Park Ridge, Ill: American Association of Neurological Surgeons, 1997, p 157)

upon 54 brain abscesses and only 32 brain tumors. Ballance (Fig. 9-4) noted that most surgically treated cases were localized by the presence of a draining sinus. Although Barker had operated upon a patient with a temporosphenoidal abscess without external signs of its presence, most surgeons were loathe to incise the dura mater and brain to explore for an abscess. As a result, the fate of patients with brain abscesses at that time was dismal. After the beginning of the 20th century, when public health measures had lessened the incidence of communicable diseases, the number of patients with brain abscesses greatly decreased. With the advent of chemotherapeutic and antibiotic agents, pyogenic lesions of the brain were rarely encountered in the major countries of the world.

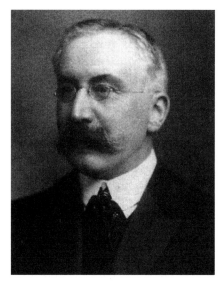

Fig. 9-4. Sir Charles Ballance (1857-1936). (From Dictionary of Medical Eponyms, *2nd ed. BG Firkin and JA Whitworth. New York: Parthenon Publishing, 1996, p 17)*

Infected Wounds of the Spinal Canal

Because wounds of the spine were considered lethal, they were treated quite conservatively, with superficial dressing. As a result, Morgagni in 1761 and other pathologists referred to peri- and epimeningitis spinalis as lethal afflictions. For that reason, surgeons paid little attention to them, especially as the victims were usually paralyzed and unable to get about. It was not until the latter part of the 19th century that such surgeons as Macewen diagnosed and attempted to treat these infections; however, success was rare.

Meningitis

As early as the primitive and pre-Renaissance times, it was recognized that certain conditions characterized by fever, headache, mental disturbances, vomiting, and impaired consciousness, called brain fever or phrenitis, resulted in a patient's fatal outcome. Avicenna had observed that, in some cases, patients with such symptoms and even a stiff neck had only an acute febrile illness, a state later called meningismus. Willis described "phrensy" as "a continual raving or a deprivation of the chief faculties of the brain, arising from an inflammation of the meninges with a continual fever." It is not clear whether Willis and other writers were differentiating meningeal and cerebral disorders. Although Cotugno had written of the cerebrospinal fluid in 1764, he did not understand its function in health and disease. Nor did Whytt, when he wrote of hydrocephalus, recognize the meningeal inflammation associated with the increased water in the ventricles. Not until 1830 did Papavoine show that such hydrocephalus could be caused by tuberculous involvement of the meninges. In the interim, Herpin had introduced the term meningitis. Its full significance was not realized until Magendie described the spinal fluid pathways. At that time, the occurrence of spotted fever, sometimes confused with typhus, was spreading from Geneva, where it apparently originated in 1805, to other parts of Europe. In that year, Vieusseux described it as an affliction of children, characterized by fever, headache, vomiting, and stiffness of the neck. Symptoms of dizziness, delirium, and stupor might follow with skin eruptions, especially purpura or erythema, which predicated its designation as "spotted fever." Cranial nerve palsies, often causing diplopia and/or deafness, were frequent complications. The disease might fulminate, with death ensuing within a few hours. The mortality rate was as high as 80%, although generally it was much lower.

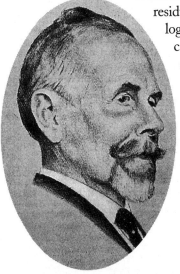

Recovery from spotted fever was usually slow, especially if it was complicated by pneumonia. The most common residual effect was deafness, although other neurological disabilities at times persisted. The causative organism was established by Weichselbaum in 1887 as the meningococcus.

The technique of lumbar puncture, introduced by Quincke (Fig. 9-5) in 1891, made it possible to determine the characteristics of the spinal fluid, in particular its constituent cells, chemistry, and serological reactions. These examinations introduced at the turn of the century were supplemented later by bacteriological, serological, and immunological tests that enabled the clinician to define the precise nature of the various meningitides.

Gowers noted that meningitis might be caused either by extension from the disease adjacent to the brain, such as infection of scalp, cranium, air sinuses, or the brain itself, or by blood-borne systemic infec-

Fig. 9-5. Heinrich Quincke (1842–1922). (From The Founders of Neurology, *2nd ed. Haymaker W, Schiller F, editors. Springfield, Ill: Charles C Thomas, 1970, p 500)*

tions, such as measles, scarlet fever, smallpox, tuberculosis, syphilis, or septicemia (endocarditis). When pathogens were identified, it became apparent that three major organisms—*Hemophilus influenzae, Neisseria meningitidis,* and *Streptococcus pneumoniae*—were responsible. The signs and symptoms of these infections were similar to the manifestations of other meningitides (headache, vomiting, and stiffness of the neck); however, more specific signs of meningeal irritation were described later. In 1882, Kernig noted that a person with meningeal irritation was unable, with the hip flexed, to fully extend the leg at the knee. A few years later, Brudzinsk reported that in such cases, if the head was passively flexed on the chest, the legs flexed.

In 1899, Slawyk described *H. influenzae* meningitis, the most common cause of meningitis in children under the age of seven years. Staphylococcic and streptococcic meningitides were rarely found except in surgical wounds or debilitated patients, and constituted the usual responsible organisms. Treatment of these infections was disappointing until chemotherapeutic and antibiotic agents were introduced.

In the latter part of the 19th century, a number of endocranial conditions resembled the meningitides, including serous effusions, arachnoiditis, pericranial infections, and meningismus. At that time, it was difficult to differentiate these various conditions, but when lumbar puncture became common at the end of the century, the spinal fluid contents identified the etiological agent in most of these conditions. It was another 35 years, during which time a number of therapies were introduced, before chemotherapy and later antibiotic drugs practically eliminated the disease.

Secondary Meningeal Infections

Many systemic infections known to the ancients have, at times, secondarily involved the central nervous system. If the primary disease was lethal, the neural complications were rarely recognized until postmortem examinations became common. For this reason, secondary infections of the central nervous system were not recognized or, if recognized, the relationship was misinterpreted. A few conditions closely related to the systemic disorder had an obvious association.

Thrombosis of the Vascular Sinuses

Infected, thrombosed vascular sinuses were recognized early by pathologists; however, no therapy was attempted until Zaufal in 1880 recommended ligating the jugular vein and cleaning out the septic, thrombotic coagulum in the sinus. The result of such a procedure is not given.

Tuberculous Meningitis

Although systemic tuberculosis has been recognized since the dawn of history, it was only in the last 200 years that involvement of the nervous system has been noted. Earlier, tuberculous disease of the brain and its coverings was called "phrenitis" or "cephalitis," acute hydrocephalus, or febrile hydrocephalus. Whytt noted the ventricular dilatation of children who, after a few weeks, succumbed. He considered the disorder to be a simple hydrocephalus. A half century later, Deh demonstrated the tubercular cause. Although Vieusseux in 1789 reported meningeal lesions in association with tubercles in the lung and abdomen, he failed to comprehend their association. Odier, the following year, noted "hydrocéphalie combinée avec l'inflammation des meninges" and suggested that the thickening of the meninges was the cause of the hydrocephalus. At the beginning of the 19th century, such "inflammation of the membranes" was called "meningitis" by Herpin. In 1817, Coindet suggested that ventricular dilatation was the result of inflammation of the walls of the ventricles and the meninges. Senn realized that hydrocephalus might be simple or the result of a tuberculous process. Senn suggested that the latter type, usually associated with some degree of ventricular enlargement, was analogous to tubercles involving other parts of the body.

Syphilis

Although syphilis was recognized in Europe beginning in the 15th century, the neurological syndromes attributed to it were not established until the early part of the 19th century. In 1822, Bayle identified general paresis, which was named two years later, and described the thickening of the leptomeninges, adhesions between the meninges and cortex, granular ependyma, and internal hydrocephalus. Tabes dorsalis was described by Romberg in 1849, although the typical pupillary changes were not published by Argyll Robertson until 1849. Their relationship to syphilis was suspected but not established until 1903, when Metschnikoff and Roux infected chimpanzees. Two years later, Schaudinn and Hoffmann demonstrated that *Treponema pallidum* was the cause of syphilis. The following year, the complement fixation test was devised by Wassermann and became a routine examination for syphilis. Although Salvarsan (arsphenamine) was effective in treating systemic syphilis, it had little effect on paresis and tabes dorsalis. Wagner-von Jauregg in 1918-1919 showed that malarial therapy arrested general paresis. However, when the antibiotics were introduced, penicillin was found to be even more satisfactory and replaced the other therapies.

Rabies

In the earliest available literature, "mad dogs" are mentioned, but their association with human disease dates from the ancient Greeks, including Democritus in 500 BC and subsequently Aristotle. Celsus in 100 AD described human rabies in the following manner: "a most heart-rending malady, in which the patient is at once tormented with thirst and a dread of water. When thus afflicted, there is scarcely a shade of hope. The sole remedy consists of throwing him unawares in a pond; and if he cannot swim, he should be allowed to drink in the water as he sinks and to be elevated alternately; if he can swim, he should be repeatedly kept under water that he may be compelled to drink; for this is the way to remove both the thirst and the hydrophobia."

Further advances came only in the 19th century when the virus was transmitted to the rabbit and dog by contaminating wounds with spittle. Later investigators could not consistently transmit the disease by subcutaneous or intravenous inoculation. Dubove in 1879 explained the difficulty by presuming that the virus had to be transmitted along nervous pathways to the central nervous system. Pasteur, aware that the virus propagated only in the nervous system, inoculated directly into the brain in 1881 and obtained consistent transmission of the disease.

Within three years after Pasteur had introduced his vaccine, neurological complications were reported. The neurological sequelae, usually occurring between the 10th and 15th day after the start of the inoculations, consisted of mononeuritis, polyneuritis, transverse myelitis (at times of the Landry type), and meningoencephalitis. These neurological difficulties usually began suddenly and peaked within 48 hours. The spinal fluid had a lymphocytic pleocytosis and an elevated total protein. The course was variable: either death (in 25% of cases) or recovery, often complete. The pathological changes consisted of a diffuse perivascular or perivenular demyelination in the brain and spinal cord. A duck embryo vaccine proved to be safer than that of brain tissue and had fewer neurological complications.

Tetanus

Tetanus has been recognized since ancient times. After an open wound, Hippocrates noted that the lower jaw was primarily involved in one of three ways. The first and simplest way was characterized by such rigidity of the lower jaw that the mouth could not be opened. The neck was rigid, the eyes teared, the face flushed, and the limbs could not be brought together. In great suffering, the victim usually died within three weeks; if the victim survived longer, recovery was common. The second form was characterized by opisthotonos and such violent and painful spasms of the back muscles that unless held by assistants, the patient fell from the bed. The arms were usually flexed rigidly. Some patients were unable to speak. Death occurred by the third day; however, if the victim survived 16 days, again recovery was common. The third and less dangerous form was confined to the muscles at the site of the wound, but might involve the entire body. After a time, the spasms relaxed and might be absent for several days as the condition abated.

The Hippocratic writers believed that a cold was a precipitating factor. Although the condition was considered quite serious, if the spasms lasted more than four days or the victim had a fever, the outlook for recovery was good. Patients were treated with hot baths, lotions, and ointments.

The Romans added little to the clinical picture. Soranus stated that tetanus might follow blows to sinews or muscles. He wrote, "The seizure is more likely to occur at the time when the wounds appear to be clean and free of foreign matter or about to form a scar." He added that the attacks might occur sooner, when the wounds were still in a stage of inflammation. He observed that at the onset of the disorder, the affected person had difficulty in moving the neck, frequent gaping, impaired swallowing, pain in the temples increased by opening the mouth, salivation, and a sardonic grin. As the condition progressed, pain in the neck increased, the jaw muscles tightened, causing the teeth to clench, the neck retracted, and cramps developed in the legs and arms. Soranus recognized that "patients hardly ever recover . . . if the spasm supervenes upon a wound or if the stiffness originates in the spine." However, if the spasm was unrelated to a wound (a misdiagnosis), recovery might occur. A century later, Aretaeus concluded, "This is an awful disease, horrible to watch and incurable."

The condition was sporadic in rural areas until Arthur Nicolaier discovered the bacillus of tetanus in 1884, which prompted the use of carbolic acid in wounds by 1905. Not long after, the use of antitoxins and toxins practically eliminated the condition.

Diphtheria

Diphtheria ("askara" or "serunke" in ancient Hebrew) was so feared that a warning blast of the shofar was given whenever a case was discovered. The pharyngeal condition was known to the Romans as the Syriac ulcer. In the 6th century, Aetius wrote that a late sequel was palatal paralysis. Schedef, in 1492, described an epidemic in Spain called "garotillo" which lasted for 150 years and in the 17th century spread to Italy and later to the New World. Heberden noted that the disease was less common in persons after adolescence. In a classical American paper, Samuel Bard in 1771 described "angina suffocativa" and its late developing paralyses. The disease was named "diphtheritis" by Pierre Bretonneau in 1826. To relieve the croup, he performed a tracheotomy in 1825 with a successful result. Trousseau elaborated upon the clinical findings. When von Behring in 1894 developed a toxin-antitoxin mixture, the disease lost its terror and almost disappeared in the 20th century.

Pertussis

The "suffocating cough of children" was called "whooping cough" by Sydenham. He noted that seizures occasionally accompanied the cough, especially in infants. These convulsive phenomena were common in the Copenhagen epidemic of 1775. Although the causative organism was isolated in 1906 by Bordet and Gengou, it has not been demonstrated in the central nervous system, even in children having cerebral manifestations. Accordingly, the pathogenesis of seizures is still obscure.

Measles

Although measles was well known to Arab physicians in the Dark Ages and to later physicians, neurological complications were reported first by Lucan in 1790 and subsequently by other authors. The sequelae, occurring within a week of the outbreak of the rash, consisted of impaired consciousness, generalized seizures, and focal neurological deficits such as paresis, ataxia, and myoclonus. Meningismus, headache, and vomiting frequently developed. Fever was the rule, with a high temperature in the terminal stages. Gowers reported that myelitis and polyradiculitis were rare complications. The brain shows perivascular demyelination with inflammatory cells about the blood vessels.

Poliomyelitis

In the middle part of the 19th century, sporadic cases of an acute febrile illness accompanied by paralysis, particularly of the limb musculature, were reported by Heine. The clinical manifestations—an acute febrile illness with headache, nausea, and vomiting, followed by signs of meningeal irritation and after a few days muscle spasm, pain, and paralysis of limb muscles—were typical; however, abortive and nonparalytic cases, especially at non-epidemic times, caused confusion. Charcot and Joffroy recognized that the paralysis was due to damage to the anterior horn cells of the spinal cord—the lower motor lesion. In 1890, Medin analyzed the epidemiology of the disease.

Fifteen years later, Wickman recognized that nonparalytic cases might carry the causative organism in the intestinal tract. When monkeys were shown to be susceptible to intracerebral inoculation, it was established that the infective agent was a filterable virus against which effective vaccines could be prepared.

Brucellosis

Brucellosis, variously also termed "undulant fever" or "Malta fever," has been recognized in various forms since antiquity. Hippocrates is said to have described a prolonged febrile illness that was probably brucellosis. Hughes compiled a bibliography of the condition from ancient times, in which he described the clinical features including the neurological complications. In 1897, Bang of Copenhagen isolated the small bacillus responsible for the contagious abortion by cattle, which he termed *Brucella abortus*. Twenty years later, this organism was shown to be a variety of that causing Malta fever (Evans).

Carrión's Disease

Graphic evidence that *verruga peruana* existed centuries ago is given by a Chancay figurine in the Lima Museum of Paleopathology. The febrile stage was described by Oroza-Eppinal in 1873; twelve years later, Daniel Carrión, a student, inoculated himself from a skin lesion and died 38 days later. The disease has been known in South America as Carrión's disease, displacing the previous term "Oroya fever." The micro-organism, transmitted by the sandfly, was identified by Alberto Barton in 1905 and named *Bartonella bacilliformis*. The clinical course of the disease is characterized by a pre-eruptive stage of malaise and an eruptive stage having a nodular, angioblastic, generalized cutaneous rash due to involvement of the reticuloendothelial system. Even before the disease was clearly identified, neurological complications were recognized by Alarco and studied in detail by Monge and Mackehenie. In 1945, Lastres y Quinones coined the term "neurobartonellosis" to describe the neurological syndromes commonly produced by cerebral involvement and rarely by spinal cord lesions.

Malaria

Although malaria has been known for ages, involvement of the central nervous system has been recognized only in recent times. Parasites in humans were identified in the latter part of the 19th century, and the reproductive cycle was identified in 1897 by Ross. In the literature of the 19th century, such terms as "malaria nervosa," "malaris comatose," or "febris perniciosa comatosa" were used to describe the cerebrovascular complications of malaria. Intracranial hemorrhage, thrombosis, and meningeal reactions have been responsible for epilepsy, myelosis, and other diseased states of the central nervous system.

Helminthiasis

From the beginning of medical history (the *Ebers papyrus*), worms have been believed to cause illness in humans. In 427 BC, an epidemic in Sicily was thought to be due to the outbreak of trichinosis. In the Hippocratic writings, both cysticercosis and hydatid cysts were referred to by writers of that time, and in the succeeding centuries, Aristotle, Aretaeus, and Galen recognized that parasites caused disease although the symptoms were not defined. About a millennium later, Rhazes described the manifestations associated with brain cysts; the nature of the invading worm and its proclivity to infest the nervous system were not recognized until postmortem examinations became common during the Renaissance period and parasites in the brain were noted. The patients' clinical symptoms—convulsions, mental disturbances, headache, and progressive coma—were much the same for all types of parasites.

Cysticercosis

From ancient times, the pig has been known to host a parasite that might be transmitted to man. As a result, Semitic and other peoples have considered pork unclean. Although the Greeks and Romans knew of worms that inhabited the gastrointestinal tract, they were unaware that a parasite might invade the brain. That was discovered much later, when autopsies became common. In the 16th century, Paracelsus noted cysticerci in the brains of persons suffering from seizures. A short time later, Paranoli described fluid-filled vesicles in the corpus callosum of a man who had died in a "fit." In 1558, Rumler found vesicles attached to the dura mater of a man who suffered from epilepsy. In the next century, Malpighi gave a full description of the clinical manifestations and pathological findings of cerebral cysticercosis. The vesicles were named "cystercus" by Laenneus, who recognized that they contained the encysted larvae of the pork tapeworm, *Taenia solium*. The clinical manifestations of such infestations—convulsions, headaches, and/or mental disturbances—were described by Griesinger in 1862, and by Lombroso and Haller in 1879. In the latter part of the 19th century, while operating on the brain for epilepsy or a suspected brain tumor, surgeons occasionally encountered such parasitic lesions. The neuropathological findings of both the acute and chronic (calcified) lesions were analyzed by Askanasy in 1890.

Echinococcus (Hydatid) Cysts

Large watery collections in the liver, termed "hydatid cysts," were described in antiquity. Hippocrates in his 55th *Aphorism* noted that when the liver contained water and burst, "the belly is filled with water and the patient dies." Later Roman and Arab writers referred to such cysts. In view of the nomadic habits of the Arabs, it is surprising that parasitic infestations were not more common. The only writer of the Moslem era to refer to hydatid cysts was Albucasis, who lived in Cordoba in the Western Caliphate. When "sectio cadaveris" became legal, reports of such lesions were common. Perhaps the ban on postmortem examinations may explain the failure to describe such lesions.

In 1694, Redi recognized the nature of such watery cysts. About a century later, Morgagni reported on watery cysts that he discovered in the brain. In 1782, Goeze described the composition of the cyst, its tapeworm head, and its suckers and hooklets, thus differentiating it from the other watery sacs found in the brain. Rudolphi in 1808 named the parasite "echinococcus." Guesnard and Chaussier described such cysts in the spinal column and cranial bones. Abercrombie noted that all brain cysts at that time were considered to be hydatid cysts; various other cystic lesions, such as colloid cysts of the choroid plexus, cystic tumors, and porencephalic cysts, were not differentiated until the latter part of the 19th century. The life history of the parasite was described in detail by Leuckart in 1895.

In 1834, Abercrombie suggested that the cysts might be excised; however, Guesnard apparently was the first surgeon to remove such a cyst. A few years later, Verdale operated upon a cyst successfully. In 1872, Westphal exposed a mass eroding the skull, evacuated a cyst, and the patient recovered. Subsequent reports described various surgical techniques—tapping the cyst, open drainage, removal of the cyst wall, extirpation of the intact cyst, aspirating the contents of the cyst, and formalizing the wall and contents of the cyst. In the middle of the 20th century, other techniques were introduced to remove the cyst intact.

Schistosomiasis

Schistosomiasis, formerly called "bilharzia," is an infestation of the blood fluke, a species of which is endemic in many parts of the world. Woodruff believed that this disease was rampant in Egypt in early times and probably spread to other Middle East countries. *Schistosoma japonicum,* a frequent contaminant of seafood, is pathogenic for man and is the cause of cerebral schistosomiasis. The earliest report of the latter was made in 1890 by Yamagiwa, who described the ova in the brain. Sporadic cases were reported later; in 1930, a patient was operated upon by Percy Sargent, who resected a granulomatous mass from the parieto-occipital lobe, following which the patient made a satisfactory recovery. The first description of such a granulomatous lesion in the spinal cord was by Muller and Stender in the same year.

Paragonimiasis

Endemic in the Far East and Southeast Asia, paragonimiasis was generally considered a benign pulmonary infestation manifesting itself by hemoptysis. It was recognized, however, that parasites might spread to the nervous system, causing seizures, general debility, and death. The involvement of the central nervous system took one of three forms—cerebral abscesses, meningitis, or spinal paragonimiasis. Although the disease was described in 1878, the first report of cerebral infestation was in 1887 by Otani in Japan. His patient was a 26-year-old man who had had a cough and hemoptysis for a year before he developed seizures and became comatose. At postmortem examination, the patient was found to have cystic lesions in the right frontal and occipital lobes containing adult worms. Paragonimiasis meningitis less commonly occurs and is often misdiagnosed as tuberculous meningitis. Spinal paragonimiasis, also rare, in the absence of pulmonary paragonimiasis was frequently confused with a spinal cord tumor. The cysts containing the worm and eggs were usually extradural. Fortunately, bithionol, an antihelminthic drug used for animals, has proved to be an effective remedy in man.

Cerebral Trichinosis

Probably responsible for outbreaks of brain fever in ancient times, cerebral trichinosis was first mentioned in modern times by Glazier in 1881 as causing a meningeal reaction. A quarter of a century later, Frothingham reported larval infestation of the brain in an autopsy. In spite of its prevalence in other parts of the body, cerebral involvement is rare. Another rare infection caused by taenia is that of coenurosis, which was first reported in the brain by Brumpt in 1912. The clinical pathological findings are very similar to those of cysticercosis. Other helminths are even less commonly found in the central nervous system.

Cerebral Amebic Abscess

Amebic infestation of the gastrointestinal tract has a long and ill-defined history. Its spread to the nervous system probably occurred in early times, but its manifestations were termed "phrenitis." The earliest verified case was reported by Morehead in 1838, although the organism was not identified until 1875 by Lorsch. When signs of meningeal involvement appeared in a person with gastrointestinal disturbances, the individual was suspected to have worms, although the parasite in the meninges was not demonstrated until Kartulis's report in 1904. Eight years later, Legrand, after extensively reviewing the subject, concluded that cerebral infestation (which occurred in 1%-5% of systemic amebiosis) traveled via meningeal vessels. Orbison et al maintained that the dissemination was by septicemia or through the vertebral veins. Cerebral abscesses, the usual result of infection, varied in size, odor, and consistency, although a rough, fibrous wall was common to all. The symptoms usually began with fever, headache, mental disturbances, and occasionally vomiting. Focal convulsions ushered in the disorder in 15% of cases, and cranial nerve palsies occurred in 25%. In about one third of the cases, the cerebrospinal fluid had an increased cell count.

Inflammatory Disorders

Progressive Ascending Paralysis

In this category are Landry's disease, Landry-Guillain, Guillain-Barré syndrome, and acute immune mediated polyneuritis. These well-recognized syndromes are characterized clinically by an initial viral-like respiratory illness followed in a few days to a week by a progressive, ascending paralysis with loss of reflexes and sometimes a variable amount of sensory impairment. The syndrome was first described in 1859 by Landry. More than 50 years later, Guillain and associates elaborated upon the clinical findings and the pathological alterations—usually a segmental inflammatory demyelination of the spinal roots and peripheral nerves. The syndrome has been given many names, including the Guillain-Barré syndrome.

Polyarteritis Nodosa

Polyarteritis nodosa, a disorder of the arterial system recognized by von Rokitansky in 1852, may manifest itself by various neurological disturbances, depending upon the cerebral vessels affected and the stage of the vasculitis. In 1866, Kussmaul and Maier wrote of a "previously unrecognized arterial disease" which they called "periarteritis nodosa," a term used until the more generalized reaction of vessel walls was recognized. The protean neurological involvement of peripheral neuropathy, present in approximately 10% of cases, was commonly preceded by pain localized to the zone of one or more involved nerves. Cerebral manifestations such as headache, confusional states, transient hallucinations, seizures, and focal disturbances (e.g., hemiparesis, aphasia, and hemianopsia) may result from thrombotic or hemorrhagic lesions. Various systemic vasculitides may induce peripheral or central nervous system manifestations such as hypersensitivity or connective tissue disease.

Lupus Erythematosus

The cutaneous manifestations of lupus erythematosus—a butterfly rash on the cheeks and over the nose—were well known after the description by Biett.

Fifty years prior to that, Kaposi had reported that the central nervous system might be implicated. In about one third of cases, confusional and psychotic states accompanied by headaches or other nervous dysfunctions were present. Seizures and such neurological complications as hemiplegia, cranial or peripheral neuropathy, and ataxia were less frequently encountered.

The usual cerebral pathology consisted of vascular hyalinization with endothelial proliferation, principally of the small vessels. Thus, although occlusion or thrombosis was infrequently found, microinfarcts, particularly in the cerebral cortex and brainstem, were often present, perhaps due to vasculitis on a complex immune basis. Subarachnoid hemorrhage occurred, usually as a terminal event.

Thrombo-Angiitis Obliterans
(von Winiwarter-Bürger Disease)

In 1879, in the gangrenous amputated leg of a man, von Winiwarter found that the arteries and veins had intimal proliferative processes with fibrinous thrombosis and the formation of small vessels. Twenty-nine years later, Bürger described a presenile occlusive vascular disorder of adults which he considered to be of an inflammatory nature. He noted no cerebral involvement, but Cserna in 1926 found evidence of intimal thickening of the cerebral vessels; Jager six years later reported four additional cases. Some investigators considered the vascular changes to be arteriosclerotic, but reporters later confirmed the distinctive character of the lesions. The brains were characterized by diffuse atrophy with whitish, shrunken, tortuous vessels, often filled with vitreous matter in the watershed areas. The larger arteries (e.g., the carotid artery or the middle cerebral artery) were occluded, but the distal arteries had anastomoses. Intermittent paresis, aphasia, and sensory or visual field disturbances were the common clinical findings. A number of toxic and autoimmune factors have been suggested as causative agents.

Takayasu's Disease

The aortic arch syndrome, termed the "pulseless disease," is the result of constriction of any large artery arising from the aorta. While in general, the aortic arch vessels are affected, any large branch may be involved. The condition was described by Davy in 1839; later, Savory and Kussmaul in 1856 independently recognized the syndrome. Takayasu in 1908 described wreath-like anastomotic shunts of arterioles and venules about the optic disc. The surrounding vessels had lumps which moved from day to day. Takayasu made no note of the patient's pulses, but Onishi, discussing a similar case, stated that "no radial pulses were felt . . . and the arms were cold."

The condition occurs much more commonly in women than in men; in the majority of patients, it occurs in the third or fourth decades of life, particularly in persons of Oriental descent.

The disease begins with localized inflammatory lesions producing muscle and joint pains, fever, and debility resulting in weight loss over a period of months or years. More specific neurological manifestations are headache, visual disturbances, sensory alterations, and less often hemiplegia. Retinal microaneurysms and arteriovenous shunts are present in the more advanced cases. Evidence of cerebral vascular insufficiency may result from carotid or brachycephalic stenosis. Strokes, intracerebral hemorrhages, and arterial hypertension are common lethal factors.

The aortic lesions have variously been described depending upon their locus and severity. The pathology consists of a ring around the aortic orifice of an artery either partially or completely occluding the lumen. The lesion may be in an acute, intermediate, or sclerosing state.

Spinal Arachnoiditis

Toward the end of the 19th century, a disorder characterized by progressive sensory and motor paresis and pathologically by sclerotic and cystic meninges with softened areas in the spinal cord was described by Schwartz, who believed it to be a syphilitic affliction. A few years later, in 1903, Spiller reported a cystic arachnoidal mass compressing the spinal cord. Subsequent writers considered this condition to be a chronic spinal arachnoiditis or a chronic inflammatory arachnoidal reaction resulting from injury, chemical irritation, or infection.

10

The Evolution of Neurosurgery

Surgical Care of Head Wounds

The Management of Trauma

Wounds of the head in war and civilian life were common in the 18th and 19th centuries. But only victims of scalp injuries were likely to survive—persons sustaining wounds that penetrated the calvarium and lacerated the cerebral cortex were almost certain to succumb within a few days. The common blunt injuries of the head producing a short period of unconsciousness and a bruise on the scalp were usually handled by the local physician with soothing applications. If a laceration required stitching, a surgeon called in to repair the damage might advise boring the head. Many surgeons believed that all head injuries were potentially serious and advocated trephining to prevent further mischief.

In his book of observations on head injuries, Pott, an avid advocate of prophylactic trephining, devoted practically his entire text to the discussion of lesions of the coverings of the brain (scalp and cranium) and only a few pages on subdural and cerebral wounds. This stemmed from Pott's appreciation that wounds of the brain were hazardous and likely to be fatal. In a book on head injuries a hundred years later, Phelps discussed the damage to the cerebral coverings in less than 10% of the more than 500 pages of text material. The major part of the book dealt with the effects of trauma on the encephalon. No longer was the skull case opened to prevent mischief from blood or purulent matter, but, as Phelps wrote, "the justifiable use of operation in head injury is very limited . . . depressed cranial fractures, uncomplicated epidural hemorrhages and, rarely, subdural lesions." To treat intracranial abscesses and gunshot wounds, the operator explored the brain in as aseptic a field as possible. Surgeons were becoming more conservative as they became aware of the many functions of the cerebral cortex and subcortical ganglia.

Advances in Individual Countries

Perhaps the progress in understanding the disorders of the nervous system was less spectacular than the advances in the basic sciences. Yet, they were essential for the foundations of clinical neurology. These developments occurred in many different countries of the world so that it is expedient to trace their evolution in the individual lands. This does not imply that the advances were made independently; there was much overlapping and integration as the neurosciences evolved.

France

In the 18th century, Paris was the leading medical center of Europe and its main attraction was surgery. Would-be surgeons came to dissect the many cadavers and to see the more than 20,000 patients being publicly demonstrated by a number of great physicians and surgeons. Although practically all French surgeons occasionally operated upon the head, only a few had extensive experience gained in the hospitals of Paris or on the battlefields of Europe. In the 18th century, the common concept of cerebral concussion implied that a blow to the head put the spirits therein in great disarray; however, some surgeons had more practical concepts regarding the loss of consciousness after a cephalic injury. Pourfour du Petit, an army surgeon, believed that coma following a head injury might be the result of compression of the cerebral hemispheres by a blood clot, a condition that should be differentiated from the unconsciousness resulting from concussion. Another surgeon who sharpened his skills on cadavers, Pierre Dionis, asserted that although trephination cured all head injuries in Rome, Avignon, and Versailles, "ils perissent tous à l'Hôtel-Dieu de Paris à cause de l'infection de l'air." Dionis acknowledged that trephining was ordinarily an elective procedure, but admitted that in the case of serious head injuries, it might have to be done promptly. He provided illustrations of his instruments, including some quite modern-looking trephines. Another of the great French surgeons, Jean-Louis Petit, held that, as some of his medical colleagues asserted, trephining was not always fatal. He admitted that a person might recover from a skull fracture without an operation but he taught that "the fracture itself indicates the trephine, not only to elevate any bone that may be depressed and remove splinters, but to give egress to blood collected between the dura and bone." A modern concept! In addition to the broken skull, Petit believed that other signs such as continuing coma, hemorrhage from the mouth, nose, or ears, paralysis, or convulsions indicated the trephine. He did not believe that trephining cured convulsions, but that it removed the cause of the fit. He maintained that an immediate loss of consciousness was evidence of concussion; a delayed coma indicated cerebral compression as the result of extravasation of blood into the extradural, subdural, or intracerebral spaces, a concept that had been recognized but not understood by the Arab surgeons of the 10th century.

A considerable amount of experimentation was being done in the 18th century. Quesnay wrote extensively on head injuries; he drove nails through the brain from side to side, noting that such wounds healed without trouble. He advised trepanning head-injured persons, but not in hospitals because of the "unwholesome state of [the] air." It is interesting to read his comment, made in 1743, that brain tumors might be surgically excised, although Benjamin Bell condemned the suggestion in the next century. A.C. Lorry (1726-1783) made serial punctures of the brainstem in dogs and concluded that the medulla oblongata was the seat of vital functions, thus anticipating M.J.P. Flourens in locating the respiratory center in the medulla. Later, Saucerotte confirmed that hemispheric lesions caused a contralateral paralysis and a compressive blood clot caused similar symptoms. He ascribed opisthotonos, hyperesthesia, and nystagmus to cerebellar lesions and also, but erroneously, forelimb paralysis.

In the 18th century, Littré's famous case of a man who, after a head injury, at autopsy had no evidence of hemorrhage or cerebral compression (although the condition of the cervical cord is not noted) stimulated interest in traumatic unconsciousness. The French Academy in 1760 offered a prize for the best study of this phenomenon. A number of theories were advanced—a transient anemia of the brain, refuted by Witkowski's demonstration that concussion might be induced in a cardiectomized frog, and distortion of the brain shown by movement of threads in the concussed brain—but a satisfactory explanation was not offered. Moreover, the plight of the head-injured was little improved since the infirmaries lacked sanitation and were overcrowded with patients having fresh and draining wounds lying in bed with others having infected, weeping wounds and hacking coughs. It is no wonder that cranial surgery fell into disrepute.

The French Revolution changed the course of operative surgery. Because the army required surgeons, essentially military medical schools were established in Paris, Montpellier, and Strasbourg. Napoleon's plan to develop an institute of medical sciences was introduced in the newly created University of Paris. That military era was dominated by Dominic J. Larrey, who devised the system of "flying ambulances" to treat the wounded on the battlefield. He was followed by G. Dupuytren, a difficult personality but a brilliant operator and fascinating lecturer who became surgeon-in-chief of the Hôtel-Dieu at the age of 38.

In the middle of the 19th century, a number of general surgeons in Paris were writing voluminous treatises on operative surgery. In the company of these giants, Paul Broca, surgeon to the Hôpital Necker, introduced modern neurosurgery. He localized intracranial lesions on the basis of the clinical findings and plotted their location by craniometric techniques. Using such criteria, he operated upon a brain abscess successfully. However, he is most renowned for his localization of the speech area in the left third frontal convolution.

England

In the 18th century, the physicians and surgeons of the British Isles were following independent careers. Although a considerable number of competent physicians practiced, only a few added to the knowledge of neurological disorders. Whytt identified a number of disorders not previously recognized; he described cataplexy or *stupor vigilans*. Periodic headaches (migraine) he considered to be due to a "cephalic sympathy." He discussed a number of other disorders, such as giddiness or vertigo, melancholy, mania, nightmares, and muscular spasms. He is best known, however, for his discussion of hydrocephalus.

Water between the skin and pericranium, and between the pericranium and the skull, Whytt called external hydrocephalus. Those watery collections within the skull—between the skull and dura mater, the two maters, and (the most common) within the ventricles—he termed internal hydrocephalus (dropsy of the cerebral ventricles). He noted that the ancient Greeks and Romans had referred only to water on or beneath the skull but not within the brain. Whytt admitted that later authors—among them Wepfer, Petit, and Le Dran—had recognized internal hydrocephalus but had given summary descriptions; he categorized Le Dran's description as being "in such a manner as would make one believe he had never seen the disease." Whytt gave a clear description of the three stages of the disorder and admitted that he had "never been so lucky as to cure one patient who had those symptoms," probably because most such cases were tuberculous meningitis, which was not identified until Papavoine's description of "arachnitis tuberculeuse" 60 years later.

In addition to this monumental work, a number of lesser lights were illuminating the disorders of the nervous system. Huxham in 1757 noted palatal paralysis in diphtheria, although he ascribed it to "diphscarletina." Fothergill in 1773 wrote an account of facial neuralgia. Pott's description of pressure paralysis of spinal caries, Underwood's report of infantile paralysis or poliomyelitis, and J. Haslam's account of general paresis in 1798 all attested to the interest in the disorders of the nervous system.

In England, until the 18th century, would-be surgeons apprenticed to a practicing operator. In 1763, the first systematic course of lectures on surgery was given at St. Bartholomew's Hospital; the surgeons began instruction at Guy's Hospital in the latter part of that century. Early in the 18th century, William Cheselden gave a course in anatomy in his home and later at St. Thomas Hospital. His success so irked the barber-surgeons that they filed a suit against him for having a corpse in his home. Merely censured, Cheselden continued his teaching at the hospital. His text *Anatomy of the Human Body* was the popular and standard textbook on the subject for years.

The wars of Europe in the late 17th century provided the military surgeons experience in treating cranial wounds; deeper injuries of the brain were dressed and left for nature to take its course. Some surgeons, such as Percivall Pott, realized that the symptoms arising as the result of a head injury were due not to the broken bone, but to the damaged brain. Even by surgeons of that era, this concept was slow to be accepted, for many still thought that spirits motivated the brain and that a blow to the head put them in disarray. Others had a more modern view of the signs and symptoms of a head injury. Harken to the comments of Turner in 1732:

> Of the first sort are stupidity and coma, upon the fall or blow, or a Delirium presently after, hemorrhage or bleeding at the ears or eyes, as well as nose and mouth, vomiting, convulsions, faltering in the speech, and palsy of the limbs—I call these, with some others of the like kind, conjectural signs, because it is very possible the same symptoms may happen to supervene upon concussion only of the brain, with effusion of blood upon its substance, yet without a fracture: Nor is any so truly pathognomonic . . . although the vomiting and sopor give us more especially great suspicion . . .
>
> The real signs, and such as give us indisputable evidence are, if there is no wound, when, by pressing one of the fingers round about the hairy scalp, we find such depression or dent and sinking therein, as lets them in below the surface of other parts of the cranium; and when by such inquiry, the bones being separated, we plainly perceive them to give way, with a crackling under our said fingers, the case is then indubitable.

Crepitation was later applied to the sign.

In the latter part of the 18th century, the treatment of a person who had suffered a head injury with a short period of unconsciousness consisted of bleeding and purging. If the patient's condition was not improving, the skull might be perforated beneath the site of a scalp bruise. If the scalp was lacerated and the underlying bone intact, the scalp was sutured and the patient was bled; if a fracture was present, the trephine was at once applied, matter removed, and the patient bled and purged. This was the routine that Pott used and recorded in 1768. Pott considered that a cracked skull should be trephined to provide free space for blood and discharges as soon as possible, for "the space of time in which it may prove beneficial is very short." The operation was performed not because "the bone was broken . . . [but] the reason . . . springs from other causes . . . the nature of the mischief which the parts within the cranium have sustained." He defined the reasons for operating upon the head-injured person: first, to relieve pressure of extravasated fluid within the head; second, to allow matter between the skull and dura mater to escape; and third, to prevent such complications.

John Hunter began his study of surgery under Pott at St. Bartholomew's Hospital, but served two years as a military surgeon in the Spanish campaign of 1762-1763. Upon his return to London, he carried out research in pathological anatomy and collected specimens which were subsequently housed in the museum named after him. He recognized that cranial fractures alone were not lethal and that the trephine should only be used if the brain was compressed by bone, blood, or pus. Other equally famous surgeons of that era frowned upon an operation for uncomplicated traumatic unconsciousness. Abernethy, in his discussion of injuries of the head, pointed out that fracture of the skull with minimal depression of the bone "does not derange the functions of the brain." However, he admitted that "there are doubtless some depressions of the skull that it would be absurd not to elevate by an immediate operation." Extravasations between the dura mater and the cranium were the only reasons for trephining. Abernethy considered that attempts to evacuate subdural clots offered little chance of relief unless the clot was fluid.

Until the beginning of the 19th century, the treatment of head injuries was judged only by the clinical outcome. Few brains of the victims were examined after death to determine the nature and lethality of the lesion. Morgagni's reports of sanguinous, purulent, or aqueous collections in the extra- or subdural space suggested that they could be drained or evacuated; however, the difficulty in localizing the lesion deterred even brave operators. At that time, the differentiation between cerebral concussion and compression in head-injured patients was difficult, although Bell attempted to distinguish the two by the character of the pulse and respiration. No wonder that at the beginning of the 19th century, Astley Cooper, the most popular surgeon in London, condemned operating on a person with a closed head injury and entertained his attentive clinic by his caustic remark, "If you were to trephine, you ought to be trephined yourself in turn."

This disagreement stemmed from the lack of insight into the basis of traumatic coma and the failure to recognize the septic state of many hospitals at that time. In spite of considerable experimental work by French surgeons, it was not generally accepted that contusion or compression of the brain was responsible for the comatose state. Many, especially army surgeons, attributed coma to a cracked skull, which should be bored and the bony spicules removed. Other surgeons believed that coma was due to blood and debris beneath a fracture. If the dura mater or brain were injured, the outcome was considered serious due to the bad air of hospitals and operating rooms. As a result, in St. Bartholomew's Hospital, where Pott had regularly trephined the head-injured, not a single case was operated on between 1861 and 1867. Yet, in the fresh air of the countryside, broken skulls were bored without ill effects. Surgeons were just beginning to realize the cause of the dreaded complication of infection.

A curious custom—shaving the head—was perpetuated by the belief that removal of thick hair aided in the reduction of the body temperature. "It permits the effective application of the ice-cap, which next to trephination, under indicated conditions, is most nearly a directly curative resource."

By the middle of the 19th century, some surgeons were aware of the effects of bleeding, either within the brain or between its membranes. Hutchinson, in clear language, described the syndrome of an extradural clot due to middle meningeal hemorrhage (previously known but not explicitly described) in these words:

> The importance of an interval of lucidity between the accident and the occurrence of symptoms has long been recognized as the chief indication of a ruptured meningeal artery. Whenever there is clear testimony as to complete immunity at first, and the symptoms have come on suddenly, then we may, with tolerable confidence, infer the existence of hemorrhage. . . . Our inferences as to the side on which the blood clot lies will be helped by observation of the hemiplegia (if it has been present), by the dilation of one pupil, and the examination of the scalp. The hemiplegia will be on the opposite side; a fixed dilated pupil will, I think, generally be present on the same side, and a puffy swelling in the scalp will often be found directly over the fracture.

By the end of the 19th century, the fractured skull was being relegated to a secondary place and primary consideration was given to the condition of the brain and the possibility that increased intracranial pressure might be due to hemorrhage. This raised the question of whether a compressed brain should not be relieved by a decompressive technique, even though a frank hemorrhage might not be present. In the 20th century, this issue was debated in the case of any patient who did not regain consciousness and recover uneventfully.

Germany

Prior to the 15th century, the people of Germany relied upon homespun remedies, charms, and the services of traveling bone-setters for their medical care. The casualties of warfare in the early 16th century were treated by wound surgeons, trained to suture lacerations, set fractures, and amputate limbs. A few, such as Brunschwig and Gersdorff of Strasbourg, had extensive military experience with such wounds. However, 50 years later, Wirtz of Basel criticized the abuses of the wound surgeons and advised soothing applications and suturing of lacerations so that healing might occur by first intention. Wirtz used the cautery only for amputations and advocated compression to stop bleeding of vessels. At the beginning of the next century, Wilhelm Fabry (1560-1624) improved wound surgery by using the tourniquet to arrest bleeding in amputation, but did not advance the treatment of head injuries. He repaired scalp wounds and trephined fractured skulls, but considered lacerations of the brain to be lethal and left them to their fate.

The outstanding German surgeon who brought wound repair into general surgery was Lorenz Heister, born in 1683. After obtaining his medical degree, he served in the Dutch army for a short time. In 1710, he was appointed Professor of Surgery at the University of Altdorf; 10 years later, he went to the University of Helmstedt where he remained until his death. Heister composed a number of clearly written and well-illustrated books on anatomy and surgery which were translated into several languages. One widely circulated book was *A general system of surgery*.

Of wounds of the head, Heister wrote, "No wounds are attended with more danger than those which are inflicted upon the head." Even if the wound appeared to be slight, "we can never promise a cure." Although he considered the state of the bone to be an important issue, he realized that the wound should be dressed carefully to keep it "from the injuries of the air." He trephined to remove bony fragments and to perforate corrupt or fissured bone until bleeding diploë was encountered. Depressed bone had to be raised by an elevator, tripes, or hooked augur or holes drilled in adjacent solid bone and fragments elevated with a chisel. Heister elevated the indented skull of infants (derby hat fracture) by pulling upon a piece of leather glued to the depressed bone; if necessary, an augur might be used to elevate the bone.

An extradural hematoma was well described by Heister in these words:

> It is well known that the bones of the cranium are often fissured and the adjacent blood-vessels, lacerated by external injuries, without any apparent fracture or depressure of them; so that if the extravasated blood be not removed by the trepan, by pressing on the brain it will greatly injure, if not totally destroy its several functions. The consequences of neglecting this instrument in such cases will be restlessness, delirium, convulsions, vertigo, apoplexies, stupidity, with a loss of the senses, speech, and voluntary motion, and, at last, death itself. This instrument therefore ought never to be neglected in urgent cases of this nature.

Heister realized that a bleeding vessel or clot compressing the brain caused pain, loss of consciousness, and death. Consequently, in the case of a head-injured victim suspected of intracranial hemorrhage, the prognosis was guarded. If a senseless person had no external wound, the head should be shaved to inspect the scalp and palpated for soft spots which might indicate swelling or bleeding. The victim might rub a sore spot on one side of the head; if one arm was not moved, it might indicate an injury to the other side of the head. If an injured locus of the scalp was found, such as a bruise or hematoma, some surgeons advised immediately trephining, but Heister waited to see the effects of repeated medical treatment such as clysters, smelling salts, bleeding, or purging. If not effective or if the patient's condition worsened, Heister advised trephining to let out grumous blood. If there seemed to be blood beneath the dura mater, he would carefully incise that membrane. If blood was not found at the first trephining, other holes should be made; Heister cited several authors who had eventually found blood and effected a cure. He recognized that contusions of the brain might be responsible for comatose states similar to those caused by large hemorrhages.

Besides traumatic injuries, Heister discussed a number of other conditions for which the surgeon might operate. Although internal hydrocephalus in newborn babies was generally incurable, fluid between the skull and scalp, diagnosed by softness of the scalp, might be relieved by cathartics, diuretics, and compresses to the swollen head. If conservative measures failed, cupping or scarification was advocated by some surgeons. Heister considered temporal arteriotomy to be a desirable procedure for bleeding when treating diseases of the eye or head such as vertigo, headache, epilepsy, and plethoric states. However, even in these disorders, bleeding should be the last resort.

Heister was quite conservative in treating spinal injuries. He recognized that the spinous processes or laminae might be damaged without injury to the spinal marrow or cord. In such cases, the back should be immobilized with compressed paste-board; healing was rapid. However, if the vertebral body was broken, the spinal marrow was almost always bruised or compressed, causing paralysis of the limbs and viscera below the injury. In such cases, death ensued shortly. Although Heister admitted that some surgeons operated upon fractured vertebrae, removed or replaced the broken bones, cleansed the wound, and applied balsam dressings, he could promise no benefit.

Heister described many causes of wry neck, which he cured by cutting the tight neck muscles near the clavicle and applying digestive ointments as recommended by Roonhuys, Tulpius, Meek'ren, and others. Heister warned that puncturing a nerve might cause a painful and disabling result.

Although French physicians had sparked the advances in medicine in the first part of the 19th century, after the Franco-Prussian War of 1870 new and well-equipped German institutes were built in which neuroscience was advancing.

Italy

In the 18th century, the scientists of Italy were so engaged in cultural activities that medical advances were limited. Early in the century, Antonio Pacchioni (1665-1726) described the granulations along the cerebral sinuses to which his name has been given. Antonio M. Valsalva, at the same time, was defining the air sinuses of the cranium which adjoin the intracranial cavity.

The greatest contribution to understanding the nervous system of that time was made by Giovanni Morgagni (1682-1771), who received his medical education at Padua in Italy. His later studies were made at the autopsy table, not just to discover diseased parts but to correlate clinical symptoms of the patient with the postmortem findings. His painstaking reports were compiled and published in 1761. In this monumental work, *De sedibus et causis morborum per anatomen indagatis*, he integrated neurological syndromes with the autopsy findings. With his special interest in vascular disease, Morgagni described extradural and subdural hematomas, aneurysms with or without subarachnoid hemorrhage, and intracerebral hemorrhages. Apoplexy, he stated, was of two types, one with blood in the brain (sanguinous) and the other with serum in or about the brain (serous). The first of these, he considered to be the result of bleeding from the choroid plexus into the ventricles or brain. The second, which he said was characterized by excessive serum in the brain, caused ill-defined and heterogeneous disorders, some now considered related to heart disease and some to various disturbances of the brain such as infarction, meningitis, epileptic seizures, or cerebral embolism. He denied, as previously thought, that apoplexy was a diseased condition of the cerebral substance, but maintained that it was primarily due to changes in the blood vessels. Subdural hematomas were known to Morgagni, who wrote: "When the cranium was open'd, I found and demonstrated blood effused to the quantity of half a pound, betwixt the dura and pia mater; or rather between the dura mater and another little membrane which membrane, being made somewhat thick with extravasated blood."

Morgagni confirmed that paralysis was caused by a cerebral lesion on the opposite side of the brain, that a cerebral syphilitic gumma simulated a tumor, that suppuration within the brain was often a sequela of middle ear disease (not the reverse as previously thought), and that postmortem examination of the entire body was a valuable aid to the physician.

Although Morgagni was particularly interested in vascular disease, he wrote of many other neurological subjects, especially head injuries and brain wounds. His clinicopathological approach was not accepted at first, but as its value was appreciated, physicians began to include pathological findings in their discussions of cases. As a result, the examination of the brain became a routine part of a case report. Thus, Matthew Baillie in 1793, using beautiful illustrations by William Clift, presented pathology as an independent subject.

In the latter part of the 18th century, Italian scientists were intrigued by the electrical stimulation of nervous tissue. Leopoldo Caldani (1725-1813), professor of anatomy at Bologna and later at Padua, studied the effect of electrical charges upon the spinal cord and the cerebral cortex, noting the production of convulsive movements. Other investigators (e.g., Luigi Rolando) also reported such responses, but the results were probably due to the spread of current to the peripheral musculature. However, Galvani had demonstrated animal electricity generated by the contact of muscle with metal, or two dissimilar metals.

Frapoli in 1771 described the course of the nutritional deficiency giving rise to pellagra. Domenico Cotugno (1736-1822) in 1774 noted the fluid about the spinal cord. Since his report was published under another title, the discovery was not widely recognized until Magendie's paper on the subject some 50 years later.

Spain

At the time of the Renaissance, many great universities sprang up in the cities of Europe. In Spain, the University of Salamanca was founded in 1243 and a century later the school at Valladolid. In 1550, at the latter university, which was considered at a par for surgical training with the schools at Montpellier and Bologna, the first chair of anatomy was established. Cranial and spinal surgery advanced when B. Hidalgo de Aguero introduced a dry method ("via particular") for treating wounds so that they would heal without suppuration. Only in the case of depressed skull fractures, which he considered dangerous, would he trephine within a day or two of injury. Hidalgo de Aguero's technique was first to clean the wound, wash it well with lukewarm water and, rather than applying an ointment of egg-white or using the cautery, put on a dry dressing. Wounds made by cutting instruments, he asserted, would heal primarily or with the application of "digestives." He advised against stretching or separating the scalp from the underlying pericranium, although he drained the wound to let out bloody fluids. Thus, Hidalgo de Aguero favored the dry treatment of simple wounds and elevated depressed fractures, but was opposed to the indiscriminate use of the trephine in fracture cases.

This conservative treatment was not practiced by some other Spanish surgeons of that time. Francisco Arceo of Guadalupe, Mexico, wrote a book on wounds in 1574, which went through several editions and was translated into four other languages. He recognized that superficial scalp lacerations might heal by primary intention. If complicated by cranial fractures with other problems such as meningeal tears and hematomas, they required trephining. Arceo was aware that fractures and contusions might occur without an external wound.

Andrés Alcazár studied medicine in Salamanca but practiced in Guadalajara. In his *Chirurgiae libri sex,* published in 1575, he discussed the neurological abnormalities produced by head injuries in considerable detail. He used a trephine with a coronal guard (abapriston) to prevent plunging when he had penetrated the skull. Based upon an extensive army experience, Dionisio Daza Chacón wrote a book entitled *Practica y teorico de cirurgia,* which is said to contain the richest personal experience of that age. He advised trephining all hematomas and abscesses and all cases of dural penetration by bony fragments, for he considered medical measures to be ineffective. However, he realized the dangers of operating upon such patients, especially those with extensive fractures or in poor general condition. Some surgeons were quite conservative in the treatment of head wounds, but a number of prominent Spanish surgeons—Cristobal of Montemayer, Arceo, Alcazar, and Daza Chacón—trephined head injuries.

In the 17th century, the practice of medicine in Spain, as in other European countries, was changing. Bitter dissension between the erudite surgeons of the long robe and the barbers of the short robe almost eliminated the surgeons. New colleges of surgery, quite independent of the universities, were being established by royal decree—the Colegio Real de San Carlos in Madrid, the Colegio Real de Cirugia de Barcelona (1748), and the Colegio Real de Cirugia de Cadiz—all with professors trained in Italian and French medical centers. As a result, the Spanish surgeons were becoming more conservative in the treatment of head injuries. Ribes at the San Carlos University in Madrid maintained that the evacuation of intracranial blood was the only reason to trephine.

In 1723, Juan de Roda y Bayas discussed the treatment of cranial wounds, noting their gravity and the seriousness of the usual forms of treatment. It is of interest that he referred to a report of Hidalgo de Aguero concerning 436 casualties with only 20 deaths, but it is not clear if these were all head wounds and, if so, their degree of brain involvement.

Although great advances were being made in medicine during the 19th century in Europe and in the United States, Diego de Argumosa, the first professor of surgery at Burgos and later at San Carlos in Madrid, admitted in 1856 that trephining, abused in the previous century, had fallen into unwarranted disuse. As a result, compressive lesions of the brain due to depressed bone, blood, pus, or tumor (exostoses or fungi), which should have been surgically handled, were being neglected. It required a number of medical discoveries in the last half of the 19th century (e.g., anesthesia and aseptic techniques) to revive surgical practice.

Perhaps the first chair of neurological surgery was established in 1895 at Madrid for Manuel Otero Acevado, who studied with Chipault in Paris and Jaboulay in Lyon. In 1898, he was named "Professor de Cirugia Nerviosa" at the University of Madrid. His interests were in the peripheral and vegetative nervous systems.

Japan

About the 7th century AD, the early indigenous medical cults of Japan were being replaced by Chinese health practitioners who thought in terms of yang and yin, and whose therapies consisted of herbs, acupuncture, and moxibustion. But these Chinese practices, introduced by traveling medicine men, gradually were lost as the result of civil war and apathy of the people. So for almost a thousand years, the Japanese peasants received folk remedies for their colds and gastrointestinal upsets. Wounds and fractures were treated as the Chinese and later the Hindus practiced. Not until the arrival of Portuguese traders in the south of Japan in the 16th century did a few Iberian medical missionaries bring herbal and arboreal medicines and introduce medical and surgical European practices. As trade relations were established, the writings of Paré, and later of Heister, were translated into Japanese. Unfortunately, the Japanese Shogunate government banned trade with outside countries in 1587. Although a few local Japanese physicians continued to practice the new therapies, medicine in general remained at a low level. For 200 years contact with the outside world was limited and information on Western medical advances was nonexistent. Occasionally an autopsy on a beheaded criminal was permitted; from such exhibits, Japanese physicians and medical students became aware that their old texts had many errors. In 1771 Sugita, using a copy of *Tafel anatomia* (a Dutch text written by J.A. Kalmus in 1647), noted the many fallacies of the older Japanese works on anatomy. As a result, Kalmus' treatise and the surgery of Heister were translated into Japanese. However, there was no evidence that disorders of the nervous system were described at that time. It was not until 1859 that the Japanese government permitted a limited public dissection of a beheaded man in Nagasaki. But again, the brain and spinal cord were not examined. However, under the Meiji regime, autopsies were allowed and a crude form of surgery became common. Until the latter part of the 19th century, the brain was considered sacred and untouchable, although scalp and skull wounds were debrided and sutured. As further evidence of the sanctity of the brain, a paper by Hashimoto published in 1885 on surgical practices in Japan makes no reference to brain surgery. However, it must be admitted that at that time, even in the Western countries, surgery on the head was largely confined to repair of wounds, usually of the scalp and skull.

The first Japanese reference to trephining and debridement of an infected war wound was in 1877. In the Japanese-Chinese war of 1894, the mortality rate from head wounds was 57.3%—about the same as that on the European battlefields at that time.

At the beginning of the 20th century, Japanese surgeons with anesthesia and aseptic techniques began to operate on the brain for epilepsy, localizing the focus either by a scalp scar or by the signature of a focal or Jacksonian seizure. The Russo-Japanese war of 1904-1905 gave an impetus to surgery on the brain with better technical and instrumental techniques.

Keiji Sano states that in Japan the first brain tumor diagnosed on the basis of clinical findings was resected in 1907 by H. Miyaka, who, in discussing the case, pointed out that the slow progress in brain tumor surgery was not lack of technical skill but difficulty in determining where to operate. For that reason, surgery on the brain in Japan did not advance rapidly until radiographic methods of localizing lesions with ventricular air were introduced.

Russia

Until the 9th century, medical care in Russia consisted of folk and herbal remedies. In those days, the Russian people were so healthy, according to W. M. von Richter, that physicians were not needed. Therefore, priests and secular friends tended to the common ailments of the peasants. Foreign physicians brought in to care for the nobility, if unsuccessful, were condemned to death—a practice which did not make the profession more attractive. Epidemics such as the bubonic plague of 1348-1351 decimated the population. When the practice of medicine was being stimulated by the introduction of printing in the Mediterranean countries, Russia suffered from a dearth of publications. The first Russian medical books described hydrotherapy and herbal medicine in the beginning of the 17th century. Czar Feodor in 1654 established a five-year course to train physicians, mainly to provide surgeons for the army; however, it was soon abandoned. A half century later, Peter the Great erected a military hospital and medical school, which stimulated the development of medical services in several Russian centers. A few medical texts of the ancient physicians, including Hippocrates' *Aphorisms*, were printed. In order to obtain better trained medical men, Peter the Great sent a number of Russian students to Padua for training and imported German and Dutch surgeons for the military services. In spite of this, in the next 70 years during the succession of a number of rulers, medical practice declined. During the reign of Catherine II, some hospitals were established, but even at these centers the quality of the medical care was "shocking." There were five university medical centers, but in general the training was poor. Only at the Medical Academy founded in 1835, where the brighter students were trained, was the teaching at all satisfactory. Unfortunately, the Russian people, bankrupted by the Napoleonic and Crimean Wars, hampered by the ruling despots, and lacking the stimulus of enlightened teachers, were not enthused by the medical advances in the other countries of Europe and regarded the medical profession with disgust and scorn.

Although occasional operations were performed on the brain by Russian general surgeons in the 19th century, surgery of the nervous system was not championed by Pirogoff, the outstanding St. Petersburg surgeon. Yet, as interest in surgery of the brain and spinal cord increased, monographs were written on the subject by Russian surgeons in the late 1890s. Perhaps the most innovative advance came from the development of a stereotactic instrument for locating the cortical fissures and subcortical ganglia of the brain. This guide was devised in the late 1880s by D.N. Zernov, professor of anatomy at Moscow University. In 1889, he demonstrated his encephalometer, which consisted of an aluminum basal ring fastened to the skull by ear plugs and skull pins in a nasion-inion horizontal plane. Equatorial and meridian arches provided a means of determining polar coordinates based upon an encephalometric map of the cranial sutures, cortical sulci, and certain subcortical structures. Zernov's pupil, Altunov, made maps so that adjustments could be made for brachio-cephalic and dolichocephalic heads of different sizes. In 1907, Rossolimo de-vised a modified form termed a "brain topograph" which consisted of a hemi-sphere with perforations at intervals and mounted on a base. The convexity of the hemisphere was marked by lines indicating the major sulci so that an exploring needle could be passed through a perforation to any desired cortical or subcortical point. Although Rossolimo wrote that the instrument was used successfully, it apparently was abandoned when large bone flaps were reflected, exposing an extensive cortical surface. The Horsley-Clarke technique was introduced more than 10 years later.

Fat Emboli and Neurosurgical Trauma

When the Hippocratic physicians wrote in discussing fractures, "convul-sions are more apt to occur if reduction takes place," they were probably refer-ring to fat emboli, although not recognized as such. Centuries later, in 1672, Richard Lower found fat globules obstructing many of the pulmonary vessels of a crush victim. The first recognized case of cerebral fat emboli was reported by Wagner in 1865. In 1878, Czerny described the clinical picture of cerebral fat emboli (confusion, drowsiness, hyperthermia, focal motor symptoms or signs, and coma) and emphasized the importance of ophthalmoscopic exami-nation of the retinae in confirming the diagnosis. At the beginning of the next century, Hamig reported that lipuria may occur without cerebral symptoms. In 25% of such patients, there is a free interval of hours or days before the clinical manifestations appear. In 1880, Scriba described fat emboli in the cerebral ves-sels along with petechial hemorrhages and ischemic foci in the white matter. Although emboli usually occur after blunt trauma to the head produces frac-tures and soft tissue injury, they may complicate many other conditions (e.g., sickle cell anemia, burns, acute infections, and electroconvulsive therapy), par-ticularly in the young and the old.

Repair of Cranial Defects—Cranioplasty

Although skull boring was a common practice in some tribes, apparently, for an unknown reason, at times the defect was repaired. In Peruvian calvaria, defects in the skull have been found with gourds, portions of shell or bones, as well as beaten gold or silver filling the holes on occasion. That the patient sur-vived the plating is indicated by the osseous proliferation about the margins of the graft. In some South Sea islands, coconut shell was used to repair cranial defects, although the mortality rate of the operation was as high as 50%. In the Middle Ages in Europe, unscrupulous surgeons pretended to put the precious metal provided by their patients for repair of the cranial defect in the hole, but dropped it into their own pockets. Religious bigotry of that time was also present; in 1670, a skull defect in a Russian was repaired with a piece of bone taken from a dog's skull, but the ecclesiastical nobility decreed that the bone of a dog was not befitting the head of a Christian gentleman, and so under threat of excommunication, the graft was removed. With the advent of anesthesia and aseptic techniques, repair of skull defects using various types of graft gained favor. Autogenous bone was transposed to cover the defect. Periosteal flaps were slid into place and the donor site closed or allowed to granulate in. Many extracranial bones were used to repair the cranial defect; tibial osteoperiosteal grafts, ribs, ilia, and scapulae all had proponents for a time, but there were dis-advantages of each, including inadequate donor bone and fracture at the donor site. Autogenous bone was preserved and subsequently reimplanted in the skull. In World Wars I and II, many heteroplastic grafts were used as metals of the desired consistency and strength to be shaped to the contour of the skull became available.

Surgical Management of Brain Tumors

Although tumors of various types were known to the Greek and Roman physicians, there is no evidence that they were aware of such lesions in the brain. In fact, ancient peoples so confused the manifestations of intracranial neoplasms with parasitic infestations and infections that the earliest growths were probably lost among the phrenitides. Isolated reports of brain tumors in the ancient literature are vague; unless they caused an unsightly cranial defor-mity, it was not until autopsies became common in the 16th century that tumors were recognized. Even after the legalization of autopsies, the brain was rarely examined. If a mass was found, it could be inspected only by the naked eye and so was usually considered to be an inflammatory lesion of tuberculous or syphilitic origin and, much less commonly, neoplastic. In 1761, Morgagni in *De sedibus* classified masses in the brain as either inflammatory or sarcomatous, the latter being the general term for a fleshy tumor. After that time, although pathologists recognized the neoplastic nature of some brain masses, clinicians still classified brain tumors as vascular, parasitic, diathetic or constitutional (cancerous, syphilitic, or tubercular), and traumatic. Even the early pathologists, who used the microscope to examine specimens hardened by chromic acid, cut into thin sections on microtome, and stained with carmine, described cerebral masses as inflammatory or sarcomatous. Sarcomatous masses consisted mainly of the parenchymatous cerebral growths, which later would be called gliomas.

The symptoms of brain tumors were myriad. This stemmed from two main factors: first, until the latter part of the 18th century, the cerebral hemispheres were considered to be equipotential, so that manifestations of a cerebral distur-bance had no localizing significance, and second, all lesions of the brain were considered to be inflammatory in nature, either tubercular or syphilitic, and so were treated medically before the possibility of a neoplasm was considered. This meant that all subjects not responding to such therapy were in a severely debilitated state by the time a new growth was suspected. Because the outlook for a person with a cerebral neoplasm was so bleak, even if operated upon, surgical intervention was rarely recommended. As a result, even a patient harboring a benign tumor was considered to have a cancer and nature was allowed to take its course.

It was not until the 17th century, when autopsies became common, that an occasional brain tumor was

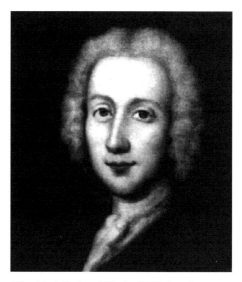

Fig. 10-1. Robert Whytt of Edinburgh (1714-1766). (From the National Library of Medicine)

disclosed which pathologists considered operable. Although Willis had listed headaches, seizures, and coma as signs of a brain tumor, a century passed before doctors ventured to make such a diagnosis. Morgagni in 1761 wrote of their symptomatology and demonstrated that some extracerebral neoplasms were easily removed—at least, at autopsy. The difficulties in diagnosing and localizing such lesions were formidable obstacles for the surgeon. In a 1768 publication, Whytt (Fig. 10-1) wrote that vomiting and headaches often heralded a tumor within the head, and others shortly emphasized that persistent, intolerable headaches might be due to an intracranial neoplasm. That the first evidence of some brain tumors was a seizure or convulsion was known to Morgagni. In the early 19th century, a number of writers discussed the occurrence of seizures as the first manifestation of a brain tumor. After the demonstration by Macewen and the Maida Vale physicians that a tumor causing focal convulsions might be excised, surgeons were encouraged to explore the brain of convulsing patients; unfortunately, neither finding a tumor nor relieving the epilepsy was common.

The only objective finding indicative of a brain tumor was the swelling of the optic disc caused by the increased intracranial pressure. Although long known that the eye was the window to the brain, it required the ophthalmoscope, invented by Helmholtz in 1851, to reveal the optic disc. Two years later, Türck observed that the papilla was swollen when the pressure within the calvarium was increased as the result of a brain tumor. Von Graefe called the condition "Staungspapilla" and differentiated it from papillitis resulting from inflammation of the nerve head. Schwalbe in 1869 showed that the subarachnoid space extended about the optic nerve, the sheath of which was distended by cerebrospinal fluid under pressure, and the central retinal vessels, especially the veins, were compressed. The view was generally accepted that the swollen disc was due to elevated intracranial pressure obstructing the venous return.

However, in the 19th century, it was recognized that these clinical evidences of a brain tumor might also occur in the course of a number of other disorders of the brain. At that time, many mass lesions found in the intracranial cavity were of an inflammatory nature due to tuberculosis, syphilis, or pyogenic organisms causing abscesses. A significant number were the result of such parasitic infestations as hydatid cysts and cysticercosis. Consequently, less than half of the lesions were neoplastic. As the achromatic microscope was just being developed, the identification of these tumors as benign or malignant rested upon the gross appearance of the mass; a fleshy or infiltrating lesion was considered a sarcoma. Because of this, the pathological reports of brain tumors in the early 19th century are open to question.

The localization of cerebral lesions at that time was vitiated by the prevailing concept that the cerebral cortex was inexcitable and equipotential. There was increasing evidence around this time in favor of focal cortical function. Consider that Robert Todd, seeking the locus which might give rise to minor epileptic episodes, noted upon stimulating the cerebral cortex "nothing like convulsions but slight convulsive movements of the muscles of the face" such as "caused by the stimulus of galvanism acting upon the nerves of the face." In France, neurologists, stimulated by Dax of Montpellier, Bouillaud of Paris, and Broca of aphemia fame, were propounding that speech mechanisms were localized in the left inferior precentral convolution. The proof that there was a cortical localization of function came when Fritsch and Hitzig showed that the frontal cortex of dogs could be excited to produce discrete movements of the limbs and if that area of cortex were excised on one side, a paralysis of the opposite limbs resulted. This was further confirmed by Ferrier's studies of the cortical excitability of primates three years later. Using faradic current, he showed that muscular responses could be elicited by stimulating the parietal, precentral, superior temporal, and parietal cortices, but most readily, the precentral gyrus, his "motor-region." As a result of these studies, Ferrier placed the cortical center for vision in the supramarginal and angular gyri, hearing in the superior temporosphenoidal convolutions, touch in the hippocampal formation, smell in the cornu ammonis, and taste nearby.

These early studies of the localization of function were handicapped by poor techniques to assess the sensory modalities and the lack of anatomical verification of the lesions. As a result, more refined studies modified some of Ferrier's conclusions.

To localize the excitable zone on the overlying human scalp required mapping the Rolandic fissure based upon surface landmarks. Broca used a flexible square, one arm of which passed just below the nose and the other was passed at a right angle to the external auditory canal. The other arm at right angles ran over the vertex to the opposite ear. This latter line was a rough approximation to the location of the underlying Rolandic fissure. In 1878, Lucas Championniere devised the first of a number of more accurate guides to that fissure. His appliance was based upon the midline from the nasion to the inion. At a point two centimeters posterior to its midpoint, another line was drawn at an angle of 67 degrees laterally to indicate the site of the Rolandic fissure. Subsequently, a number of elaborate schemas were devised to mark on the scalp the cortical surface sulci. When large bone flaps were reflected later, such systems were no longer necessary and so were abandoned.

Using such landmarks, the surgeon could define the site of a brain lesion. However, the signs of a brain tumor might be mimicked by other afflictions of the brain. Gowers pointed out that two states were likely to lead to diagnostic errors. One was a systemic disorder such as anemia, kidney disease, or lead poisoning. The second was a disturbance of brain function such as hemiplegia or idiopathic seizures. In the differential diagnosis, the mode of development of the symptoms was important, for tumors usually had a slow course and rarely a sudden or rapid onset, such as that characterized by vascular disease or infections of the brain. In the 19th century, general paresis of the insane was sufficiently common to require consideration. If the typical picture was tremor of the lips and face, expansive delirium without headache, optic neuritis, or vomiting, a course of mercury was given. Chronic cerebritis or encephalitis (now considered a viral infection) could be ruled out by such a therapeutic regime. Several acute disorders (e.g., cerebral aneurysm, brain abscess, and meningitis) required long observation of the disorder. Tuberculomas and parasitic infestations might be suspected if there was evidence of pulmonary or abdominal disease. When considering these conditions, the neurologists of the 19th century prescribed mercury rubs for a therapeutic test in all patients. As a result, the patient often was blind and in dire straits before a diagnosis of brain tumor was seriously entertained.

Tumors of the Skull

Because cranial neoplasms caused erosion or proliferation of the involved bone, evidence of their presence remained long after death of the individual. On that basis, Moodie identified cranial tumors of prehistoric man and illustrated the abnormalities in such age-old skulls. In the Middle Ages, tumors of the base of the skull producing obvious facial deformity were mentioned by a number of writers; Veiga in 1506 referred to such a tumorous lesion. When surgery became common, cranial tumors causing facial disfigurement were operated upon in the 18th and 19th centuries, particularly by such French surgeons as Petit and Delbeau. The osteomas causing facial deformities most commonly arose in or about the frontal, ethmoidal, or maxillary sinus and less commonly elsewhere. They might be asymptomatic or compromising air-containing structures, vessels, or nerves, causing various complaints. Tumors at the base of the skull frequently involved cranial nerves producing sensory or visual disturbances. A number of rarer bone tumors—osteoid-osteomas, fibromas, and chondromas—have been reported. These skull tumors have been attributed to an embryonal, traumatic, or infectious etiology.

Bony tumors of the crown of the head, when of appreciable size, were quite disfiguring even after death. Malpighi and Morgagni described a number of such cranial growths later called "osteoma," a term suggested by Hooper in 1826. They were often a manifestation of an underlying tumor of the meninges.

Extracerebral Tumors

Some tumors peculiar to the intracranial cavity were attached to the coverings of the brain. Because they often infiltrated and stimulated the adjacent bone to proliferate, calvarial thickenings have been identified by paleopathologists in prehistoric skulls. Other tumors arising at the base of the brain eroded or absorbed the adjacent bone as they grew; the effects were still apparent in skulls examined centuries after the death of the individual. Such changes were quite obvious if the tumor was in a confined space such as the sella turcica or the internal auditory meatus. Occasionally, a calcified tumor often attached to the skull was found within the cranial cavity.

In the Renaissance period, as autopsies became frequent, thickenings and masses attached to the coverings of the brain, called "fungus durae matris," were described. Many were neoplastic, although other lesions, mainly inflammatory, were included in that designation. At the beginning of the 19th century, Richard Bright described a lobulated fungating tumor arising from "the arachnoid lining the dura mater." Four years later, Cruveilhier called these new growths "tumeurs fungueuse" or "tumeurs cancereuses des meninges." However, the malignant nature of these lesions was questioned by Lebert, who first stated that he had only found fibroblastic elements, but later admitted that some lesions were cancerous. He believed that the benign tumors arose from the membranes at the base of the skull, but physicians were uncertain of their classification. Virchow agreed with Lebert that the fungus durae matris was noncancerous and that brain-sand tumors (psammomas) were benign, but he believed that the larger tumors were sarcomatous. At about the same time, Wilhelm His defined the lining membrane of cavities which arose from mesenchymal cells as endothelium rather than epithelium. Accordingly, Golgi, who was interested in tumors with psammoma bodies, suggested that they be called endotheliomas. This term appealed to the pathologists of Europe, who adopted the designation with the qualifying term "dural." However, when endothelial tumors other than those arising from the meninges were described, the term "dural endothelioma" was questioned.

Although the dural origin of these tumors had been assumed, evidence was accumulating that the pacchionian bodies were of leptomeningeal derivation. Rainey, Luschka, and others had favored this origin before Key and Retzius in 1876. So when Cleland of Glasgow in 1864 demonstrated that two small psammomatous tumors were easily dislodged from the dura mater, he called them "villous tumors of the arachnoid," for he thought that they originated from

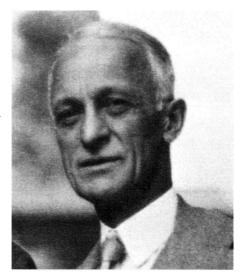

Fig. 10-2. Harvey W. Cushing (1869-1939). (From the collection of A. Earl Walker)

the pacchionian granulations. Some 40 years later, M.B. Schmidt of Strassburg stated that the cellular structure of small meningeal tumors resembled that of the endothelial cells of the arachnoidal villi and that the same psammomatous concretions were seen in such tumors and in the brains of the elderly.

Although these tumors in the 19th century were called fungus durae matris, psammomas, sarcomas, or endotheliomas, Harvey Cushing (Fig. 10-2) coined a noncommittal name for them—meningioma. He recognized that they could be subdivided into various histological types such as psammomatous or meningotheliomatous.

When operative excisions became common, neurosurgeons noted that these tumors seemed to have certain sites of predilection. Cushing and Eisenhardt, in particular, categorized the common topographical site of the meningeal tumors; prior to their monograph, few such distinctions had been made.

In the posterior fossa, the majority of meningeal tumors were found in the region of the cerebellopontine angle or "lateral recess," but their differentiation from acoustic nerve tumors was difficult. It was not until histological confirmation was possible that the nature of recess tumors could be certain. The same difficulty arose with parasellar tumors. It was probably Krogius in 1896 who reported a meningeal tumor involving the gasserian ganglion, although the sketch of that tumor suggested that it arose in the middle fossa. A few years later, Dercum, Keen, and Spiller reported on a tumor of that region which was probably an endothelioma, although it may have been a neurinoma. The first meningeal tumor of the suprasellar region was found at autopsy in

1899 by James Stewart. Later, these tumors having a characteristic clinical history were reported with greater frequency.

Most early tumors of the base of the frontal lobe were considered sarcomas. Cruveilhier termed a case "tumeur cancereuse" in 1835 and Cleland found a case in a cadaver being dissected and reported it as a "villous tumor of the arachnoid." The earliest case to be treated surgically was that of a 35-year-old woman, who in 1885 consulted Francesco Durante because of memory impairment, change of personality, and loss of smell in the left nostril for a year or more.

Suspecting a left frontal tumor, Durante made an osteoplastic frontal bone flap and scooped out a lobular tumor about the size of an apple. Because the tumor had penetrated the left cribriform plate, Durante inserted a drain through the left nostril and closed the wound. A cerebrospinal fluid leak stopped after a short time, and the patient was well for almost 12 years, when she had a recurrence and underwent reoperation. The tumor was diagnosed as a "fibrosarcoma." Subsequent operations for such olfactory groove tumors were infrequently reported.

Tumors of the optic nerve sheath were rare and even when exposed, it was difficult to decide if they were primarily of the orbital or intracranial cavities. One of the earliest was reported by Pagenstecher and illustrates this dilemma. The patient, a 30-year-old woman, underwent the removal of an eye, presumably for a psammomatous meningioma involving the optic nerve. Twenty-five years later, another operation was performed in this patient for a recurrence in the orbit, at which time a walnut-sized intraorbital tumor was removed and the foramen cauterized. Unfortunately, meningitis caused an early death. An autopsy revealed a "hazel-nut" sized tumor within the skull extending from the optic foramen. An even earlier case was reported by Dusaussy in 1875. The patient was a 50-year-old man, blind in the left eye from an unknown cause, whose eye had been proptosing for six years. An exenteration was carried out and a chestnut-sized tumor was removed in one piece. A cerebrospinal fluid leak developed and death from meningitis ensued. A residual tumor the size of a large bean was found encircling the nerve within the skull; it was diagnosed as an "angioblastic sarcoma."

Fungating tumors developing on the lateral convexity of the intracranial cavity often had an overlying cranial deformity indicative of their presence. Such tumors of the lateral sphenoidal ridge (pterional tumors), with a thickening of the overlying bone suggesting leontiasis ossea or osteitis deformans, were usually slow growing. One patient operated upon by Horsley was well 12 years later. Global pterional tumors are often much larger than their symptomatology would suggest. In 1731, Caspart described and illustrated such a tumor in his dissertation. He speculated upon the possibility of surgical excision of these masses. In 1879, Bramwell wrote of an extensive sarcoma of the dura mater without evidence of paralysis.

Parasagittal tumors were fairly common, but often were difficult to remove surgically. An early case was reported by Bright in 1831 in which the tumor was adherent on the right side along the anterior four inches of the longitudinal sinus. Henschen described a bilateral parasagittal tumor in a woman who had a spindle cell sarcoma partially removed by Lennander of Upsala in 1893. Three years later, the patient died and a tumor was found in the area of the sinus. In 1922, Cushing proposed the term "parasagittal meningiomas" for these tumors, which frequently had a history of Jacksonian seizures beginning in the foot or leg and a progressive spastic paresis of the leg.

Hyperostotic convexity swellings described as fungus durae matris, hemicraniosis, or perforating skull tumors were obvious lesions. Kaufman in his dissertation described such a case, in which Heister applied caustic lime with a fatal result. A quarter of a century later, Olaf Acrel operated upon another case which also ended fatally. In 1774, Louis reviewed the fungating tumors of the dura mater.

Peritorcular Tumors

Peritorcular tumors lay along the lateral sinus and were hazardous operative risks because of their vascular involvement. When aseptic surgery became the accepted practice and progressive paresis and focal epilepsy were recognized as indicating a tumor of the convexity of the brain, the surgical exposure was bloody and traumatic to the adjacent brain. Hence, excision of these tumors, because of their late diagnosis and large size, carried a high incidence of mortality. If the patient survived, the long-term result was often satisfactory in terms of seizures and the neurological condition of the patient. The earliest reported operation for a peritorcular tumor was carried out on March 4, 1887 by Birdsall and Weir. The patient's history of homonymous hemianopsia, "neuroretinitis," and unsteady gait predicted the site of the lesion at the occipital pole. It was attached to the tentorium, where bleeding could not be controlled even with packing, and the patient died within a few hours. The second case, reported in 1906 by Oppenheim and Krause, involved a mass which Krause (Fig. 10-3) successfully removed.

Tumors of the Cerebral Hemispheres

It is impossible to say with certainty who described the earliest neoplasms of the cerebral hemispheres because, until the latter part of the 19th century, all varieties of space-occupying lesions—tumors, cysts, abscesses, granulomas, and metastases—were classified as brain tumors. In isolated cases, these lesions could be identified with reasonable certainty, but many were so vaguely described that their nature cannot be ascertained. However, as most were

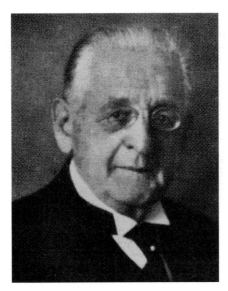

Fig. 10-3. Fedor Krause (1857-1937). (From A History of Neurosurgery. *Greenblatt SH, Dagi TF, Epstein M, editors. Park Ridge, Ill: American Association of Neurological Surgeons, 1997, p 468)*

treated with mercury rubs and potassium iodide for some time on the suspicion of syphilis, the hope of successful treatment of a neoplastic lesion was dismal. Prior to the localization of the motor cortex in 1870, surgeons who were bold enough to open the skull would only operate if there was external evidence such as a hyperostosis or scalp scar of a lesion.

In a treatise on diseases of the nervous system published in 1871, Hammond of New York discussed the treatment of brain tumors without mentioning the possibility of surgical intervention. On the other side of the Atlantic, an English physician stated, "The symptoms connected with tumours of the brain are very obscure . . . giddiness, headache, sickness, convulsions and blindness." Although a reference is made to one patient being cured, no indication of surgical treatment was made.

At that time, tumors of the brain were described in generic terms as infectious (syphilis or tuberculosis), sarcomatous, carcinomatous, fibrous, parasitic (cysticercosis or echinococcosis), or mixed (i.e., vascular tumors, cholesteatomas, or neuromas). When the interstitial cells of the nervous system were defined by von Kölliker and Dieters, von Monakow noted that they resembled the cells of certain previously described infiltrating tumors of the brain. As these tumors were of varied morphological structure, von Monakow recognized that they could be classified on the basis of their consistency. He called the hard and infiltrating glial tumors "glioma durum." Golgi concluded that these interstitial cells, which he called astrocytes, made up the firm tumors. However, this cell type was variously described as radiating or stellate cells by von Kölliker, fibrous astrocytes by Dieters, brush cells by Bell, and spider cells by Jastrowitz. As a result, such tumors were called gliomas by Golgi in 1884, astromas by von Lenhossek in 1895, amebic giant cell gliomas by Lotmar, and astrocytomas by later pathologists. The other common type of brain tumor—soft, cellular, often necrotic, and infiltrating—general pathologists referred to as sarcomas or, if considered as infiltrating glial tumors, they were designated generically as malignant gliomas.

When metallic impregnations were developed in the late 19th century, these soft infiltrating tumors were found to be composed of various cell types. Some were characterized by a perivascular irradiation of the tumor cells which contained blepharoplasts. Besold considered these tumors to be a perithelioma or sarcoma but later they were shown to be of ependymal origin and called ependymomas. Another brain tumor composed of small, regularly arranged cells was recognized as a distinct type by Robertson in 1900, who called the primary cell a "mesoglia." Rio del Hortega in 1921 named this cell type oligodendroglia, and tumors composed of such small cells with round, darkly staining nuclei, faintly staining cytoplasm, and delicate protoplasmic cell processes were called oligodendrogliomas.

In the 20th century, further subgroups were described, such as medulloblastomas and spongioblastomas, and a number of classifications based upon biohistological cell type, degree of malignancy, and histology were proposed.

Surgery for Brain Neoplasms

Many writers point to the removal of a brain tumor by Godlee, and its localization by Bennett on clinical grounds, as the beginning of the modern era of neurological surgery. This feat excited English medical circles when its report in 1885 was hailed as the "first in medical history." Yet, this was not quite the milestone that the English indicated, and were it not for the prominence of London neurology at that time, the incident might have been forgotten.

The patient was a 25-year-old man who had suffered from severe headaches and vomiting for four years. On examination, the patient's intelligence, speech, hearing, and senses seemed to be in order. He had, however, bilateral papilledema, paralysis of the left hand, and weakness of the left leg. At times, he had clonic jerkings of the paralyzed muscles. Bennett diagnosed the condition as a tumor in the upper third of the Rolandic fissure. After trephining in this area, Godlee opened the dura mater and in the cortex exposed a tumor, part of which he excised with a spoon. The dura mater and scalp were closed. The patient recovered from the anesthetic but on the fourth day the wound had signs of inflammation and broke down. The patient died of meningitis about four weeks after the operation.

When the details were presented before the Medical and Chirurgical Society of London, Hughlings Jackson and Ferrier commended the authors highly for their demonstration that a small lesion of the brain could be accurately localized and surgically removed. That the patient succumbed to sepsis in a few days was passed off as an unfortunate surgical complication. But Macewen of Glasgow pointed out that he had been making clinical localizing diagnoses of brain lesions, including tumors, for eight years and that in 1879 he had successfully removed a tumor from the brain of a patient who was still alive.

That local jealousies existed is evidenced by the fact that Bramwell, in his

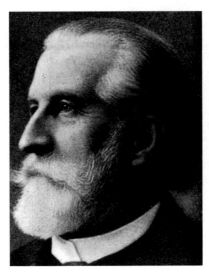

Fig. 10-4. Ernst von Bergmann (1836-1907). (From A History of Neuro-surgery. *Greenblatt SH, Dagi TF, Epstein M, editors. Park Ridge, Ill: American Association of Neurological Surgeons, 1997, p 157)*

book on brain tumors published in 1888, does not mention Godlee's case but credits Macewen with the first successful operation for tumor. Von Bergmann (Fig. 10-4) refers to both Macewen's operation and that of Durante (an olfactory groove meningioma removed in May 1884) as preceding the Bennett and Godlee case. Starr, in his book on brain surgery published in 1893, merely lists the Maida Vale case, although American reports are abstracted. A report of a patient operated upon in San Francisco in 1886 by Hirschfelder is given prominence as the first successful American operation, although the patient died within a week of a wound infection. However, Keen's patient, operated upon for a convexity meningioma in 1887, who survived for over 30 years, is usually acclaimed as the premier in America.

It is unfortunate that Bennett's patient had an infiltrating glioma or sarcoma, for irrespective of the surgical result, the patient would probably have died within a few months from his malignant tumor. Had the lesion been a fungal tumor (meningioma) or an abscess, a successful outcome of the case (especially if an infection had been drained) would have greatly advanced brain surgery.

Tumors of the Cerebral Blood Vessels

Tumors of the brain composed of vascular elements were practically unknown until autopsies became common. Virchow in 1851 described the fine telangiectatic lesions of the cerebral cortex; some 12 years later, he asserted that such vascular anomalies were developmental neoplasms. Later observers held that they were developmental anomalies which were often asymptomatic but might cause focal disturbances such as partial seizures or neurological defects.

As these tumors were more frequently reported, pathologists attempted to classify them on the basis of arterial or venous composition. The venous angiomas were of various degrees or types (simple, serpentine and racemose, or circoid). Cutaneous nevi or port wine marks on cutaneous segments corresponding to a cephalic angioma, such as Kalischer's early case, were recognized. Occasionally, the cortical lesion had sufficient calcification to be seen in x-ray photographs of the head. The venous plexus, although appearing to be a superficial vascular plexus, was usually wedge-shaped with a tongue penetrating to the ventricular wall. Although of congenital origin, the lesion might not produce symptoms until late in life.

Arterial angiomas with arteriovenous communications may be congenital or secondary to trauma or disease of a congenital venous anomaly. The early diagnostic criteria were based upon the clinical findings of: 1) an intracranial bruit, first mentioned by Steinheil; 2) increased extracranial vascularity, described by Emanuel and Isenschmidt and manifested by dilated scalp vessels, hypertrophy of the carotid arteries, diminished or abolished bruit upon carotid compression, and cardiac hypertrophy, all the result of increased blood volume; 3) unilateral exophthalmos which rarely pulsated; and 4) often focal epilepsy. The lesion, composed of pulsating arteries or veins, was usually wedge-shaped with the apex at the ventricular margin. The vessels (small arterioles and venules separated by glial tissue) had well-defined walls which might be thickened and calcified.

Surgical repair of these lesions was not attempted until well into the 20th century. At that time, ligation of the feeding vessels and excision of the vascular mass were possible when transfusions of whole blood were available.

Pituitary Tumors

From the time of the Greek philosophers, the pituitary gland was thought to secrete a mucous substance which passed out through the nose. Not until the Renaissance period was this concept questioned by Vieussens and Sylvius, who believed that the "glans pituitam excipiens" of Vesalius was in some fashion related to the fluid about the base of the brain. Lower, however, was the first to suggest a more modern view: "whatever Serum . . . [comes] through the infundibulum to the glandula pituitaria distills not upon the palate but is poured again into the blood and mixed with it." However, that such mixing was related to the skeletal changes depicted by artists in sculpture and paintings was entirely unknown. Not until Marie in 1886 wrote of the bony proliferations in acromegaly and Minkowski, a year later, showed their relationship to pituitary abnormalities was the hypophysis recognized to modulate growth. In 1900, Benda clarified the issue when he demonstrated that the pituitary tumors causing acromegaly were adenomas composed of eosinophilic cells. Because some tumors of the hypophysis were not associated with acromegaly, the concept was not generally accepted. However, Babinski in 1900 and Fröhlich in 1901 demonstrated that other types of pituitary tumors were associated with the hypodevelopment of the skeleton. A few years later, Marburg described the nonsecreting pituitary chromophobe adenomas which gave rise to a hypopituitary state. The situation was clarified by Cushing in 1909. He showed that acromegaly was the result of hyperpituitarism caused by the secretion of an acidophilic adenoma in an adult, and the glandular disturbance associated with a nonsecreting chromophobe tumor was due to hypoactivity of the pituitary. The adiposogenital syndrome which Fröhlich had described was recognized as the pre-adolescent form of pituitary hypofunction. At about the same time as these cases were being discussed, Osler reported the death of a patient suffering from an acute myxedematous condition, tachycardia, glycosuria, melena, and mania who had reddish-purplish stria on the flanks, bloated face, irritability, and diarrhea. A postmortem was not obtained. The clinical picture resembled Robb's and Cushing's later description of pituitary basophilism. After the mid-20th century, the various pituitary secretory factors were identified and the classification changed from a histological to an endocrinological basis.

Parasellar Neoplasms

Parasellar neoplasms have been recognized for centuries. Many different lesions, such as solid masses, cysts, calcified tissue, and vascular anomalies, develop from the various tissues in or about the pituitary fossa. Until the beginning of the 20th century, these conditions were not differentiated but lumped together as pathological curiosities. Even in the 19th century, pathologists, who became acquainted with such tumors much earlier than clinicians, had difficulty in classifying them. A tumor of the optic chiasm was recognized by Hegmann in 1842, but was not distinguished from the endotheliomas until Hudson in the next century clarified their histological characteristics. Although Michel in 1873 noted their association with von Recklinghausen's disease, the relationship was not well established. Ophthalmic surgeons exenterated them with the globe; Dandy, while unroofing the orbit, excised the tumor with parts of the optic nerve and chiasm.

Tumors Involving the Third Ventricle

Tumors arising from the tissues surrounding the third ventricle region are a mixed group of dysembryonic origin, some derived from intra- and some from paraventricular structures.

The most distinctive tumors of the third ventricle were colloid cysts. Wallman in 1858 was the first to report marble-sized, thin-walled cysts containing a tenacious yellow jelly-like material. Subsequently, isolated cases were described until Weisenberg reviewed the literature and summarized the symptomatology. He emphasized the early headaches, loss of vision, and change in consciousness upon cephalic postural changes which were thought to be the result of obstruction of the foramina of Monro. Dandy in 1930 was the first to make the diagnosis of such a case.

The early reports of other intraventricular tumors are difficult to classify, even with the autopsy reports. In 1879, Falkson described an imbecilic boy of 16 years with severe loss of vision, headache, papilledema, and extraocular palsies, who at autopsy was found to have a large, oval, cystic tumor attached to the floor of the third ventricle. Histologically, the tumor had many epithelial lined cysts with "sarcomatous" and cartilaginous areas. It was considered of pineal or choroid plexus origin but probably was a teratoid pineal tumor. A few years later, Richards reported a 50-year-old man who became progressively demented and was committed to a mental hospital where he died after 10 months. At autopsy, a tumor the size of a golf ball was easily lifted out of the third ventricle. It was a rather gelatinous, solid, encapsulated mass that was diagnosed as a sarcoma. Dandy was able to collect a dozen such cases from the literature. The majority of these tumors were of epithelial origin (pearly tumors, dermoids, or teratomas) but they probably included choroid plexus papillomas, meningiomas, and gliomas, although the latter were diagnosed as sarcomas. These were all autopsied cases. The first patient successfully operated upon was Dandy's case 2, a 6-year-old girl who had a negative posterior fossa exploration.

Pineal Tumors

Although the pineal gland has been known for centuries, tumors of that region were rarely recognized by the early pathologists. Even Gowers refers only to one case—a cystic tumor occupying the third ventricle. In 1875, Weigert described a pineal teratoma occurring in a 14-year-old boy. However, the clinical manifestations of a pineal tumor were slow in developing. In 1896, Gutzeit called attention to the association of pineal tumors and pubertas praecox, which Pellizzi in 1910 named "macrogenitosomia praecox." These disturbances were striking, but many pineal tumors—teratomas and dermoids—produced only intracranial hypertension and impairment of vertical gaze (Parinaud's syndrome). Basing the diagnosis on these signs, Krause attempted to reach these tumors by a cerebellar approach; Horsley operated upon them supratentorially, but the results were dismal failures.

Tumors of the Lateral Ventricles

The rare tumors arising within the lateral ventricles caused symptoms of increased intracranial pressure—headache, dizziness, and vomiting. Focal manifestations (e.g., epilepsy, hemiplegia, and ataxia) were less common and often had false localizing signs. However, some intraventricular tumors (e.g., sarcomas, meningiomas, dermoids, or papillomas) were readily recognized at autopsy and at surgery in the late 19th century.

The red granular appearance of papillomas of the choroid plexus is so characteristic that they were easily identified, although earlier they had been confused with the calcified cholesteatomas described by Virchow. The earliest case, reported by Guerard in 1832, was a 3-year-old girl whose tumor was discovered at autopsy. After that report, 50 years elapsed before Audry in 1886 could collect 25 cases from the world literature. In 1930, Van Wagenen garnered another 22 cases. Although these tumors were benign, their diagnosis was difficult because localizing signs were few and progressive hydrocephalus was the only manifestation of their presence.

Beginning in the middle of the 19th century, pathologists reported small or larger cysts or solid tumors of the lateral ventricles. Henning and Wagner in 1885 described a large intraventricular mass in a baby which was probably a dermoid. Epidermoids with a sheen were identified by Broca and others. The first of the rare intraventricular tumors, now termed meningiomas, was discussed by McDowell in 1881.

Tumors of the Corpus Callosum

In the 17th and 18th centuries, the corpus callosum was considered to include not only the midline commissure but its extension over the lateral ventricle to the white matter, now termed the centrum ovale. As a result, its tumors included neoplasms considered hemispheric. The early custom of examining the brain by making a horizontal section through the cerebral hemispheres probably explains the frequency with which tumors of the corpus callosum were noted when autopsies became common in the 17th century. Platter is said to have reported a callosal tumor. Wepfer's case of 1675 concerned a 23-year-old woman who experienced a sudden sensation of something bursting in the head and urinary incontinence. She recovered from this episode, but about six months later her left leg became so weak that she was unable to stand on it. Then, her left side became weak; she became dizzy and developed a headache and impaired vision in the right eye. The hemiplegia gradually improved until 18 months later, when she became delirious and died. A cystic tumor in the posterior part of the corpus callosum extended to the right lateral ventricle and the internal capsule. In 1856, von Rokitansky found a callosal lipoma in a brain with agenesis of the corpus callosum.

Subsequent reports of single cases and series of cases appeared in the literature. Bristowe in 1886 postulated a corpus callosum syndrome consisting of progressive hemiparesis with vague motor impairment of the opposite side, apathy, headache, vomiting, and drowsiness. However, a definite syndrome was not established until psychological studies of patients who had had section of the corpus callosum for the relief of seizures were reported.

Brainstem Tumors

Neoplasms originating in, invading, or displacing the brainstem were not often reported in the 19th century. Diathetic tumors (tuberculomas and syphilomas) involving the brainstem were noted both singularly and confluent with meningeal involvement. A hypertrophic, and usually distorted, pons indicated the rare glioma of the pons, well illustrated by Gowers. A few other intramedullary tumors were not identified. Of the extra-axial tumors, pineal neoplasms were mentioned by pathologists as causing hydrocephalus. At the base of the rhombencephalon, cystic lesions in the cerebellopontine angle, solid tumors, granulomas (diathetic), parasitic cysts, and other tumors were found. Of these lesions, those in the cerebellopontine angle were the best known. From the descriptions, the histological nature of many of these lesions (neuromas, meningiomas, and epidermoid cysts) cannot be ascertained.

Cerebellar Tumors

Although tumors of the posterior fossa were known to pathologists in the 18th century, intrinsic cerebellar neoplasms were less common. In the latter part of the 19th century, Wilks reported on a number of gliomas of the pons, hydatid cysts in the cerebellum, soft gelatinous tumors, tuberculomas of the pons, and a cerebellar cyst in a 21-year-old woman who had suffered headaches, diplopia, and unsteady gait for only a few days. This woman had a cyst in the left cerebellar hemisphere. Wilks described another case of a girl with neck pains for a few days who stopped breathing and was given artificial respiration for eight hours; she had an infiltrating glioma of the medulla oblongata. Maunsell removed a hydatid cyst from the cerebellum in 1888; according to Starr, the first successful operation on a cystic cerebellar tumor was performed by McBurney on March 15, 1893.

The early operative mortality rate of operations on posterior fossa tumors was high because the surgical approach was bloody, the cerebrospinal fluid dynamics were not understood, and the surgical technique for operating about vital brainstem structures was crude. Horsley and Krause both recommended that the patient undergo operation in a lateral position (Fig. 10-5). Later, a headrest was devised for the patient's face to rest upon and yet allow the anesthesiologist access to the mouth and respiratory passages. To lower the intracranial pressure and decrease bleeding, de Martel in 1913 devised a chair so that the patient could be operated upon in the sitting position. Krause used an osteoplastic flap to expose the posterior fossa, but most neurosurgeons made a craniectomy. To reduce the intracranial pressure, which was usually quite high, Krause punctured the posterior horn of the lateral ventricle to allow fluid to drain during the operative procedure. In the early 20th century, Cush-

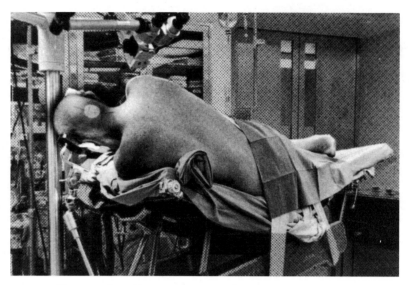

Fig. 10-5. Operative arrangement for the lateral approach to the cerebellopontine angle. (From the collection of A. Earl Walker)

ing emphasized the necessity of a meticulous layer-by-layer closure of the wound to prevent leakage and infection.

The first tumors of the cerebellum to be reported by pathologists were solid tuberculomas, cystic lesions, and sarcomas. Some of the latter were called meningeal sarcomas on the basis of their dissemination in the subarachnoid space about the spinal cord and cerebral hemispheres. A friable mass usually was found in the vermis. The histological resemblance of these tumors to the adrenal medulla led to their designation as neurocytomas. Some years later, Cushing and Bailey termed these disseminating lesions medulloblastomas, presumably developing from undifferentiated, bipotential (both neuroblastic and spongioblastic) cells of the fetal external granular layer of the cerebellar cortex, which is prominent early in life.

The other common cerebellar tumor is an astrocytoma; this neoplasm is often cystic, with or without a mural nodule, and tends to develop in a cerebellar hemisphere. It presents a little later in life than medulloblastomas, in children in their early teens, and even if not completely removed, might not cause symptoms for many years.

The third type of tumor of the cerebellum arising from the cells lining the ventricles—ependymoma—was not identified until the 20th century.

Acoustic Nerve Tumors

The clinical manifestations of neoplasms of the acoustic nerve are so distinctive and the morbid appearance of the growth so typical at the autopsy table that this type of neoplasm should have been recognized quite early in medical history. Yet, according to C.G. Lincke, who compiled the early literature in 1837, the first report of such a pathological lesion was made by Sandifort of Leyden in 1776. The autopsy findings of this typical case were summarized as follows: "and so this little body, hiding in the recess of the brain, is to be considered as the cause of deafness in this case." However, the first description of the clinical manifestations of such a tumor seems to have been reported by Leveque-Lasourie almost 50 years later. His patient was a 38-year-old woman who suffered from vertigo, then headache, impaired vision, and tinnitus followed by deafness of the left ear; she eventually became unstable on her feet, developed numbness of the extremities, dysarthria, and deviation of the protruded tongue, and died. Examination of her brain revealed a fibrous tumor "supposedly arising from the acoustic meatus" attached to the petrous bone. Because the precise relationships of the tumor to the acoustic nerve and auditory canal were not clearly described, as Cushing states (1922), this lesion may have been a meningioma, although the chronology of the symptoms suggest an eighth nerve tumor. Abercrombie's case of 1828 is no more certain. A patient seen by Charles Bell in 1830 probably had an acoustic nerve tumor, although the history is somewhat atypical. The patient was a woman who had "an unusual sensation on the left side of the tip of the tongue" for approximately a year. This feeling spread over the left side of her lower face and jaw, although the motor power of the face and jaw was preserved. However, the senses of taste and feeling on the left side of the tongue and cheek were absent. In the course of the next year, the patient lost her hearing in the left ear and developed a left facial weakness and paralysis of the left temporal and masseter muscles. She died approximately two years after the onset of her symptoms. At postmortem a tumor about the size of a pigeon's egg, containing yellow fluid, was found in the left cerebellopontine angle from the fundus of which a thin strand representing the fifth cranial nerve emerged to enter the base of the cranium. The seventh cranial nerve ran about a centimeter from its origin to enter the tumor. The internal acoustic meatus was filled with a membranous portion of the tumor. A case reported by Boyer in 1834 of a tumor extending into an enlarged auditory canal was more certainly of acoustic nerve origin.

Perhaps the most remarkable case was reported by Cruveilhier in 1835. The patient was a 26-year-old woman who had suffered excruciating vertex headaches and progressive deafness of the left ear. She had convulsive contractions of the left side of the face and progressive loss of vision. The clinical findings and differential diagnosis were discussed in great detail by Cruveilhier. At autopsy, a hard tumor was found in the left cerebellopontine angle and was beautifully illustrated by Chazal. Oppenheim made the first topographical diagnosis and, although he considered that the tumor arose from the cerebellum, his accompanying sketch indicates a typical acoustic tumor. An earlier case presented by G.F. Stevens was correctly diagnosed, but the patient refused to undergo operation. Subsequently, postmortem examination confirmed "a fibrosarcoma projecting into a dilated internal acoustic meatus." These tumors were variously termed acoustic tumors, neurofibroma or fibrosarcoma, and recess tumors. In 1902, Henneberg and Koch not only introduced the term "cerebellopontine angle tumor" but also described a case of bilateral tumors of the acoustic nerves.

As pathologists noted the ease with which some of these tumors could be removed from their beds at autopsy, von Monakow concluded that acoustic nerve tumors should be favorable for surgical excision. However, the few daring surgeons who attempted to resect these tumors encountered many problems. In the first place, the surgical approach to the cerebellopontine angle was bloody and not a few surgeons were unable to reach their goal before the patient succumbed to the shock of blood loss. Both suboccipital and transtemporal approaches were explored. The direct route through the pyramidal bone and middle ear used by otologists proved difficult and was abandoned. The lateral suboccipital approach was bloody and, when the dura mater was opened, the cerebellar hemisphere herniated and had to be excised to expose the tumor. As a result, a number of surgical approaches were used, including craniectomies, double flaps across the lateral sinus which might be ligated, transtentorial approaches, and a lateral suboccipital craniectomy sufficient to expose the cerebellar hemisphere. When the tumor was seen, finger dissection was both bloody and traumatic to the cerebellum and brainstem, so that at the turn of the century, of eight patients operated upon by outstanding surgeons, only three survived. Because of this high mortality, Cushing advocated a bilateral exposure to allow greater room, careful control of bleeding from the scalp, relief of intracranial pressure by ventricular puncture, and an intracapsular gutting of the tumor; using this technique in the 20th century, he was able to operate upon these tumors with a permissible mortality (Fig. 10-6). By 1903, Horsley had removed six such tumors, some successfully. But the operative mortality rate remained high.

Tumors of the Foramen Magnum

Neoplasms of the craniocervical junction were not recognized until the 19th century. Todd in 1849 described a 16-year-old girl who complained of pain in the head and stiffness of the neck. She had a completely flaccid paralysis of the left arm and dragged the left leg in walking. The day after admission to the hospital, she lost the use of the left leg completely, although she still had con-

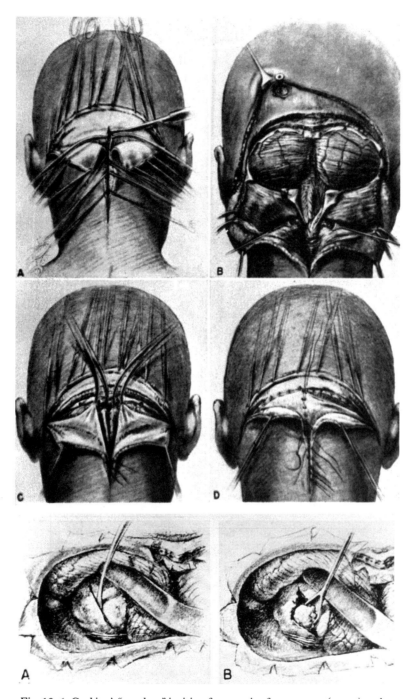

Fig. 10-6. Cushing's "crossbow" incision for posterior fossa surgery (upper) and his exposure of a cerebellopontine tumor (lower). (From the collection of A. Earl Walker)

siderable sensation in the paralyzed limbs. The next day, her right arm was weak and she was incontinent. The paralysis was worse the following day, and her respirations were gasping. The only muscle below the neck that could be moved was the right sternocleidomastoid. Her heart ceased. Todd commented, "It was impossible to conceive a more easy or gradual mode of cutting the thread of life." At autopsy, an enlarged odontoid process was found eroding the dura mater and "a fibrocartilaginous growth compressed and flattened the spinal cord on the left of the median fissure."

The Evolution of Surgical Techniques for Removal of Brain Tumors

As interest in the surgery of the brain developed, the management of persons suspected of harboring a tumor underwent radical changes. The early practice of a six months' trial of mercury rubs and iodides, while the victim of an intracranial neoplasm observed his paretic limbs become weaker, his eyesight fade, and his general health deteriorate as the result of vomiting and seizures, was reduced by Horsley to three months as quite adequate to eliminate the possibility of an infective process. Anesthesia, although an asset to the patient, was often a trial and tribulation for the surgeon operating upon the central nervous system. To obtain a smooth induction of anesthesia required time; this irked the surgeon accustomed to performing his procedure in a few minutes. Victor Horsley's anesthesiologist complained that Horsley would begin his operation before the patient was fully anesthetized, would have completed his task, and would be out the door by the time the patient was in a state of surgical anesthesia. In fact, some surgeons insisted that the induction of anesthesia was more of a procedure than the surgical operation. Each of the early anesthetic agents—ether, chloroform, and nitrous oxide—had disadvantages, such as respiratory disturbances, bleeding, and cardiac depression. Particularly if ether was used, further problems were the accumulation of mucus in the throat, increased bleeding, and impaired breathing. To avoid this complication, Horsley used chloroform for anesthesia in spite of its greater danger. For intracranial operations requiring meticulous handling of neural tissue, when local anesthesia became available in 1884, some surgeons preferred to inject the reagent and operate rather than to wait for the anesthesiologist to put the patient to sleep.

The preparation of the scalp for an operation followed the antiseptic regime of shaving the head a day or two before the proposed operation, shampooing the scalp, and covering it with gauze wrung out of a 2.5% solution of carbolic acid for one or two days. At the time of the operation, the scalp was washed and lavaged with a 1:1000 mercuric chloride solution, shaved, and scrubbed with a soft brush. Cushing wrapped the field with a bichloride sheet before the operation; however, some operators used the general surgical preparation of ether and iodine for the scalp preparation.

The position of the patient—standing, lying, or sitting—apparently depended upon the length of the operative procedure. Bleeding was less when a patient was standing, as seen in medieval illustrations of the scalp being incised and a lesion, real or fancied, being excised. Many trephining scenes, however, show the victim lying in various positions. Not until the modern era of long operations was the comfort of the patient and the convenience of the operator considered paramount. Ways of decreasing bleeding and improving the airway were devised. Horsley designed an extension to the operating table for the head to rest upon. Other surgeons used pillows under the shoulders to allow adequate respiratory excursions and a horseshoe-shaped headrest to permit the anesthesiologist access to the mouth and nose. Because bleeding was profuse with the patient in the horizontal position, Cushing had the head of the operating table slightly elevated. Later surgeons devised a chair so that with the patient sitting, an attached head-holder could be fixed by pins inserted into the skull.

The cruciate incision used from ancient times to expose a lesion was inadequate to allow inspection of large traumatic and inflammatory lesions of the brain. Moreover, when sutured, such wounds often broke down at the corners. As a result, Horsley made a semi-lunar or horseshoe incision, leaving intact the vascular supply to the flap, a technique adopted by most surgeons thereafter.

Bleeding from the scalp incision was a problem for brain surgeons. A number of ingenious techniques were devised to control the scalp vessels. Bands of various materials—rubber tourniquets, pliable tubing, and even steel rings— were tied around the cranium. Toward the end of the 19th century, sutures were placed along the scalp incision by Lampshear on one or both sides, or across the base of the horseshoe incision. A fitted plate conforming to the shape of the skull and the incision was secured to the scalp by sutures to compress the margin of the incision. Some surgeons tried to tie bleeding vessels as the scalp was cut. If the hemorrhage was severe, Charles H. Frazier (Fig. 10-7) exposed the carotid arteries in the neck so that they might be occluded by temporary ligation. Chipault devised serrated spring clips to grasp and compress the scalp margins; T-shaped clamps or gauze pads were applied along the cut edges. Frazier compressed the margin of the incision while hemostats were being applied to the galea and turned back to stop the bleeding. Cushing had his assistants digitally compress the margins of the scalp incision as he placed the hemostats on the galea. Subsequently, angled hemostats and spring clips were devised to compress more accurately the scalp margins. To constrict the vessels, Mayer injected "Adrenalin" along the site of an incision for hemostasis and easier application of clips or clamps.

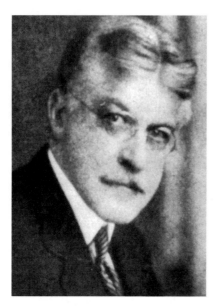

Fig. 10-7. Charles Harrison Frazier (1870-1936). (From the collection of A. Earl Walker)

When the cranial opening was made, bleeding from the diploic vessels was troublesome, for the usual clamping technique was not feasible. Spicules of various substances were used to plug the diploic channels, but were abandoned when hemostatic bone wax was introduced by Horsley about 1886, and P.W. Squire concocted a mixture of beeswax, almond oil, and salicylic acid which could be sterilized and rubbed into the open diploic channels.

Locating the site of the surgical exposure posed a problem. The earlier blind trephinations which might expose an extensive clot on the surface of the brain were replaced by carefully planned incisions and perforations based upon scalp maps of the motor cortex. Unless a cutaneous or osseous abnormality suggesting an underlying lesion was visible, only lesions causing paresis or focal seizures, presumed to lie along the Rolandic fissure, could be localized by scalp markings indicating the central sulcus. These methods used mechanical guides (encephalometers) devised by Cuban, French, German, Italian, and Russian surgeons. The English operators drew linear graphs upon the scalp based upon Reid's line, the midline, and the calculated Rolandic fissure.

It should be understood that at that time the trephine opening was only two or three centimeters in diameter, so that placement of the opening had to be planned quite accurately. Not until the late 19th century were large bone flaps reflected which exposed much of the convexity of the cerebral hemisphere so that the chance of finding a lesion was greatly increased.

The earliest tumors of the brain to be recognized were those that produced an obvious swelling or deformity of the skull. The lump on the head which Acrel incised in 1768 proved at autopsy to be a bloody tumor eroding the skull. Six years later, Louis described such masses as fungi of the dura mater, some of which were probably of infectious origin. Several reports at the beginning of the 19th century also confused neoplastic and inflammatory lesions of the skull. Cruveilhier differentiated the two conditions and described the growths as cancerous tumors of the meninges. However, Lebert in 1845 questioned their malignancy and called the lesions "fibroplastic tumors." The uncertainty of their nature in the latter part of the 19th century is reflected in the various terms applied to these lesions. Virchow called them sarcomas, a term used as late as 1885. However, some pathologists questioned their malignancy; Golgi in 1869 suggested the term endothelioma. Cleland noted their resemblance to pacchionian granules and referred to them as villous tumors of the arachnoid. Surgeons considered their encapsulated nature and the ease of their resection by finger dissection as an indication of their benignity. In 1888, Weir and Seguin asserted their favorable outcome if removed in toto. Horsley believed that they could be shelled out and completely removed. Von Bramann recognized that the overlying attached dura mater, infiltrated bone, and capsule adjoining the tumor should be excised.

After anesthesia and aseptic techniques were developed, surgeons realized that such intracranial tumors should be operable, but found their surgical instruments and operative techniques too crude to use on the delicate brain tissue. Moreover, a trephine opening was rarely large enough to expose the entire surface of the tumor. To obtain a wider exposure, in 1889 Wagner, using a scalpel, hammer, and chisel, resected a flap of scalp and skull hinged upon muscle so that it could be replaced. With a large osteoplastic flap, the surgeon could cut the dura mater about an attached tumor or reflect the dura mater to explore much of the lateral cortex. Thus, masses (usually firm and encapsulated) attached to the dura mater were quite accessible to the surgeon's scalpel. Accordingly, his palpating fingers could outline the dural attachments of the tumor and guide scissors to cut the dura mater about the tumor. The resulting cavity, the walls of which bled profusely, was packed with a hot sponge or gauze. If necessary, the packs might be left in place and the scalp margins loosely sutured over them. In two or three days, the packing could usually be removed without incurring further hemorrhage. If the wound did not have to be packed, the scalp margins were loosely approximated and a drain left to allow bloody fluid to escape. After such a cranial operation, most patients were in a state of shock; if they survived, as the blood pressure rose, further bleeding might require additional packing.

If there was no evidence of a tumor when the skull was trephined—which happened in almost half of the cranial operations in those days—the surgeon had a dilemma. He had to consider a number of possibilities. A tumor might be present in the underlying brain tissue. Some other diffuse process might exist in the cerebral hemisphere. More likely, the lesion, whatever its nature, was located in some other part of the brain. At that point, the majority of surgeons would neither open the dura mater nor insert a needle to feel for a resistant mass or to tap a cyst. Amidon found that of 100 operations for brain tumors in the late 19th century, the dura mater was opened by injury or intent in only 31 cases. Von Bergmann had reported that the diagnosis was inaccurate in 31.2% of cases and Oppenheim in 27.5% of cases. Most surgeons still regarded the brain and its membranes with the same reverence as they looked upon the heart and pericardium—regions never to be approached with trocar or scalpel. Although Middeldorpf in 1856 had advocated making brain punctures, it is not clear that he had ever done so. Weir in 1887 was the first to needle the brain to locate a tumor. Only a few 19th century operators such as Frazier punctured the exposed cortex. Roberts commented that many patients died of brain abscesses or tumors because the surgeon feared to needle or incise the brain. In 1898, David Ferrier wrote "the treatment of intracranial tumours forms a rather melancholy chapter in therapeutics."

Even if the dura mater was opened, increased pressure within the brain caused the cortical tissue to extrude, rupture, and bleed profusely. If the arachnoid was spared, bleeding from the cortical veins might be a problem for the surgeon of the late 19th century. Most operators preferred to occlude smaller vessels, often difficult to ligate, with the cautery—a technique abhorred by some surgeons such as Horsley. Bennett and Godlee used galvanic electrocautery; others (Roberts) applied a hot needle to the bleeding point. Horsley sprayed a sublimate or saline solution heated to between 110° and 115°F over the bleeding vessels and applied gentle pressure with a soft sponge to arrest oozing. Some operators used a hot dry sponge (Krause) or hot air blast (Kenyon) to control bleeding from the surface of the cortex.

Having controlled the bleeding, the surgeon still had problems. The swollen brain, unless the tumor was superficial, made it almost impossible for the operator to feel a tumorous mass. Accordingly, in many cases, the scalp was sutured without finding a lesion. If a tumor was apparent, usually the surgeon removed a small portion with a spoon or finger. If the neoplasm appeared to be encapsulated, the surgeon might pass a finger about its margin until the mass could be enucleated and removed. At times, scalpel and finger dissection caused so much bleeding that hot packs were ineffective until the patient's blood pressure fell. In such cases, large feeding vessels were tied with catgut or silk sutures. The bleeding tumor bed was filled with hot, dry or wet, absorbent cotton or iodoform gauze. Horsley emphasized that well-oxygenated blood promoted hemostasis and lessened venous oozing. Muscle, although used in prehistoric times, was not applied to bleeding points until the early part of the 20th century. By that time, silver clips had been devised and astringent solutions introduced. The electrosurgical unit, the sucker, and biological materials came later.

Although packing the tumor bed with plain or iodoform gauze for one or two days was a common practice at the end of the 19th century, the prolonged pressure was likely to cause edema or necrosis of the underlying brain and predispose to infection. Accordingly, Frazier applied pressure only in dire emergencies; Cushing preferred to irrigate with saline solutions. If bleeding persisted, the vessels were sought and tied off or a pack was left in place for a day or two. The scalp margins were loosely approximated with widely spaced running sutures. Unfortunately, such tumor excisions were usually fatal or, if the patient survived the operation, a septic complication might develop.

This despairing outlook was due to several factors—the difficulty in diagnosing and localizing a tumor, the swelling of the brain, the infiltrating nature of many lesions, and the profuse bleeding encountered during the craniotomy and excision of the tumor. This pessimistic outlook for surgical intervention is illustrated by White's review of 100 autopsied cases of brain tumor at Guy's Hospital. Of these, 45 were of tubercular origin, many associated with tuberculosis of other organs. Thirty-six patients had neoplasms—24 gliomas, 10 sarcomas, and two gliosarcomas. In one third of the cases, the lesion was unexpectedly found at operation or autopsy. Only nine were judged to be operable (five in the cerebellum and four in the frontal or occipital lobes). The first intracranial tumors successfully removed were those by Macewen and by Durante. Macewen's patient was a male who had a small left orbital tumor excised early in life; however, he continued to suffer headaches and had a convulsion beginning in the right side of the face and extending to the right limbs and entire body with loss of consciousness. Upon re-exploration, the bony medial wall of the left orbit was thickened over an en plaque tumor of the dura mater, which was removed. The patient lived eight years more and died of nephritis. At autopsy, no tumor was found. Durante's patient had proptosis of the left eye and, at operation, a tumor was found infiltrating the lamina cribrosa. The tumor and the atrophic frontal lobe were resected. Some bleeding was controlled by a pack which was removed in 10 days. The patient lived some years before a second operation for a recurrence was performed.

Thus, the pioneering surgeons of the 19th century overcame difficulties in localizing a surgical lesion, opening the bony calvarium, incising the dura mater to expose a pathological state, arresting bleeding before the patient was in shock, closing the wound, and applying a dressing.

The experiences of these pioneering neurosurgeons exemplify the trials of physicians throughout the world who dared to explore the nervous system in the latter part of the 19th century. A three-volume text edited by Chipault relates the experiences of the surgeons who operated upon the nervous system in those days.

11

Neuroscience Comes of Age

The Beginning of Clinical Neurology

In the 18th century, the disorders of the nervous system were the province of any physician. It was not until the middle of the next century that disorders of the brain and spinal cord became segregated and were considered a special unit. At that time, the mental and neurological disturbances were cared for in various ways by physicians especially interested in such disorders. In France, the neurologists were developing quite independently of the madhouse doctors. In Germany, the specialties were combined. In England, neurology stimulated by John Hughlings Jackson and William Gowers split from the alienists. In the United States, the field was neuropsychiatry, to some extent predicated by the therapeutic poverty of neurology. The disciples of the two fields separated as the specialties developed, however, and confined their practice to either psychiatry or neurology.

As neurology became independent of psychiatry and medicine, the specialists settled the disorders of their practice. Although at first there was some overlap, such as the epilepsies, the fields soon became quite well defined. By the end of the 19th century, psychiatric and neurological societies were meeting independently with little overlap of subjects. The domain of neurology consisted of a number of disorders well known for ages, such as epilepsy and the traumatic disorders of the brain and spinal cord, and many disorders only recognized in the 19th century as originating from the nervous system. The semeiology and pathology of these neurological disorders established the foundation of neurology.

Advances After the Renaissance

After the Renaissance of arts and literature, many advances in medicine were made. Harvey defined the circulation of the blood as it passed from the vena cava through the heart and lungs to reach the aorta. Beginning in the 17th century, Willis expounded on the cerebral circulation, von Haller (1753) demonstrated neural irritability, and Morgagni (1761) described the morbid changes in the nervous system. With these advances, clinicians began to define the illnesses that they encountered at the bedside in pathological rather than symptomatic terms. Thus, paralysis was not an entity but the manifestation of a disordered state of the brain or spinal cord. The dropsies of the cerebral ventricles were evidence of tuberculous meningitis, hydrocephalus or, rarely, other disorders; the apoplexies of the 17th century were the result of cerebral hemorrhage, thrombosis, or even cardiac disturbances. The falling sickness of earlier ages, although usually a manifestation of epilepsy, might be a sign of a brain tumor, heart disease, or metabolic upset. Thus, many disorders of the nervous system, known to the earlier physicians by their symptoms, became disease entities.

In the early 19th century, the anatomical and physiological knowledge acquired previously was applied to bedside practice. Andral, in his clinic for neurological disorders, integrated his clinical examinations with postmortem findings in order to determine the true nature of the morbid entity (Table 1). Guillaume Benjamin Amend Duchenne (Fig. 11-1) walked the wards of Parisian hospitals and applied electrodes to stimulate the muscles and nerves of patients suffering from such neurological disorders as locomotor ataxia, muscle palsies, and neural intoxications. He studied the responses of the denervated muscles in poliomyelitis and of the abnormal fibers of pseudohypertrophic muscular dystrophy. The findings were correlated with the later pathoanatomical studies of Charcot and Cornil. Duchenne's accounts of the electrical responses of patients suffering from progressive muscular atrophy, which Aran had described earlier, led to their names being attached to the disorder. Duchenne also defined glosso-labio or bulbar paralysis. In his later years, Duchenne developed a dementia and died practically unknown.

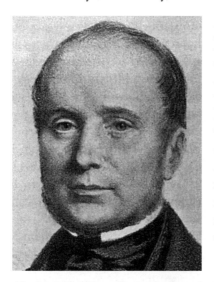

Fig. 11-1. Guillaume Benjamin Amend Duchenne (1806-1875). (From The Founders of Neurology, *2nd ed. Haymaker W, Schiller F, editors. Springfield, Ill: Charles C Thomas, 1970, p 431)*

TABLE 1

TERMS USED BY HALL AND ANDRAL

Marshall Hall (1836)	G. Andral (1844)
Congenital Anomalies	
Anencephalic fetus	
Hypertrophic brain	Hypertrophic brain
Atrophic brain (congenital hemiplegia)	Cerebral atrophy
Infections	
Meningitis and encephalitis	Abscess of brain
Myelitis; ascending paralysis	Purulent meningitis
Tuberculosis of the brain	Tuberculous meningitis
Hydrocephalus	Hydrocephalus
Neoplasms	
Scirrhous or encephaloid tumors	Gliomas, fibromas, cystic,
Neuromas	multiple
Vascular Lesions	
Apoplexy, cerebellar and cerebral	Cerebral and cerebellar hemorrhage
Softening (congestion)	Softening (cerebral or
Hyperemia	cerebellar)
Spinal hemorrhage	Subdural hematoma
Syndromes	
Convulsive, hemicrania, hydrophobia, hysteria, chorea, paralysis agitans, intoxications, trigeminal neuralgia, uremia, delirium	

Another French neurological giant who embellished the specialty was Jean M. Charcot (1825–1893). The best and most popular clinic in Paris at that time was Charcot's clinic, the Sâlpetrière (Fig. 11-2), which attracted students from near and far. Much of Charcot's work was published in collaboration with his assistants at the Sâlpetrière—C.J. Bouchard on miliary cerebral aneurysms, Pierre Marie on muscular atrophy, Richer on hysteria, Gilles de la Tourette on hysteria (1884), and Pitres on the cortical motor centers (1895). Many were reported in his lectures at the Sâlpetrière. Charcot is renowned for his description of amyotrophic lateral sclerosis in 1874, which was named after him (Charcot's disease), progressive muscular atrophy (Charcot-Marie-Tooth disease), the dystrophic arthritic changes in tabes dorsalis (Charcot joints), and the intention tremor of multiple sclerosis. Charcot was a skilled artist and with Paul Richer published two monographs on demonomania in art.

A famous pupil of Charcot, Pierre Marie (Fig. 11-3) was a professor at the Paris faculty. In 1886, Marie and Charcot described peroneal muscular atrophy, a subject on which Tooth in England had written his thesis the same year. In

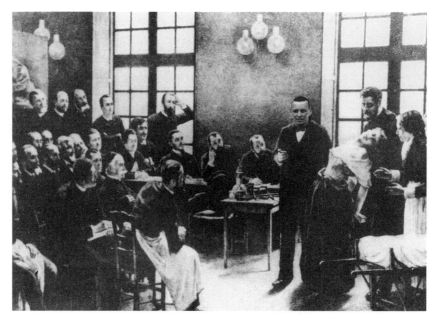

Fig. 11-2. Charcot's clinic at La Sâlpetrière. (From the collection of A. Earl Walker)

the 1890s, Marie described pulmonary hypertrophic osteoarthropathy (1890) and hereditary cerebellar ataxia (1893). Five years later, he defined the type of arthritis deformans later called Strümpell-Marie disease. On the basis of his experiences in World War I, he wrote on wounds of the brain, spinal cord, and peripheral nerves. Although Bernard Mohr had noted metabolic disturbances caused by pituitary dysfunction in 1840, it was not until 46 years later that Pierre Marie suggested the eosinophilic adenomatous basis of acromegaly. Earlier, Krebs and Fritsch had suspected such a causation but an enlarged thymus in their patient had confused the issue. Marie's report resolved the problem. Later, Fröh-

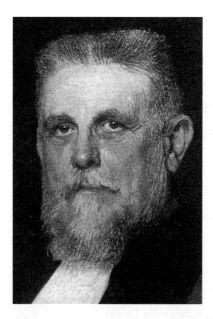

Fig. 11-3. Pierre Marie (1853-1940). (From The Founders of Neurology, *2nd ed. Haymaker W, Schiller F, editors. Springfield, Ill: Charles C Thomas, 1970, p 477)*

lich described the hypopituitary state as the adiposito-genital syndrome.

A number of other outstanding neurologists in Paris were clarifying the disorders of the nervous system at the end of the 19th century. These included Jules Dejerine (1849-1917), who wrote on aphasia, tabes dorsalis, muscular atrophy, interstitial neuritis, olivopontocerebellar atrophy (with Thomas), the thalamic syndrome, parietal lobe disorders, and other neurological diseases during his tenure as clinical chief at the Sâlpetrière; Georges Gilles de la Tourette (1857–1904), who described tics; Fulgence Raymond (1844–1910), an outstanding clinical lecturer; Joseph F. Babinski (Fig. 11-4), Chief at La Pitié and known for his elucidation of the toe, pupillary, defense, and pilomotor reflexes; André Thomas, known for his studies of the cerebellum; A. Souques, known for describing hysterical disorders of the nervous system; and Paul Richer, the artist of the Sâlpetrière known for his anatomical art, neurological illustrations, and statuary.

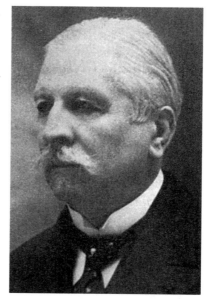

Fig. 11–4. Joseph F. Babinski (1857-1932). (From The Founders of Neurology, *2nd ed. Haymaker W, Schiller F, editors. Springfield, Ill: Charles C Thomas, 1970, p 398)*

In England, at the beginning of the 19th century, several physicians published results of neurological studies. Richard Bright wrote of unilateral convulsions, brain abscesses secondary to otitis media, pressure palsies, and cerebral hemiplegias, which he illustrated. James Parkinson accurately described in 1817 the shaking palsy named after him. During the same era, Richard Bentley Todd lectured on postconvulsive hemiplegia or paresis, Charles Bell demonstrated the sensory functions of the posterior spinal roots and the sensorimotor function of the portio dura of the facial nerve (paralysis of which was named Bell's palsy), and Robert J. Graves noted pinpoint pupils in cerebral disease.

In 1836, Marshall Hall (Fig. 11-5), a brilliant English investigator who had demonstrated that the reflex arc was quite independent of the brain and had introduced a physiologically sound method of resuscitating drowned persons, published his lectures delivered the previous year entitled *The Nervous System and its Disorders*. Although devoid of pathological confirmation and of illustrations, his clinical accounts were far ahead of the practices of his time. The revised table of contents (Table 1) gives evidence of the clinical knowledge of

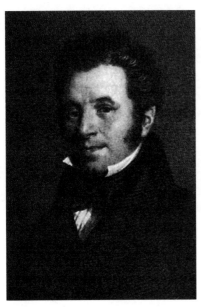

Fig. 11-5. Marshall Hall (1790–1857). (From The Founders of Neurology, *2nd ed. Haymaker W, Schiller F, editors. Springfield, Ill: Charles C Thomas, 1970, p 222)*

this outstanding physician. A comparison with the conditions discussed by Riverius and Willis in the 17th century and those of Hall and Andral in the 19th century indicates the trend toward an anatomico-pathological classification of disease.

In the second half of the century, a center for patients with paralysis and epileptic disorders was established in London, where several physicians, including an outstanding neurologist named John Hughlings Jackson (1835-1911), specialized in the diagnosis and care of patients with nervous diseases. On the basis of careful clinical observation, Hughlings Jackson conceived of the brain as a multilayered organ controlling the neural activities. As the pyramidal tract in the early part of the 19th century was thought to originate from the corpus callosum, he localized the second level in the frontal cortex. As Hughlings Jackson believed that the higher motor centers exerted both excitatory and inhibitory influences upon the next higher or lower level, he was able to explain the occurrence of unilateral seizures followed by paresis. Obviously, he was handicapped by incomplete knowledge of the function of the subcortical ganglia and their fiber connections.

Probably the greatest neurologist of the latter part of the 19th century was William R. Gowers (1845–1915), after whom a spinal cord tract was named. He wrote an encyclopedic manual on diseases of the nervous system in which he introduced a modern clinicopathological classification of neurological disorders. Gowers and Hughlings Jackson were among the founders of The National Hospital for Epileptics and Paralysed at Queen Square, London. Many famous neurologists attended The National Hospital in the late 19th and early 20th centuries and would-be neurologists from all parts of the world flocked to learn of the afflictions of the nervous system.

In Germany and the neighboring countries, the nervous system was being investigated both in the laboratory and on the hospital wards. The first clinically oriented monograph on nervous disorders is generally accredited to Moritz H. Romberg (Fig. 11-6). His textbook was divided into two sections, the first related to sensory and the second to motor disorders. Following the example of the earlier writers, Romberg gave extensive histories of the patients but rather scanty accounts of the objective findings. Techniques for examining the sensory modalities of touch, pain, temperature, and two-point discrimination were described. Reflexes were poorly understood and so only a few, such as the corneal, were examined. Romberg noted, however, that a tabetic person with his eyes closed "began to sway and to stumble" when standing—a sign of posterior column dysfunction to which his name has been attached. No illustrations brightened his histories, nor were attempts made to correlate the clinical findings with their pathological substrate. Although the greater part of the text deals with peripheral nerve and spinal cord disorders, there is a section on cerebral paralysis in which Romberg discusses a number of pathological states—general paresis, tumors of the base of the brain, pontine gliomas, aneurysms, meningitis (chronic), softenings of the subcortical nuclei and white matter, and dis-

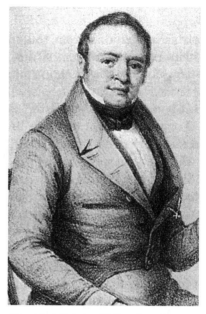

Fig. 11-6. Moritz H. Romberg (1795-1873). (From The Founders of Neurology, *2nd ed. Haymaker W, Schiller F, editors. Springfield, Ill: Charles C Thomas, 1970, p 507)*

turbances of the mind. Although the gross pathological changes are described, no mention is made of microscopic findings; yet the microscope and histological techniques were being developed at that time. Romberg admits that "the attempt has often been made to discover detached foci of innervation in the brain, but it has invariably failed." Although Romberg distinguished the motor disturbances of paralysis and incoordination, he made no attempt to define their origins. Similarly, he discusses the disturbances of speech, mentation, and other higher mental functions without attempting to correlate them to anatomical lesions. It is apparent, as Spillane comments, that Romberg was "the emerging clinical neurologist."

A number of outstanding German physicians, some psychiatrists, followed Romberg. In 1880, Wilhelm H. Erb (Fig. 11-7), professor at Heidelberg, introduced electrodiagnosis and electrotherapy as aids to the diagnosis of neurological disease. Theodor H. Meynert (Fig 11-8), professor of neurology and psychiatry at Vienna in the last quarter of the 19th century, advanced the basic knowledge of the brain and mental afflictions resulting from disease. Karl Wernicke (1848–1905), professor of psychiatry at Berlin and Breslau, was an active investigator and writer on the higher mental functions and their

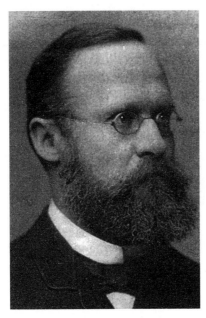

Fig. 11-7. Wilhelm Heinrich Erb (1840-1921). (From The Founders of Neurology, *2nd ed. Haymaker W, Schiller F, editors. Springfield, Ill: Charles C Thomas, 1970, p 436)*

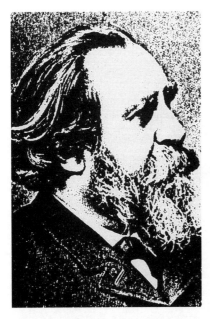

Fig. 11-8. Theodor H. Meynert (1833-1893). (From the collection of A. Earl Walker)

anatomical correlates, especially those related to speech. Nikolaus Friedreich (1825-1882) of Würzberg wrote on agoraphobia, pseudosclerosis, and the significance of the knee jerk. Heinrich Quincke (1842–1922) described angioneurotic edema and in 1891 introduced lumbar puncture as a diagnostic procedure, and Hermann Oppenheim (1858–1919) of Berlin wrote several textbooks on neurology and in 1900 described amyotonia congenita.

The treatment for disorders of the nervous system was limited in the latter part of the 19th century. Only a few measures to improve the general well-being of individuals and a few specific pharmacological preparations were available. The patient was advised to avoid excessive work, worry, extremes of cold, and smoking. A sea voyage, spas such as Turkish baths, light diet, ice bags to the head, heat to the limbs, and for congestion of the brain, blisters to the occiput, leeches to the head and, rarely, bleeding were prescribed. The earlier therapies such as bleeding, counter-irritation, and electrotherapy were largely abandoned. Pharmacological therapy was rampant—for tonics, strychnine, arsenic, iron, and quinine were prescribed; for fever, diuretics were prescribed as well as mild laxatives; and for the tremor of Parkinson's disease, hyoscamus was the most effective medication. A course of potassium iodide and mercury rubs was given; however, the multiple drug and herbal preparations of the 17th century were no longer prescribed for all unusual and persistent illnesses as well as those suspected to be associated with venereal disease.

In the first half of the 19th century, although knowledge of the workings of the brain and spinal cord had advanced considerably, surgery of the nervous system both in the hospital and on the battlefield was hazardous and attended with high mortality. A number of developments were occurring, however, which promised to bring operations upon the nervous system from a crude manual exercise to a skilled art. Anesthesia, known to the Greeks and Romans who used mandragora and to the Chinese who prescribed scopolamine, was greatly improved by the introduction of gaseous and volatile agents which could be controlled. With such anesthetics to relax the patient, time-consuming and delicate operations could be performed; however, the specter of infection hovered over the surgical field.

When Louis Pasteur (1822-1895) introduced limited heating of wine, he not only saved that industry in France, but he initiated the antiseptic treatment of wounds. At that time, Lister was contemplating means of preventing the formation of "laudable pus" in wounds so that they might heal by first intention. Aware that pasteurization could not be used, Joseph Lister tried a number of chemicals and, fortunately, hit upon carbolic acid as a means of preventing putrification. In 1867, after two years of experimentation and clinical trials, he published his findings in *Lancet*. The report was received with mixed reactions. Ernst von Bergmann followed Lister's theory, however, and blended the antiseptic method into a steam-sterilizing ritual.

Finally, the demonstration that much activity of the brain was initiated in the cerebral cortex stimulated daring operators to explore the secrets of the brain and to cut away diseased tissue. Victor Horsley is often said to have sired such brain surgery; other pioneers such as Pierre Paul Broca in France, von Bergmann in Germany, William Macewen in Scotland, and William W. Keen in the United States deserve mention. Although all were general surgeons, they found operating upon the nervous system particularly appealing, and in later years, devoted much of their skill to neurosurgical procedures.

Pierre Paul Broca (1824-1880), who founded brain surgery in France, antedated the other patrons by a few years. Although his surgical exploits on the brain were overshadowed by his anthropological explorations and clinical localization of the speech center in the third left frontal convolution, he did much to advance operative practices. He was the first to operate successfully upon a brain abscess using cranial topography for localization of the lesion.

In 1860, Ernst von Bergmann (1836-1907) graduated in medicine from the University of Dorpat. Subsequently, he served in the Russo-Austrian and Franco-Prussian wars, gaining valuable surgical experience in treating the casualties, especially in handling head wounds. At the conclusion of these hostilities in 1870, he wrote an extensive account of his experiences treating head injuries and his use of antiseptic surgery in the care of wounds for Pitha and Billroth's handbook of special surgery.

In 1882, von Bergmann succeeded Langenbeck as head of the surgical department at the University of Berlin. Four years later, he introduced steam sterilization and shortly thereafter developed an aseptic operating technique. In a treatise published in 1888, von Bergmann discussed the surgical treatment of brain diseases, congenital anomalies, brain abscesses, brain tumors, epilepsy, and intracranial hypertension. He differentiated between the malformations of the neural axis consisting of a fluid-filled sac—meningocele—and those containing neural tissue—encephaloceles and meningomyeloceles. The former he could cure by ligating the neck of the cystic mass and suturing the skin margins; the latter, often associated with hydrocephalus even if surgically repaired, usually terminated fatally. At that time, encapsulated brain abscesses, often secondary to ear infections, were the most common brain tumor. Von Bergmann recognized that a "running ear" due to otitis media might lead to periphlebitis and an extradural empyema with lateral sinus thrombosis and an intracerebral abscess. Even though Peyronie had advocated puncturing the brain to aspirate an abscess, von Bergmann preferred to drain such lesions. He recognized that patients with brain abscesses had a better outlook than those with an infiltrating brain neoplasm, which was usually difficult to define and rarely completely removed with finger dissection or gutting. Encapsulated growths would be readily extirpated by finger dissection, and, if bleeding could be controlled, the patient survived. Von Bergmann referred to seven surgically treated cases, of whom three patients lived for some years. For the treatment of seizures, he excised "spasmic centers" but he admitted that the results of these operations were disappointing.

Von Bergmann's contribution, somewhat revised, was reprinted as a book. The 1888 text is divided into five sections which give a general idea of the surgery being done at that time. The English edition, published as volume VI of Wood's medical and surgical monographs, consisted of pages 767 to 968 of that monograph. Devoid of illustrations, it contained 101 citations to the European and American literature. Von Bergmann attempted to report on the literature of the medical world, for each surgeon operating upon the nervous system had treated only a few cases. Accordingly, he refers to his own cases and the reports in the literature. The text discusses only the surgery of the brain— that of the spinal cord and peripheral nerves was covered by others; however, von Bergmann relates surgical care of congenital anomalies, abscesses, tumors, and epilepsy.

It is noteworthy that von Bergmann pays little attention to personal experiences, augmenting his descriptions with rather detailed case histories of previous cases, some treated successfully and some succumbing. He refers to the different types of congenital anomalies, asserting that only the meningoceles were operable. These were mainly frontal and often misdiagnosed as cysts. Deep abscesses due to trauma or infected skull wounds usually involved the ear. Other abscesses were metastatic or tuberculous. Von Bergmann used a chisel and mallet to cut his cranial opening.

Victor Alexander Haden Horsley was born on April 14, 1857 in London, England. He received his medical education at the University of London. After passing the Royal College of Surgeon's examination, he served as house officer at the University College Hospital. His scientific curiosity was manifested at this time by his interest in anesthesiology; he had his associates put him to sleep with various anesthetics so that he might appreciate the reactions.

In 1884, Victor Horsley, at the age of 27 years, was appointed professor superintendent of the Brown Institute in London, where he was welcomed by the research team of Schafer and Charles Beevor, who were exploring with electric current the functions of the cerebral cortex. While there, he formulated a bone wax to plug bleeding diploic vessels at the cut margins of bone.

In 1886, Horsley was appointed surgeon to The National Hospital for Epileptics and Paralysed, Queen Square, London. On May 25, 1886, he performed his first human neurosurgical operation on a 22-year-old epileptic man who had suffered a compound fracture of the skull at the age of seven years. Horsley removed a cerebral scar from the posterior part of the superior frontal gyrus. The patient's mental status improved and his fits ceased. A year later, Horsley excised a tumor from the spinal canal, for which he is justly renowned. Although not the first such operation, as has been declared, it was a notable achievement. At the International Medical Congress in Berlin in 1890, he presented his decompressive operation for the relief of inoperable brain tumors and the results of 44 intracranial operations with only 10 deaths, some due to malignant gliomas. This was an amazing record for a time when brain operations were thought to be usually fatal.

At the beginning of the century, Horsley turned to medical politics and became an ardent, almost fanatic, crusader for medical, social, and educational reforms. But his aggressive, imperious, and uncompromising attitude made him many enemies. These political activities usurped his time so that he had little left for scientific and medical papers in his later years. Consequently, his operative achievements in the 20th century are not recorded. At the outbreak of World War I, he requested active duty. Finally, he, the leading neurological surgeon of the British Empire, was assigned to the Mediterranean Expeditionary Force and died in Mesopotamia of heat stroke on July 16, 1916. The seriousness of his last illness, like the importance of his work and life, was not fully appreciated until too late.

Sir William Macewen was born in 1848 on the island of Bute at the mouth of the river Clyde. His medical education at the University of Glasgow brought him in contact with Joseph Lister, professor of surgery, whom he highly esteemed. Macewen was among the first to use the neurological examination to localize surgical lesions. In 1876, he diagnosed a brain abscess which, after the boy's death, was found where he predicted. In 1879, he localized and removed a

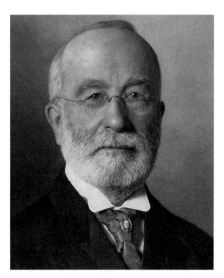

Fig. 11-9. William W. Keen, Jr. (1837-1932). (From A History of Neurosurgery. *Greenblatt SH, Dagi TF, Epstein M, editors. Park Ridge, Ill: American Association of Neurological Surgeons, 1997, p 177)*

subdural hematoma; the same year, he extirpated successfully a meningioma with an overlying hyperostosis. These were operated upon five years prior to Bennett's exploration of the brain tumor diagnosed by Godlee, which was acclaimed the first to be localized on neurological findings. Macewen had performed five laminectomies for paraplegia, some due to granulomatous tumors, before Horsley and Gowers reported their removal of a spinal tumor.

The "cracked pot" sound of a fractured skull is often attributed to Macewen, although he maintained that he was describing a differential percussion note heard when the lateral ventricles were distended. He was a dexterous surgeon who made a number of innovations in general surgery and whom Harvey Cushing acclaimed as the chief pioneer in craniocerebral surgery.

William W. Keen, Jr., (Fig. 11-9) a native of Philadelphia, graduated from Jefferson Medical College in 1862. He served in the American Civil War and in collaboration with Silas Weir Mitchell and George Morehouse published a monograph of their experiences with nerve wounds.

At that time, surgery was quite crude, the antiseptic techniques were just developing, and surgeons operated in bloody aprons using soiled instruments. Bleeding was controlled by tying larger vessels and applying compresses to oozing points. Head wounds frequently broke down, drained, and the patient died of pyemia. For depressed fractures of the skull, operative elevation was successful if the dura mater was not violated; if the brain was exposed, the mortality rate was about 80%. Wounds of the extremities, often involving nerves, were merely closed loosely because the risk of infection was so great. The classic monograph on wounds of the peripheral nerves by Weir Mitchell, Morehouse, and Keen detailed the sensory and motor disturbances, and also clearly described causalgia and its consequences. At the end of the Civil War, Keen visited Europe where he spent some time with Rudolph Virchow in Berlin and Claude Bernard in Paris.

Upon Keen's return to Philadelphia, he opened a practice at the Jefferson Medical College. After hearing Joseph Lister discuss his antiseptic surgical technique in September 1876, Keen resolved to adopt the technique. Using that antiseptic procedure, in 1887 he removed a brain tumor for which he is renowned. The patient was a 26-year-old man who had suffered from seizures, progressive hemiplegia, and speech impairment. In his preparation of the patient, Keen meticulously followed the antiseptic regime. The day before operation, he shaved the patient's head, scrubbed it with soap and water, and applied a corrosive sublimate dressing. The next morning, the patient's head was cleansed with ether and mercuric chloride. After scrubbing with soap and water, Keen doused his hands with alcohol and a sublimate solution. With surgical instruments boiled for two hours and sponges immersed in carbolic and sublimate solutions, the craniotomy was made with a 1½-in. trephine, and the opening was enlarged to expose a velvety outgrowth. The dura mater was cut around the tumor so that Keen could enucleate it with a finger; in so doing, he tore several veins which required ligation or compression with sponges. The dural defect was left open, and the scalp closed over a drain. On the first postoperative day, a large blood clot was removed from the wound. Because the patient's condition worsened on the 10th postoperative day, the wound was reopened, disclosing a swollen brain. The wound drained for a month. It was covered with a split-thickness skin graft and soon healed. The patient survived 30 years and, upon his death, an autopsy showed no signs of residual tumor.

In addition to removing intracranial neoplasms, Keen performed a number of other neurosurgical operations for which he devised special instruments. After his war experiences, Keen was interested in the care of head injuries, especially those complicated by subdural or extradural hemorrhages, which he thought should be evacuated early.

Keen used ventricular drainage for hydrocephalus by puncturing in the frontal, occipital, or temporal region. For spasmodic torticollis, he sectioned the first, second, and third cervical posterior roots, and at times, the spinal accessory nerve supplying the sternocleidomastoid muscle. He performed a number of linear craniotomies for craniostenosis and microcephaly, but admitted that the results were not satisfactory. He was more successful in treating tic douloureux by gasserian ganglionectomy, reporting six cases in 1890 with one death. Although Keen and Spiller had discussed the possibility of performing a retrogasserian neurectomy for trigeminal neuralgia, Keen deferred to Charles Frazier who, under Spiller's direction, perfected that procedure.

Probably as the result of his military experience, Keen was interested in spinal cord and nerve injuries, for which he advised an early operation to prevent scar formation and compression of the nerve roots. Although in their early reports, Keen and his associates did not recommend suture of divided nerves, later they approximated the cut ends with one or two sutures. Such suture of the radial nerve gave a satisfactory recovery of function.

Keen was recognized by surgeons around the world as a pioneer in brain surgery. Although somewhat overshadowed by the University of Philadelphia neuroscientists, Keen maintained his place among the leaders of neurosurgery.

The Dawn of Clinical Neurology

It is difficult to define the first rays of neurology because fragments of nerve function and dysfunction were present in the earliest writings. By the time of Hippocrates, a number of nervous disorders—paralysis, convulsions, intoxications, etc. were known. Galen added an anatomico-physiological basis to these disorders. As Vieussens, Riverius, and Willis wrote of their experimantal and clinical experiences, the Renaissance Period established a pathological basis for clinical upsets of the nervous system. Although Willis may be called the "Father of Neurology," his family was slow to develop.

In the 18th century, the disorders of the nervous system were the province of any physician. It was not until the middle of the next century that conditions of the brain and spinal cord became segregated and considered a special unit. Years had elapsed before Whytt confirmed Galen's experiments and established segmental spinal reflex activity, spinal inhibition and shock. Much of the productive investigation was carried out by individuals working in isolation. Charles Bell established the motor role of the anterior roots of the spinal cord, and Magendie the sensory paths of the posterior roots. At the time, the mental and neurological disturbances were coslesced and so the specialty was of psychiatry and neurology. In fact, for a hundred years the neurologist attended the madhouse to make a living by examining the epileptic and paralyzed to satisfy their scientific interest. They sought ways and means by which they could assess the functional activity of the nervous system. Their examinations tended to separate psychiatrists who formerly had diagnosed and treated all afflictions, organic and functional. With objective means of assessing the function, neurologists could separate the disorders of the mind form those of the brain. In a few cases, the pathological lesion affected both faculties. The special field of organic brain disorders were clearly within the province of the neurologist. However, in Italy, the two specialties combined. In Germany, the psychiatrists often interested in basic neuroscience such as neuro-anatomy, not infrequently enlisted the aid of the neurologist. In England, Hughlings Jackson and William Gowers dominated the medical field and they were able to take control and split from the alienists to develop an independent service. In the United States of America, the field neuropsychiatry was united although psychiatry predominated. By the end of the 19th century, neurology was principally confined to the organic disorders of the nervous system. As a result, these physicians limited their practice to either psychiatry or neurology.

The domain of neurology consisted of a number of disorders well known for ages, such as epilepsy and the traumatic disorders of the brain and spinal cord, as well as many conditions only recognized on the 19th century as originating from the nervous system. The abnormalities, previously not identified, led to the diagnostic understanding of neurological disease. The semeiology and pathology of these neurological disorders established the foundation and dawn of clinical neurology.

Epilogue

This account of the genesis of ideas in neuroscience terminates at the end of the 19th century, setting the stage for the tremendous explosion of new knowledge in neuroscience that has occurred during the 20th century. In this historical account are the seeds of the early advances that occurred in the areas of neurophysiology, electrophysiology, and the biochemistry of the brain.

Although a good understanding of the pathophysiological processes leading to disorders of the central nervous system was evolving, there was probably no way that anyone at the end of the 19th century could have predicted the developments in molecular biology that dominate the field of neuroscience today. It is important, however, for us to continue to reflect upon and respect the pioneering efforts of investigators throughout the history of neuroscience who have made this field of knowledge one of the most exciting and fruitful that exists in all of human endeavor.

As we approach the 21st century, neuroscience is the crown jewel of medical progress. The molecular mechanisms encoded in the human genome are being carefully analyzed. Gene therapy is a practical reality. Developmental neurobiology offers an understanding of the process of neuronal differentiation, neuronal network formation and modulation, and the promise of effective means of regeneration in the damaged nervous system. Mechanisms of disease resulting in behavioral disorders and psychosis should become elucidated as the power of new knowledge in neuroscience is applied to this difficult area. The "mind-brain" dualism that has concerned philosophers and scientists for centuries may be resolved.

Many of the existing developments in neuroscience are the direct result of advances in technology. Computer science development has given us sophisticated diagnostic and functional imaging of the nervous sytem, interactive computer-guided methods of reaching any part of the brain, and models for understanding many aspects of brain function. The technological aspects of molecular biology continue to expand, with new methodologies leading to new strategies of scientific analysis.

The volume of knowledge, the complexities of technology, and the power of the computer must not, however, seduce us away from the fundamental aspects of the endeavors exemplified by the human physicians and scientists dealing with neurological disorders that are the subject of this book. Careful clinical observation continues to be at the heart of our efforts and should not be replaced by technological methods of analysis. Those human elements that resist the impersonal dissection of current scientific methodologies should be cherished as the basis of the human condition. Hopefully, humanity, intellect, civilization, and the arts will continue to enjoy parallel and equivalent importance as we move ahead, respecting and remembering the heritage of those who gave us the beginnings of neuroscience.

Edward R. Laws, Jr.
George B. Udvarhelyi

References

Abercrombie J: **Pathological and Practical Researches on Diseases of the Brain and Spinal Cord.**
Edinburgh: Waugh and Innes, 1828 (3rd ed, 1834)

Abernethy J: **Surgical Observations on Injuries of the Head and on Miscellaneous Subjects.** Philadelphia: T Dobson, 1811

Acrel O: **Case Report in Chirurgiska Händelser, Anmärkte och Samlade uti Kongl. Lazarettet och Annorstädes, med Ansenliga Tilökningar och Bifogade Afritningar.** Stockholm, 1768

Adamkiewicz A: Die Blutgefässe des menschlichen Rückenmarkes. 1. Die Gefässe der Rückenmarkssubstanz. **Sitzungsber Akad Wiss Wien Math Naturwiss Kl 84:**469-502, 1881

Adamkiewicz A: Die Blutgefässe des menschlichen Rückenmarkes. 2. Die Gefässe der Rückenmarksoberfläche. **Sitzungsber Akad Wiss Wien Math Naturwiss Kl 85:**101-130, 1882

Adams F: **The Genuine Works of Hippocrates.** Baltimore, Md: Williams & Wilkins, 1939, 384 pp, 2 Vols (London: Printed for the Sydenham Society, 1849)

Adams J: A case of aneurism of internal carotid in the cavernous sinus, causing paralysis of the third, fourth, fifth and sixth nerves. **Lancet 2:**768, 1869

Adelmann H: The problem of cyclopia. **Q Rev Biol 11:**161-182, 1936

Adie WJ: Idiopathic narcolepsy: a disease *sui generis;* with remarks on the mechanism of sleep. **Brain 49:**257, 1926

Aëtius of Amida: Tetrabiblione, quoted by Major RH: **A History of Medicine.** Springfield, Ill: Charles C Thomas, 1954, Vol 1, pp 211-212

Albucasis: **Albucasis de chirurgia.** (J Channing, ed). Oxford: Clarendon Press, 1778, 2 Vols

Alcazar A: **De vulneribus capitis.** Salamanca, 1575

Alcmaeon of Crotona: quoted by Garrison FH: **History of Medicine. 9th ed.** Philadelphia, Pa: WB Saunders, 1928, pp 89-90

Aldini J: **Essai Théoretique et Expérimental sur le Galvanisme.** Paris: Fournier, 1804, 398 pp

Alexander of Tralles: **Practica.** (T Puschmann, trans). Vienna: Braumuller, 1878-1879, 2 Vols (1504, orig)

Alexander W: **The Treatment of Epilepsy.** Edinburgh: YJ Pentland, 1889, 220 pp

Altunov NV: **Encephalometric Investigations of the Brain Relative to Sex, Age and Skull Indices.** Moscow, 1891

Anderson J: On sensory epilepsy. A case of basal cerebral tumours affecting the left temporo-sphenoidal lobe, and giving rise to a paroxysmal taste-sensation and dreamy state. **Brain 9:**385-395, 1886/1887

Andral G: **Essai d'Hématologie Pathologie.** Paris: Fortin, Masson & Cie, 1843

Andral G: **Précis d'Anatomie Pathologique.** Bruxelles: Wahlen et Cie, 1837

Aran FA: Recherches sur une maladie non encore décrite du système musculaire (atrophie musculaire progressive). **Arch Gen Med (4th ser) 24:**4-35, 172-214, 1850

Aran FA: Revue clinique des hopitaux et hospices. **Un Med 2:**553-554, 557-558, 1848

Arceo F: **De recta curandorum vulnerum retione, et aliis eus artis praeceptis, libri ii.** Amberes, 1574

Aretaeus: **The Extant Works of Aretaeus, the Cappadocian.** (F Adams, ed and trans). London: Sydenham Society, 1856, 510 pp

Argyll Robertson D: On an interesting series of eye symptoms in a case of spinal disease, with remarks on the action of belladonna on the iris. **Edinburgh Med J 14:**696-708, 1869

Aristotle: **Aristotle's Psychology: A Treatise on the Principles of Life.** (WA Hammond, trans). London: S Sonnenschein & Co, 1902, 339 pp

Arnold DJ: Weitëre Beiträge zur Akromegaliefrage. **Virchows Arch Pathol Anat Physiol 135:**1-78, 1894

Arnold J: Myelocyste; Transposition von Gewebskeimen und Sympodie. **Beitr Pathol Anat Pathol 16:**1-28, 1894

Asclepiades of Prussia: quoted by Major RH: **A History of Medicine.** Springfield, Ill: Charles C Thomas, 1954, Vol 1, pp 164-166

Asklepios: quoted by Major RH: **A History of Medicine.** Springfield, Ill: Charles C Thomas, 1954, Vol 1, pp 102-105

Auché M: Des névrites péripheriques chez les cancéreux. **Rev Med (Paris) 10**:785-807, 1890

Aurelianus C: **On Acute Diseases and on Chronic Diseases.** (IE Drabkin, trans). Chicago, Ill: University of Chicago Press, 1950, 1019 pp

Avenzoar: **Alterser.** Venice: Teisar, 1490

Averroës: **Colliget [Book on universals].** Lugduni: J Guinta, 1531

Avicenna: **Libri in re medica omnes qui hactenus ad nos pervenere.** Venice: V Valgrisium, 1564, 2 Vols

Avicenna: **The Canon of Medicine.** (OC Gruner, trans). London: Luzac & Co, 1930

Axtell WH: Acute angulation and flexure of the sigmoid. A causative factor in epilepsy. Preliminary report of 31 cases. **Am J Surg 24**:385-387, 1910

Babinski J: Tumeur du corps pituitaire sans acromégalie et avec arrêt de dévelopement des organes génitaux. **Rev Neurol 8**:531-533, 1900

Babinski JFF: Sur le réflexe cutané plantaire dans certaines affections organiques du système nerveux central. **Compt Rend Soc Biol (9th ser) 3**:207-208, 1896

Babinski JFF: Sur le rôle du cervelet dans les actes volitionnels nécessitant une succession rapide de mouvements (diadococinésie). **Rev Neurol 10**:1013-1015, 1902

Babinski JFF: De l'abduction des orteils (signe de l'éventuil). **Rev Neurol 11**:1205-1206, 1903

Badal J: Contribution à l'étude des cécites psychiques. Alexie, agraphie, hémianopsie inférieure, trouble du sens d'l'espace. **Arch Ophtalmol (Paris) 140**:97-117, 1888

Baillic M: **The morbid anatomy of some of the most important parts of the human body.** London: J Johnson & G Nicol, 1793

Ballala of Benares: **The Narrative of Bhoja (Bhojaprabandha).** (LH Gray, trans). New Haven, Conn: American Oriental Society, 1950, 107 pp

Ballance CA: **The Dawn and Epic of Neurology and Surgery.** Glasgow: Jackson and Wylie, 1930

Bang BLF: Die Aetiologie des seuchenhaften ("infectiösen") Verwerfens. **Z Thiermed 1**:241-278, 1897

Bar-sela A, Hoff HE: Asaf on anatomy and physiology. **J Hist Med Allied Sci 20**:358-389, 1965

Bard S: **An enquiry into the nature, cause and cure of the angina suffocativa, or sore throat distemper, as it is commonly called by the inhabitants of this city and colony.** New York, NY: S Inslee & A Car, 1771

Barker AE: Notes on a case of cerebral suppuration due to otitis media diagnosed and successfully treated by trephining and drainage. **Br Med J 1**:777-781, 1888

Bartholin C: **Institutiones anatomicae.** Leiden: Hack, 1641, 496 pp

Bartholow R: Aneurisms of the arteries at the base of the brain: their symptomatology, diagnosis and treatment. **Am J Med Sci 64**:373-386, 1872

Bartholow R: Experimental investigations into the functions of the human brain. **Am J Med Sci 67**:305-313, 1874

Bartholow R: Experiments on the function of the human brain. **Br Med J 1**:727, 1874 (Letter)

Bastian HC: On the symptomatology of total transverse lesions of the spinal cord with special reference to the condition of the various reflexes. **Med Chir Trans 73**:151-217, 1890

Batten FE: Ataxia in childhood. **Brain 28**:484-505, 1905

Bechterev VM von: Acutely developing disturbances of movement in alcoholics with features of cerebellar ataxia. **Obozr Psikhiat 5**:1-4, 1900

Beck A: Die Bestimmung der Localisation der Gehirn- und Rückenmarksfunctionen vermittelst der elektrischen Erscheinungen. **Centralbl Physiol 4**:473-476, 1890

Behring AE von: Die Behandlung der Diptherie mit Dipththerie Heilserum. **Dtsch Med Wochenschr 19**:543-547, 1893; **20**:645-646, 1894

Bell B: **A system of surgery.** Edinburgh: C Elliott, 1782-1787, 7 Vols

Bell C: **Idea of a New Anatomy of the Brain Submitted for the Observations of his Friends.** London: Strahan and Preston, 1811, 36 pp

Bell C: On the nerves: giving an account of some experiences on the structure and functions, which lead to a new arrangement of the system. **Phil Trans 111**:398-424, 1821

Bell C: **The Nervous System of the Human Body.** London: Longman et al, 1830, 238 pp

Benda C: Beiträge zur normalen und pathologischen Histologie der menschlichen Hypophysis Cerebri. **Berl Klin Wochenschr 37**:1205-1210, 1900

Benivieni A: **De abditis nonnulus ac mirandis morborum et sanationum causis.** Florence: F Giuntae, 1507

Bennett AH, Godlee RJ: Case of cerebral tumour. The surgical treatment. **Trans R Med Chir Soc Lond 68:**243-275, 1885 (Reproduced by Wilkins RH (ed): **Neurosurgical Classics.** Park Ridge, Ill: American Association of Neurological Surgeons, 1992, pp 361-371)

Bennett AH, Godlee RJ: Excision of a tumor from the brain. **Lancet 2:**1090-1091, 1884

Berengario da Carpi J: **Commentaria cum amplissimis additionibus super anatomia Mundini una cum textu ejusdem in pristinum et verum nitorem redacto.** Bologna: H de Benedictis, 1521, 528 pp

Berger H: Ueber das Elektrenkephalogramm des Menschen. I. Mitteilung. **Arch Psychiat Nervenkr 87:**527-570, 1929

Bergmann E von: **Die Chirurgische Behandlung von Hirnkrankheiten. Zweite, Vermehrte und Umgearbeitete Auflage.** Berlin: A Hirschwald, 1888, 189 pp

Bergmann E von: Zur Sublimatfrage. **Therapmh 1:**41-44, 1887

Bheshagratna KK: **The Sushruta Samhita.** 1963

Bianchi GB: **Storia Del Mostra Di Due Corpi.** Turin, 1748, 139 pp

Bianchi L: La funzione dei lobi prefontale. **Arch Ital Biol 22:**102-105, 1894

Bible: **Genesis 17:3**

Bible: **Leviticus 13:3**

Bible: **Mark 9:17**

Bickers DS, Adams RD: Hereditary stenosis of the aqueduct of Sylvius as a cause of congenital hydro-cephalus. **Brain 72:**246-262, 1949

Blocq L, Marinesco G: Sur un cas de tremblement Parkinsonien hémiplégie symptomatique d'une tumeur de pédoncle cérébal. **Compt Rend Soc Biol (9th ser) 2:**105-111, 1893 (or 45:105, 1893)

Blum F: Der Formaldehyd als Härtungsmittel. **Z Wissensch Mikrosc 10:**314-315, 1893

Boerhaave H: **Praelectiones academicae de morbis nervorum.** Lugduni Batavorum: apud Petrum, 1761

Bolk L: **Das Cerebellum der Säugethiere.** Harlen: Bohn, 1906

Bonetus T: **Sepulchretum.** 1679, 3 Vols

Bonhoeffer K: Klinisch-anatomische Beiträge zur Pathologie des Sehhügels und der Regio subthalam-ica: ein Sehhügelherd. **Monatschr Psychiat Neurol 67:**253-271, 1928

Bonnier P: Le question de l'orientation lointaine. **Rev Scient Paris 2:**837-839, 1904

Bontius J: **De medicina indorum.** Lugduni Batavorum: F Hackiun, 1642

Bordet JJBV, Gengou O: Le Microbe da la coqueluche. **Ann Inst Pasteur 20:**131-141, 1906; **21:** 720-726, 1907

Bouillaud JB: Exposition de nouveaux faits à l'appui de l'opinion qui localise dans les lobules antérieurs du cerveau dont cette opinion à été sujet. **Bull Acad Med 4:**282-328, 333-349, 353-369, 1839/1840

Bouillaud JB: Recherches cliniques propres à démontrer que la perte de la parole correspond à la lésion de lobules antérieurs du cerveau et à confirmer l'opinion de M. Gall sur le siège de l'organe du lan-gage articulé. **Arch Gen Med 7:**25-45, 1825

Bouillaud JB: Recherches expérimentales sur les fonctions du cerveau (lobes cérébraux) en général, et sur celles de sa portion antérieure en particulier. **J Physiol Exp Pathol 10:**36-98, 1830

Bouillaud JB: **Traité Clinique et Physiologique de l'Encèphalite ou Inflammation du Cerveau.** Paris: JB Baillière, 1825

Bourneville S, Noir J: Hydrocéphalie. **Prog Med (Paris) 12:**17-23, 1900

Boyle R: **Experimenta et observationes physicae.** London: J Taylor, 1691, 32 pp

Bramann von: Ueber Exstirpation von Hirntumoren. **Arch Klin Chir 45:**365-400, 1893

Bramwell B: **Intracranial Tumours.** Edinburgh: YJ Pentland, 1888, 270 pp

Bramwell B: **The Diseases of the Spinal Cord.** Edinburgh: Maclachlan and Stewart, 1882, 300 pp (2nd ed, 1884)

Breasted JH: **The Edwin Smith Surgical Papyrus Published in Facsimile and Hieroglyphic Trans-literation with Translation and Commentary in Two Volumes.** Chicago, Ill: University of Chicago Press, 1930

Bretonneau P: **Des Inflammatións Spéciales du Tissu Muqueux et en Particulier de la Diphthérite, ou Inflammation Pelliculaire.** Paris: Crevot, 1826

Brewitt-Taylor CH: **San Kuo, or Romance of the Three Kingdoms.** Shanghai: Kelly & Walsh, 1925, 2 Vols

Bright R: Cases and observations illustrative of diagnoses where tumors are situated at the base of the brain; etc. **Guys Hosp Rep 2:**279-310, 1837

Bright R: Fatal epilepsy, from suppuration between the dura mater and arachnoid. **Guys Hosp Rep 1:**36-40, 1836

Bright R: **Reports of Medical Cases Selected with a View of illustrating the Symptoms and Cure of Diseases by Reference to Morbid Anatomy. Diseases of the Brain and Nervous System.** London: Longman, 1831

Broadbent WH: Cerebral mechanism of speech and thought. **Med Chir Trans 55:**145-194, 1872

Broca P: Perte de la parole; ramollissement chronique et destruction partielle du lobe anterieur gauche du cerveau. **Bull Soc Anat (Paris) 2:**235-238, 1861

Broca P: Remarques sur le siège de le faculté du language articulé, suivie d'une observation d'aphémie. **Bull Soc Anat (2nd ser) 6:**330-357, 1861

Broca P: Sur la topographie cranium cérébrale. **Rev Anthrop 5:**193, 1876

Broca P: Sur les trépanations préhistoriques. **Bull Mem Soc Anthropol (Paris) (2nd ser) 25:** 542-557, 1874

Brossard J: **Etude Clinique sur une Forme Héréditaire d'Atrophie Musculaire Progressive Débutant par les Membres Inférieurs (Type Fémoral avec Griffe des Orteils).** Paris: Steinheil, 1886

Brousse A: De l'Ataxie Héréditaire. Montpellier, 1882, No 37 (Thesis)

Brown S, Schäfer EA: An investigation into the functions of the occipital and temporal lobes of the monkey's brain. **Phil Trans R Soc Lond 179B:**303-327, 1888

Brown S: On hereditary ataxy with a series of twenty-one cases. **Brain 15:**250-268, 1892

Brown-Séquard CE: De la transmission des impressions sensitives par la moëlle épinière. **Compt Rend Soc Biol (Paris) 1:**192-194, 1849

Brown-Séquard CE: Recherches expérimentales sur la production d'une affection convulsive épiletiforme, à la suite de lésions de la moëlle épinière. **Arch Gen Med (5th ser) 7:**143-149, 1856

Brudzinski J: Un signe nouveau sur les membiers inférieurs dans les méningites chez les enfants. **Arch Med Enf 12:**745, 1909

Bruno: **Cyrurgia magna.** 1252

Bruns V von: Die chirurgischen Krankheiten und Verletzungen des Gehirns und seiner Umhullung, in von Bruns V (ed): **Handbuch der Praktischen Chirurgie für Aerzte und Wundärzte.** Tübingen: H Laupp, 1854

Brunschwig H: **Dis ist das buch der cirurgia hautwirckung der wundartzney von Hyeronimo Brunschwig.** Strassburg: J Grüninger, 1497

Brunus: Chirurgia magna, in: **Collectio chirurgica.** Veneta, 1498, pp 83-102

Bubnoff N, Heidenhain R: Ueber Erregungs - und Hemmungsvorgänge innerhalb der motorischen Hirncentren. **Arch Ges Physiol 26:**137-200, 1881-1882

Budge EAW: **The Book of the Dead.** London: Kesgan, Paul, Trenol, Trubner & Co, 1898, 354 pp

Bürger L: Thrombo-angiitis obliterans; a study of the vascular lesions leading to presenile spontaneous gangrene. **Am J Med Sci 136:**567-580, 1908

Cabanis PJG: **Rapports du Physique et du Moral de l'Homme.** Paris: Masson et Cie, 1843, Vol 1, 405 pp

Cairns H: Acoustic neurinoma of right cerebello-pontine angle. Complete removal. Spontaneous recovery from post-operative facial palsy. **Proc R Soc Med 25:**35-40, 1931

Caldani LMA: **Icones Anatomices.** Venice, 1801-1813

Canappe J: **L'anatomie des os du corps humain.** Lyons, 1541

Captaine PA: **Un Grand Medicin du XVIe siecle, Jean Fernal.** Paris: Librairie le Francois, 1925

Carville C, Duret H: Sur les fonctions des hémisphères cérébraux (histoire, critique et recherches expérimentales). **Arch Physiol (2nd ser) 2:**352-491, 1875

Casal G: **Historia natural, y medica de el principado de asturias.** Madrid: M Martin, 1762

Casserius J: Tabulae anatomicae LXXIIX, in Spigelius A (ed): **Opera que extant.** Amsterdam, 1645

Caton R: The electric currents of the brain. **Br Med J 2:**278, 1875

Celsus AC: **Translations of the Eight Books on Medicine. 2nd ed.** London: Simpkin & Marshall, 1831, 263 pp (revised by GF Collier)

Charcot J: De la maladie de Ménière (vertigo ab aure loesa). **Prog Med (Paris) 2:**37-38, 49-51, 1874

Charcot JM, Bouchard A: Douleurs fulgurantes de l'ataxie sans incoordination des movements; sclérose commençante des cordons postérieurs de la moëlle épinière. **Gaz Med Paris (3rd ser) 21**:122-124, 1866

Charcot JM, Bouchard CJ: Nouvelles recherches sur la pathogenie de l'hemorrhagie cerebrale. **Arch Phys Norm Pathol 1**:725, 1868

Charcot JM, Cornil AV: Contributions à l'étude des altérations anatomiques de la goutte. **Compt Rend Soc Biol Mem (3rd ser) 5**:139-163, 1864

Charcot JM, Joffroy A: Une observation de paralysie infantile s'accompagnant d'une altération des cornes antérieures de la substance grise de la moëlle. **Compt Rend Acad Soc Biol (5th ser) 1**: 312-315, 1870

Charcot JM, Marie P: Sur une forme particulière d'atrophie musculaire progressive, souvent familiale, débutant par les pieds et les jambes et atteignant plus tard les mains. **Rev Med 6**:97-138, 1886

Charcot JM, Pitres JA: **Les Centres Moteurs Corticaux chez l'Homme.** Paris: Rueff & Cie, 1895

Charcot JM, Richer P: **Les Démoniaques dans l'Art.** Paris: A Delahaye & E Le Crosnier, 1887

Charcot JM, Richer P: **Les Difformes et les Maladies dans l'Art.** Paris: Lecrosnier and Bebé, 1889

Charcot JM, Vulpian EFA: De la paralyse agìtante. **Gaz Hebd 8**:765-767, 1861/1862

Charcot JM: Des amyotrophies spinalis chroniques. **Prog Med 2**:573-574, 1874

Charcot JM: Des différentes formes de l'aphasie de la cécité verbale. **Prog Med (Paris) 11**:441-444, 1883

Charcot JM: Deux cas d'atrophie musculaire progressive avec lesions de la substance grise. **Arch Physiol Norm Pathol 2**:744-760, 1869

Charcot JM: Histologie de la sclérose en plaques. **Gaz Hop 41**:554-555, 1868

Charcot JM: **Leçons sur les Localizations dans les Maladies du Cerveau et de la Moelle Epinière Faites à la Faculté de Médecine de Paris. Recueillies et Publiées par Bourneville et E. Brissaud.** Paris: VA Delahaye, 1876-1880, 425 pp

Charcot JM: **Leçons sur les Maladies du Système Nerveux Faites à la Salpêtrière.** Paris: A Delahaye, 3 Vols, 1872-1873

Charcot JM: **Lectures on the Diseases of the Nervous System.** (WB Hadden, trans and ed). London: New Sydenham Society, 1877, 2 Vols

Charcot JM: Sur quelques arthropathies qui paraissent dépondre d'une lésion du cerveau ou de la moëlle epiniere. **Arch Phys Norm Pathol 1**:161-178, 1868

Chassaignac E: Mémoire sur l'écoulement séreux qui s'effectue par d'oreille à la suite des fractures du rocher. **Mem Soc Chir (Paris) 1**:542-562, 1847

Chen KKK, Ling ASH: Fragments of medical history. **Ann Med Hist 8**:185-191, 1926

Cheselden W: **The anatomy of the human body, 6th ed.** London: W Bowyer, 1741, 336 pp

Chiari H: Ueber die Pathogenese der Sogennanten Syringomyelie. **Z Hielkunde 9**:307-336, 1888

Chiari H: Ueber Veränderungen des Kleinhirns infolge von Hydrocephalie des Grosshirns. **Dtsch Med Wochenschr 17**:1172-1175, 1891

Chiari H: Ueber Veränderungen des Kleinhirns, des Pons, und der Medulla Oblongata infolge von congenitaler Hydrocephalie des Grosshirns. **Denkschr K Akad Wiss Math Nature Kl 63**:71, 1895

Chipault A: **Chirurgie opératoire du système nerveux.** Paris: Rueff & Cie, 1891, 2 Vols

Chipault A: Note sur deux instruments destinés à facilites les operations crâniennes: une pince à compresses, une pince hémostatique à demeure. **Trans Neurol Chir 2**:15-16, 1897

Chopart F, Desault PJ: **Traité des maladies chirurgicales et des operations qui leu conviennent.** Paris: Villier, 1796, 2 Vols

Clarke ES, O'Malley CD: **The Human Brain and Spinal Cord.** Berkeley, Calif: University of California Press, 1968, 926 pp

Cleland J: Contribution to the study of spina bifida, encephalocele, and anencephalus. **J Anat Physiol 17**:257-291, 1883

Cleland J: Description of two tumours adherent to the deep surface of the dura mater. **Glasgow Med J 11**:148-159, 1864

Clevenger SV: **Spinal Concussion.** Philadephia, Pa: FA Davis, 1889, 359 pp

Cobb S: Haemangioma of the spinal cord associated with skin naevi of the same metamere. **Ann Surg 62**:641-649, 1915

Constantine A: **Arch Gaschichte Med 23**:293-298, 1930

Constantinus Africanus: **Pantegni [The Total Art].**

Constantinus Africanus: **Regimen Sanitatis or Flos Medicine.**

Cooper A: **Lectures on the Principles and Practice of Surgery.** London: H Renshaw, 1839, 683 pp

Cooper A: Some experiments and observations on tying the carotid and vertebral arteries, and the pneumo-gastric, phrenic and sympathetic nerves. **Guys Hosp Rep 1:**457-475, 1836

Cords R: Einseitige Kleinheit der Papille. **Klin Monatlbl Augenheilk 71:**414, 1923

Corner GW: Anatomical texts of the Eastern Middle Ages. A study of the transmission of culture, with a revised Latin text of "Anatomia Cophonis" and translation of four texts. **Ann Med Hist 10:**1928

Corning JL: Spinal anesthesia and local medication of the cord. **NY Med J 42:**483-485, 1885

Cotugno DFA: **De ischiade nervosa commentarius.** Naples: Simoni, 1764

Critchley M: **The Divine Banquet of the Brain and Other Essays.** New York, NY: Raven Press, 1979, 267 pp

Croce GA della: **Chirurgiae . . . libra septem. . . .** Venetiis: Jordanum Zile Hum, 1573

Cruce JA: **Chirurgiae libri septum.** Venice: J Zilettus, 1573, 311 pp

Cruveilhier J: **Anatomie Pathologique du Corps Humain; ou, Descriptions, avec Figures Lithographées et Coloriées; des Diverses Altérations Morbides dont le Corps Humain est Susceptible.** Paris: JB Baillière & Fils, 1829-1842

Cruveilhier J: Sur la paralysie musculaire, progressive, atrophique. **Bull Acad Med 18:**490-502, 546-583, 1852-1853

Cserna S: Arteritis obliterans mit analogen Vëranderungen in den venen. **Arch Intern Med 12:** 213-226, 1926

Cumings JN: The copper and iron content in brain and liver in the normal and hepato-lenticular degeneration. **Brain 71:**410-415, 1948

Cushing H, Eisenhardt L: **Meningiomas. Their Classification, Regional Behaviour, Life History, and Surgical End Results.** Springfield, Ill: Charles C Thomas, 1938

Cushing H: A note upon the faradic stimulation of the postcentral gyrus in conscious patients. **Brain 32:**44-53, 1909

Cushing H: Surgery of the head, in Keen WW (ed): **Surgery: Its Principles and Practice.** Philadelphia, Pa: WB Saunders, 1908, pp 17-276

Cushing H: Technical methods of performing certain cranial operations. **Surg Gynecol Obstet 6:** 227-246, 1922

Cushing H: The basophil adenomas of the pituitary body and their clinical manifestations (pituitary basophilism). **Johns Hopkins Hosp Bull 50:**137-195, 1932

Cushing H: The hypophysis cerebri. Clinical aspects of hyperpituitarism and of hypopituitarism. **JAMA 53:**249-255, 1909

Cushing H: The meningiomas (dural endotheliomas): their source, and favoured seats of origin. **Brain 45:**282-316, 1922

Czermak JN: Ueber mechanische Vagus-Reizung beim Menshen. **Jena Z Med Naturw 2:**384-386, 1865-1866

Czerny V: **Beiträge zur Operativen Chirurgie.** Stuttgart: F Enke, 1878, 392 pp

Dale HH: The action of certain esters and ethers of choline, and their relaton to muscarine. **J Pharmacol 6:**147-190, 1914

Dalechampius J: **Chirurgie françoise. Ensemblé de quelques traictez des opérations de chirurgie facilitées et éclaircies par Jean Girault.** Paris: O de Varennes, 1610, 664 pp

Dandy W: An operative treatment for certain cases of meningocele (or encephalocele) into the orbit. **Arch Ophthalmol 2:**123-132, 1929

Dandy WE, Blackfan KD: An experimental and clinical study of internal hydrocephalus. **JAMA 61:** 2216-2217, 1913

Dandy WE, Blackfan KD: Internal hydrocephalus, an experimental, clinical and pathologic study. **Am J Dis Child 8:**406-482, 1914

Dandy WE: The treatment of carotid cavernous arteriovenous aneurysms. **Ann Surg 102:**916-926, 1935

David JP: **Dissertation sur les éffets du mouvement et du répos dans les maladies chirurgicales.** Paris: Vallat-la-Chapelle, 1779, 164 pp

Davidoff LM, Dyke CG: Agenesis of corpus callosum. Its diagnosis by encephalography. Report of three cases. **Am J Roentgenol 32:**1-10, 1934

Dax M: Lésions de la moitié gauche de l'encéphale coincidant avec l'oublie des signes de la pensée (lu a Montpellier en 1836). **Gaz Hebd Med Chir 2:**259-262, 1865

Daza Chacón D: **Práctica y teórica de Cirurgia en romance y en Latin.** Valencia, 1673 (Valladolid, 1584-1595)

de Argumosa D: **Resumen de Cirugia.** Madrid, 1856

de Cyon E, Ludwig CFW: Die Reflexe eines der Sensiblen Nerven des Herzens auf die motorischen der Blutgefässe. **Arb Physiol Anat Leipzig 1:**128-149, 1867

de Martel T: La technique opératoire en chirurgie nerveuse. **Gaz Hop (Paris) 86:**2045-2048, 1913

de Panizza B: Osservazioni sul nuevo ottico. **Giornale I 1st Lomb Sci 7:**237-252, 1855

de Roda y Bayas J: **Cirugia Rational; Breve, Sagua y Curacion de las Herida de Cabeza.** Zaragoza: P Carreras, 1923

de Sauvages: **Nosologia methodica.** Amsterdam: Sumptibus Fratrum de Tournes, 1763

Dejerine J: **Anatomie des Centres Nerveux.** Paris: J Rueff et Cie, 1890-1891, 2 Vols

Dejerine J: Contribution à l'étude anatomo-pathologie et clinique des différentes variétiés de cécité verbale. **Compt Rend Soc Biol (Paris) 44:**61-90, 1892

Dejerine J: Sur un cas de cécité verbale avec agraphie, suivi d'autopsie. **Compt Rend Soc Biol (Paris) 43:**197-201, 1891

Dejerine JJ, Roussy G: Le syndrome thalamique. **Rev Neurol 12:**521-532, 1906

Dejerine JJ, Sottas J: Sur la névrite interstitielle hypertrophique et progressive de l'enfance. Affection souvent familiale et à début infantile, caractérisée par une atrophie musculaire des extremités avec troubles marqués de la sensibilité et ataxie des mouvements et relevant d'une névrite interstitielle hypertrophique à marche ascendante avec lésions médullaires associées. **Compt Rend Soc Biol (9th ser) 45:**63-96, 1893

Delpech JM: **De l'Orthomorphie.** Paris: Gabon, 1828, 2 Vols

Delstanche: Notes relatives à un cas d'abcès intradural consécutif à une otite moyenne purulente droite. **Bull Soc Belge Otol Lar Rhin 3:**38-40, 1898

Demy G, Camus P: Sur une forme d'hypochondrie aberrante due à la perte de la conscience du corps. **Rev Neurol 13:**461-467, 1905

Dercum FX, Keen WW, Spiller WG: Endothelioma of the Gasserian ganglion; two successive resections of the ganglion; first by the extradural (Hartley-Krause) operation and second by an intradural operation. **JAMA 34:**1026-1033, 1900

Descartes R: **De homine figuris et latinitate donatus a Florentio Schuyl.** Lugduni Batavorum: F Moyardum & P Leffen, 1662

Detmold W: Abscess in the substance of the brain; the lateral ventricles opened by an operation. **Am J Med Sci (new ser) 19:**86-95, 1850

Dingwall SJ: **Artificial Cranial Deformation; A Contribution to the Study of Ethnic Mutilations.** London: John Bale Sons, & Danielsson, 1931, 313 pp

Dionis P: **Cours de'operations de chirurgie. . . .** Paris: L d'Houry, 1707

Dott NM: Intracranial aneurysms: cerebral arterioradiography: surgical treatment. **Edinburgh Med J (new ser) 40:**219-234, 1933

Dreschfeld J: On some of the rarer forms of muscular atrophies. **Brain 9:**178-195, 1886

Duane A: Congenital deficiency of abduction associated with impairment of adduction, retraction movements, contractions of the palpebral fissure and oblique movements of the eye. **Arch Ophthalmol 34:**133-159, 1905

DuBois-Reymond E: **Untersuchungen über Thiersche Elektricität.** Berlin: GE Reimer, 1848-1884, 2 Vols

Duchenne de Boulogne GBA: **De l'Electrisation Localisée, et de son Application à la Pathologie à la Pathologie et à la Thérapeutique.** Paris: JB Baillière, 1855 (2nd ed, 1861; 3rd ed, 1872)

Duchenne de Boulogne GBA: Étude comparée des lésions dans l'atrophie musculaire graisseuse progressive et dans la paralysie générale. **Un Med 7:**215-255, 1853

Duchenne de Boulogne GBA: Paralysie musculaire progressive de la langue, du voile du palais et des lèvres. **Arch Gen Med (5th ser) 16:**283-296, 431-445, 1860

Duchenne de Boulogne GBA: Recherches faites à l'aide du galvanisme sur l'etat de la contractileté et de la sensibilité électro-musculaires dans les paralysies de membranes supérieures. **Compt Rend Acad Sci 29:**667-670, 1849

Duckworth WLH: **Galen on Anatomical Procedures, The Later Books.** (MC Lyons and B Towers, eds). Cambridge, Engl: Cambridge University Press, 1962, 279 pp

Duplay A: Observations de maladies des centres nerveux; recueilliés à l'hôpital de la Pitié, dans le service de M. le professuer Rostan. **Arch Gen Med (2nd ser) 6:**478-499, 1834

Dupuytren G: **Leçons Orales de Clinique Chirurgicale Faites à l'Hôtel Dieu de Paris. Recueillies par Brierre de Boismont et Marx.** 2nd ed. Paris: Germer-Baillière, 1839

Durant W: **The Story of Civilization. Part 1. Our Oriental Heritage.** 1954, Vol 1, p 532

Durant W: **The Story of Civilization. The Life of Greece.** 1939, Vol 2, pp 95-96

Durante F: Estepazione di un tumore endocranico (forma morbosa prima e dopo l'operazione). **Boll Accad Mem Roma 11:**247-252, 1885

Durante F: **Trattato di patologia e terapie chirurgica generale e speciale.** Rome: Societa ed Dante Alighieri, 1898-1899, 3 Vols

Dutrochet RJH: **Recherches Anatomiques et Physiologiques sur la Structure Intime des Animaux et der Végétaux, et sur leur Motilaté.** Paris: JB Baillière, 1824, 233 pp

Duval M: Technique de l'emploi du collodion humide pour la pratique des coupes microscopiques. **J Anat Physiol 15:**185-188, 1879

Dyke CG, Davidoff LM, Masson CB: Cerebral hemiatrophy with homolateral hypertrophy of the skull and sinuses. **Surg Gynecol Obstet 57:**588-600, 1933

Ebbell B: Die Ält-Agyptische Chirurgie, die Chirurgischen Abschnitte der Papyrus E. Smith und Papyrus Ebers. **Skr Norske Viden Akad Oslo II Hist-Filos Kl 2:**1-92, 1939

Ecker A: **On the Convolutions of the Human Brain.** (JC Galton, trans). London: Smith & Elder, 1873

Ehrenberg CG: Nothwendigkeit einer feineren mechanischen Zerlegung des Gehirns und der Nerven vor der chemischen dargestellt aus Beobachtungen von CG Ehrenberg. **Ann Phys Chem 28:**449-473, 1833

Ehrlich P: Ueber die Methylenblaureaction der lebenden Nervensubstanz. **Dtsch Med Wochenschr 12:**49-52, 1886

Eijkman C: Polyneuritis bij hoenders. **Geneesk T Nederl Indie 36:**214, 1896

Elgood C: A medical history of Persia and the eastern caliphate from the earliest times until the year 1932. **J Hist Med 7:**194-197, 1952

Elliott TR: On the action of adrenalin. **J Physiol 31:**xx-xxi, 1904

Erasistratus, in: **Medicorum Graecorum Opera Quae Exstant.** (DCG Kühn, ed). Leipzig: C Cnoblochius, 1823, 26 Vols

Erb WH: Handbuch der Krankheiten spinalen Symptomencomplex. **Berl Klin Wochenschr 12:** 357-359, 1875

Erb WH: Ueber Schnenreflexe bei Gesunden und ber Rückenmarkskranken. **Arch Psychiatr Nervenkr 6:**792-802, 1875

Esch P: Ueber Kernikterus der Neugeborenen. **Zentralbl Gynek Leipz 32:**969-976, 1908

Estienne C: **De dissection partium corporis humani.** Paris, 1545

Estienne C: **La dissection des parties du corps humain divisée en trois livres.** Paris: Simon de Collines, 1546

Eulenburg M: Ueber progressive Muskelatrophie. **Dtsch Klin 6:**129-131, 1856

Eustachius B: **Tabulae anatomicae.** (JM Lancisius, trans). Amsterdam: R and G Wetstenios, 1722, 115 pp

Evans AC: **Studies on Brucella (Alkaligenes) Melitensis.** Washington, DC: Government Printing Office, 1925

Exsner S: **Untersuchungen über die Localisation der Functionen in der Grosshirnrinde des Menschen.** Wien: Wilhelm Braumüller, 1881

Fabricius Hildanus: **Observationum et curationum medico-chirurgicarum. Opera quae extant omnia.** Frankfurt: J Beyeri, 1646

Faivre E: Observations sur les granulations méningiennes ou glandes de Pacchioni. **Ann Sci Natl (Zool) (3rd ser) 20:**321-333, 1853

Fallopius G: **Observationes anatomicae.** Venetiis: MA Ulmum, 1561

Fallopius G: **Opera omnia. Cui nunc denum accessit tomus secundus.** Francofurti: A Wecheli, 1600, 2 Vols

Falret J: De l'état mental des épileptiques. **Arch Gen Med 16:**661-679, 1860; **17:**461-491, 1861; **18:** 423-443, 1861

Fazio F: Ereditarietà della paralisi bulbare progressiva. **Riv Med 4:**327, 1892

Feindel W (ed): **Thomas Willis: The Anatomy of the Brain and Nerves. Classics of Neurology and Neurosurgery Library.** Montreal: McGill University Press, 1983, 192 pp

Fernel JF: **Medicina.** Lutetiae Parisiorun: A Wechelum, 1554

Ferrara G: **Nuova selva di cirugia divisia in tre parti.** Venice: S Combi, 1608, 565 pp

Ferrier D: Discussion of paper by Bennett AH, Godlee RS: Case of cerebral tumour. The surgical treatment. **Br Med J 1:**988-989, 1885

Ferrier D: Experimental researches in cerebral physiology and pathology. **West Riding Lunatic Asylum Med Rep 3:**30-96, 1873

Ferrier D: On the localisation of the functions of the brain. **Br Med J 2:**766-767, 1874

Ferrier D: **The Functions of the Brain.** London: Smith, Elder and Co, 1876

Ferrier D: The localisation of function in the brain. **Proc R Soc Lond 22:**229-232, 1874

Finkelnburg FC: Asymbolie und Aphasie. **Berl Klin Wochenschr 7:**449-450, 460-462, 1870

Flechsig P: **Die Leitungsbahnen im Gehirn und Rückenmark des Menschen auf Grund entwicklings geschlichlicher Untersuchungen.** Leipzig: Wilhelm Engelmann, 1876

Fleischl von Marxow E: Mittheilung betreffend die Physiologie der Hirnrinde. **Centralbl Physiol 4:** 538, 1890

Fletcher HM: A case of megaloencephaly. **Trans Pathol Soc Lond 51:**230-232, 1900

Flourens MJP: **Recherches Expérimentales sur les Propriétés et les Fonctions du Système Nerveux dans les Animaux Vertébrés.** Paris: Crevot, 1824, 332 pp

Flourens MJP: Recherches physiques sur les propriétés et les fonctions du système nerveux dans les animaux vertébrés. **Arch Gen Med 2:**321-370, 1823

Foerster O: Motorische Felder und Bahnen, in Bumke O, Foerster O (eds): **Handbuch der Neurologie.** Berlin: Springer-Verlag, 1936, Vol 6, pp 1-357

Foix C, Hillemand P: Les synchromes de la région thalamique. **Presse Med 33:**113-117, 1925

Fontana FGF: **Richerche filosofiche sopra il veleno della vipera.** Lucca: J Giusti, 1767

Fontana FGF: **Traité sur le venin de la vipère.** Florence, 1781, 2 Vols

Foster H: **Lectures on the History of Physiology During the Sixteenth, Seventeenth and Eighteenth Centuries.** Cambridge, Engl: Cambridge University Press, 1901, 310 pp

Fothergill J: in Elliott J: **A complete collection of the medical and philosophical works of John Fothergill.** London: J Walker, 1781, 661 pp

Fothergill J: Remarks on that complaint commonly known as under the name of the sick head-ach. **Med Observ Inqu 6:**103-137, 1777/1784

Fournié E: **Recherche Expérimentales sur le Fonctionnement du Cerveau.** Paris: A Delahaye, 1873, 99 pp

Frapolli F: **Animadversionen in morbum, vulgo pellagram.** Milan: J Galcatium, 1771

Frazier CH: Remarks upon the surgical aspects of operable tumors of the cerebrum. **Univ Penn Med Bull 19:**49-70, 1906

Freud S: **Zur Kenntriss Der Cerebralen Dysplegien Des Kindesalters (Im Anschluss An Die Little 'Sah Krankheit).** Leipzig: F Deutcke, 1893, 168 pp

Freud S: **Zurr Auffassung der Aphasien, eine Kritische Studie.** Vienna: Deuticke, 1891 [**On Aphasia: A Critical Study.**] (E Stengl, trans). New York, NY: International Universities Press, 1953]

Friedreich N: Ueber Ataxie mit besonderer Berüchsichtigung der hereditären Formen. **Virchows Arch Pathol Anat 68:**145-245, 1876

Friedreich N: Ueber degenerative Atrophie der spinalen Hinterstränge. **Virchows Arch Pathol Anat 26:**391-419, 433-459, 1863; **27:**1-26, 1867

Friedreich N: **Ueber Progressive Muskelatrophie, über Wahre und Falsche Muskelhypertrophie.** Berlin: Hirschwald, 1873

Fritsch G, Hitzig E: Ueber die elektrische Erregbarkeit des Grosshirns. **Arch Anat Physiol Wiss Med 37**:300-332, 1870

Fritz K von: Asclepius, a review. **J Hist Med 2**:110-116, 1947

Fröhlich A: Ein Fall von Tumor der Hypophysis cerebri ohne Akromegalie. **Wien Klin Rundschau 15**:883-906, 1901

Froin G: Inflammations méningées avec réactions chromatique, fibrineuse et cytologique du liquide céphalo-rachidien. **Gaz Hop 76**:1005-1006, 1903

Frugardi R: **Practica chirurgicae.** 1170

Frugardi R: **The Surgery of the Four Masters.**

Funk C: The etiology of deficiency diseases. **J State Med 20**:341-368, 1912

Fürbringer P: Zur klinischen Bedeutung der spinalen Punction. **Berl Klin Wochenschr 32**:272-277, 1895

Fuster B, Gibbs E: Caracteres electroencefalográficos de la epilepsia psicomotoriz; foco de espiculas negativas de localización temporal anterior en el EEG obtenido durante el sueño normal o inducido con diferentes drogas. **Neurocirugia 4**:287-291, 1948

Gale T: **An excellent treatise of wounds made with gonneshot.** London: R Hall, 1563

Galen: **De Usu Partium [On the Usefullness of the Parts of the Body].** (MT May, trans). Ithaca, NY: Cornell University Press, 1968

Galen: **Oeuvres Anatomiques, Physiologiques et Médicales de Galien.** (Ch Daremberg, trans). Paris: JB Baillière, 1854, 2 Vols

Galen: **On the Opinions of Hippocrates and Plato.** (transl, Kuhn)

Gall F: **Sur les Fonctions du Cerveau et sur Celles de Chacune de ses Partes, Vol 2.** Paris: JB Baillière, 1822

Gall FJ, Spurzheim JC: **Anatomie et Physiologie du Système Nerveux en Général, et du Cerveau en Particulier.** Paris: F Schoell et al, 1810-1819, 4 Vols

Galvani L: De viribus electricitatis in motu musculari commentarius. Pars prima. **Bononien Sci Art Instit Acad 7**:363-418, 1791

Gama JP: **Traité des Plaies de Tête et de'Encéphalite, etc. 2nd ed.** Paris, 1835, 616 pp

Gamper E: Zur Klinik der Sensibilitätsstörungen bei Rindenläsionen. **Monatschr Psychiat Neurol 43**:21-36, 1918

Gardner WJ, Angel J: The mechanism of syringomyelia and its surgical correction. **Clin Neurosurg 6:** 131-140, 1959

Gardner WJ: Hydrodynamic mechanism of syringomyelia: its relationship to myelocele. **J Neurol Neurosurg y 28**:247-259, 1965

Gardner WJ: **The Dysraphic States from Syringomyelia to Anencephaly.** Amsterdam: Excerpta Medica, 1973

Garrison FH: **An Introduction to the History of Medicine, 4th ed.** Philadelphia, Pa: WB Saunders, 1929, 996 pp (Reprinted 1960)

Garrison FH: **Contributions to the History of Medicine.** New York, NY: Hafner, 1966, 989 pp

Gaubius HD: **Institutiones pathologiae medicinalis.** Edinburgh: A Donaldson et J Reid, 1772, 337 pp

Gay JA: Abcés sous la dura-mère guéri par le trépan. Rec périod. **Soc Med Paris 2**:170-172, 1797

Gélineau JBE: De la narcolepsie. **Gaz Hop (Paris) 53**:626-635, 1880

Geoffroy Saint-Hilaire I: **I. Histoire Générale et particulière des Anomalies de L'Organisation.** Paris: JB Baillière, 1832-1837, 3 Vols

Geoffroy Saint-Hilaire I: **Philosphie Anatomique. Tome II. Des Monstruosités.** Paris: Chez l'Auteur, 1822

Gerlach J von: **Mikroskopische Studien aus dem Gebiete der Menschlichen Morphologie.** Erlangen: F Enke, 1858, 72 pp

Gerlach J von: Über die struktur der grauen Substanz des menschlichen Grosshirns. **Zentralbl Med Wissensch 10**:273-275, 1872

Gersdorff H von: **Feldbüch der Wundartzny - sampt vilen Instrumenten der Chirurgey.** Strassburg: H Schotten, 1540, 210 pp

Glisson F: **Tractatus de natura substantiae energetica.** London: Brome and Hooke, 1672

Golgi C: Recherches sur l'histologie des centres nerveux. **Arch Ital Biol 3:**285-317, 1883; **Arch Ital Biol 4:**92-123, 1884

Golgi C: Sulla struttura sullo sviluppo degli psammomi. **Morgagni 11:**874-886, 1869

Goltz FL: Der Hund ohne Grosshirn. **Pfluegers Arch Ges Physiol 51:**570-614, 1892

Gotfredsen E: **A Dissertation on the Anatomy of the Brain, by Nicolaus Steno.** Copenhagen: Nyt Nord Forlag Arnold Busck, 1950

Gowers WR, Horsley V: A case of tumour of the spinal cord; removal; recovery. **Med Chir Trans (2nd ser) 71:**377-430, 1888

Gowers WR: **A Manual of Diseases of the Nervous System.** London: J & A Churchill, 1886-1888, 2 Vols

Gowers WR: **Epilepsy and Other Chronic Convulsive Diseases.** London: J & A Churchill, 1881 (2nd ed, 1901)

Gowers WR: Tetanoid chorea associated with cirrhosis of the liver. **Dis Nerv System 2:**656, 1888

Gowers WR: **The Border-Land of Epilepsy.** London: J & A Churchill, 1907

Gowers WR: **The Diagnosis of Diseases of the Spinal Cord.** London: J & A Churchill, 1880

Graefe A von: Verhandlungen ärztlicher Gesellschaften. **Berl Klin Wschr 5:**125-127, 1856

Graefe FWEA von: **Ueber Complications von Sehnvervenentzündung mit Gehirnkrankheiten. Graefes Arch Ophthal 7(2 Abt):**58-71, 1860

Graña F, Rocca ED, Graña L: **Las Trepanaciones Craneanas en el Perú en la Época Pre-Hispánica.** Lima, Peru: Imprenta Santa Maria, 1954, 340 pp

Gratiolet LP: **Mémoires sur les Plis Cérébraux de l'Homme et des Primatès.** Paris: Bertrand, 1854

Graves RJ: **A System of Clinical Medicine.** Dublin: Fannin & Co, 1843

Greenfield JG, Pritchard B: Cerebral infection with *Schistosoma japonicum.* **Brain 60:**361-372, 1937

Greig DM: Hypertelorism. A hitherto undifferentiated congenital cranio-facial deformity. **Edinburgh Med J 31:**560-593, 1924

Griesinger W: Fortgesetzte Beobachtungen über Hirnkrankheiten. Cysticerken und ihre Diagnose. **Arch Heilk 3:**207-240, 1862

Grünbaum ASF, Sherrington CS: Observations on the physiology of the cerebral cortex of the anthropoid apes. **Proc R Soc Lond 72:**152-155, 1903

Gudden B von: Beitrag zur Kenntniss des Corpus mamillare und des sögenannter Schenkel des Fornix. **Arch Psychiatr 11,** 1884-1885

Gudden B von: Experimental Untersuchungen über das peripherische und centralen Nervensystem. **Arch Psychiatr Nervenkr 3:**693-723, 1870

Guillain G, Barré JA, Strohl A: Sur un syndrome de radiculo-névrite avec hyperalbuminose du liquide céphalo-rachidien sans réaction cellulaire. Remarques sur les caractères cliniques et graphiques des réflexes tendineux. **Bull Mem Soc Med Hop Paris 40:**1462-1470, 1916

Gull W: Cases of aneurism of the cerebral vessels. **Guys Hosp Rep (3rd ser) 5:**281-304, 1859

Gunn MR: Congenital ptosis with peculiar associated movements of the affected lid. **Trans Ophthalmol Soc UK 3:**283-286, 1883

Gutzeit R: Ein Teratom der Zirbeldrüse. Königsberg: E Erlatis, 1896, 50 pp (Thesis)

Guy de Chauliac: **Ars chirurgica [On Wounds and Fractures].** (WA Brennan, trans). Chicago, Ill: Privately printed, 1923, 153 pp (1363, orig ms)

Guy de Chauliac: **De la practique de cyrurgie.** (N Panis, trans). Lyons, 1478

Guy de Chauliac: Treatment of wounds. **J Hist Med 19:**193-214, 1964

Hall HC: **La Dégénérescence Hépatolenticulaire.** Paris: Masson, 1921

Hall M: **Lectures on the Nervous System and Its Diseases.** London: Sherwood, Gilbert, and Piper, 1836

Hall M: **Memoirs on the Nervous System.** London: Sherwood, Gilbert, and Piper, 1837

Hall M: On a new mode of effecting artificial respiration. **Lancet 1:**229, 1856

Hall M: On the reflex function of the medulla oblongata and medulla spinalis. **Phil Trans R Soc Lond 123:**635-665, 1833

Hall M: **Synopsis of Cerebral and Spinal Seizures of Inorganic Origin and of Paroxysmal Form as a Class.** London: J Mallett, 1851

Haller A von: De partibus corporis humani sensibilibus et irriabilibus. **Comment Soc Reg Sci Gottingen 2:**114-158, 1753

Haller A von: **Elementa physiologicae corporis humani.** Lausanne: Marci-Michael, Bosquet et Socio-
rum, 1759-1766, 8 Vols
Haly Abbas: **Liber artis medicine, qui dicitur regalis.** Venetiis: B Ricius, 1492
Hamby WB, Gardner WJ: Treatment of pulsating exophthalmos. **Arch Surg 27**:676-685, 1933
Hamig G: Uber die Fettembolie des Gehirns. **Beit Klin Chir 27**:333-362, 1900
Hammett FJ: The antatomical knowledge of the ancient Hindus. **Ann Med Hist 1**:325-333, 1929
Hammond WA: **A Treatise on Diseases of the Nervous System.** New York, NY: D Appleton & Co,
1871, 754 pp
Hannover A: Die Chromsäure, ein vorzügliches Mittel bei mikroskopischen Untersuchungen. **Arch
Anat Physiol Wiss Med**:549-558, 1840
Hansen GHA, Looft C: **Leprosy in its Clinical and Pathological Aspects.** (N Walker, transl from
Norwegian). Bristol: John Wright, 1874
Harlow JM: Passage of an iron rod through the head. **Bost Med Surg J 39**:389-393, 1848
Harlow JM: Recovery from the passage of an iron bar through the head. **Publ Mass Med Soc 2**:
327-346, 1868
Harrison RG: Embryonic transplantation and development of the nervous system. **Anat Rec 2**:
385-410, 1908
Hartmann F: **The Life of Philippus Theophrastus Bombastus of Hohenheim, Known by the Name of
Paracelsus.** London: Redway, 1950
Harvey W: **The Works of William Harvey.** (R Willis, trans). London: Sydenham Society, 1847
Hashimoto T: Chirurgische Beitrage aus Japan. **Arch Klin Chir 32**:1-57, 1885
Haslam J: **Observations on insanity.** London: F and C Rivington, 1798
Head H, Holmes G: Sensory disturbances from cerebral lesions. **Brain 34**:102-254, 1911/1912
Hegmann: De Neuromate Nervi Optici. Berlin, 1842 (Thesis)
Heine J von: **Beobachtungen über Lähmungszustände der untern Extremitäten und deren Behand-
lung.** Stuttgart: FH Köhler, 1840
Heister L: **A general system of surgery in three parts, containing the doctrine and managment.** Lon-
don: J Whiston, L Davis, C Reymer, et al, 1768, 414 pp
Helmholtz HLF von: **Beschreibung eines Augen-Spiegels zur Untersuchung der Netzhaut im leben-
den Auge.** Berlin: A Förstner, 1851, 43 pp
Henneberg, Koch: Ueber 'Central'-Neurofibromatose und die Geschwülste des Kleinhirnbrücken-
winkels. (Acusticus-Neurom). **Arch Psychiatr Nervenkr 36**:251-302, 1902
Henri de Mondeville: **Chirurgie de Mâitre Henri de Mondeville.** (E Nicaise, trans). Paris: G Baillière
& Cie, 1891, 903 pp
Henrici C: **Ueber trepanation bei Gehirnabscessen.** Kiel: CF Mohr, 1880, 26 pp (Inaugural Disserta-
tion)
Henschen SE: **Klinische und Anatomische Beiträge zur Pathologie des Gehirns.** Upsala: Almquist
und Wiksell, 1890-1922, 3 Vols
Henschen SE: On the visual path and centre. **Brain 16**:170-180, 1893
Hering HF: Die Aenderug der Herzschlagzahl durch Aenderung des arteriellen Blutdruckes erfolgt
aus reflektorischen Wege. **Pfluegers Arch Ges Physiol 206**:721-723, 1924
Heroditus: **The History of Heroditus.** (GC MacAulay, trans). London: Macmillan, 1896, 2 Vols
Herophilus, in: **Medicorum Graecorum Opera Quae Exstant.** (DCG Kühn, ed). Leipzig:
C Cnoblochius, 1822, 26 Vols
Herpin T: **Des Acier Incomplete d'Epilepsie.** Paris: 1867
Hidalgo de Aguero B: **Thesoro de la verdadera cirugia y via particular contra la commún.** Sevilla, 1604
Hill L: **The Physiology and Pathology of the Cerebral Circulation. An Experimental Research.** Lon-
don: J & A Churchill, 1896
Hilton J: **On the Influence of Mechanical and Physical Rest and the Diagnostic Value of Pain.** Lon-
don: Bell and Waldry, 1863, pp 16-58
Hippocrates: **The Genuine Works of Hippocrates.** (F Adams, trans). London: Sydenham Society,
1849, 2 Vols (New York, NY: William Wood & Company, 1829)
Hirschfeld O: Removal of a tumor of the brain. **Pacific Med Surg J 29**:210-216, 1886
His W: **Die Anatomische Nomenclatur.** Leipzig: Veit Co, 1895

His W: Histogenese und Zusammenhang der Nervenelemente. **Arch Anat Physiol (Anat Abt Suppl)**:95-117, 1890

Hitzig E: **Untersuchungen über das Gehirn.** Berlin: A Hirschwald, 1874

Hoffmann H: Stereognostiche Versuche. Dissertation, Strassburg, 1883

Hoffmann J: Ueber chronische spinale Muskelatrophie im Kindesalter, auf familiärer Basis. **Dtsch Z Nervenheilk 3**:427-470, 1893

Hoffmann J: Ueber progressive neurotische Muskelatrophie. **Arch Pyschiat Nervenkr 20**:660-713, 1889

Holmes W: Repair of nerves. **J Hist Med 6**:44-63, 1951

Hooke R: **Micrographia.** London: Martyn and Allestry, 1665

Hooper R: **The Morbid Anatomy of the Human Brain; Illustrated by Coloured Engravings of the Most Frequent and Important Organic Diseases to Which That Viscus is Subject.** London: Longman, Rees, Orme, Brown and Green, 1826

Horsley V, Sharpey-Schäfer EA: A record of experiments upon the functions of the cerebral cortex. **Phil Trans R Soc Lond 179B**:1-45, 1888

Horsley V: Antiseptic wax. **Br Med J 1**:1165, 1892

Horsley V: Brain surgery. **Br Med J 2**:670-675, 1886

Horsley V: Discussion on the treatment of cerebral tumours. **Br Med J 2**:1365-1367, 1893

Horsley V: On the technique of operations on the central nervous system. **Br Med J 2**:411-423, 1906

Hudson AC: Primary tumors of the optic nerves. **Ophthalmol Hosp Rep 18**:317-394, 1912

Hughes ML: **Mediterranean, Malta, or Undulant Fever.** London: Macmillan & Co, 1897

Hulke JW: Case of recovery after evacuation of a traumatic abscess in the brain by trephining and incision. **Lancet 1**:406, 1879

Hume EH: **The Chinese Way in Medicine.** Baltimore, Md: Johns Hopkins University Press, 1940, 189 pp

Hunt JR: The role of the carotid arteries in the causation of vascular lesions of the brain, with remarks on certain special features of the symptomatology. **Am J Med Sci 147**:704, 1914

Hunter J: **The Works of John Hunter, F.R.S. with Notes.** (JF Palmer, ed). London: Longman, Rees, etc, 1835, 4 Vols

Huntington G: On chorea. **Med Surg Rep 26**:317-321, 1872

Hurry JB: **Imhotep, The Vizier and Physician of King Zoser and Afterwards the Egyptian God of Medicine.** London: Oxford University Press, 1928, 219 pp

Huss M: **Alcoholismus chronicus eller chronisk alkoholsjukdom; Ett bidrag till Dyskrasiernas Kännedom; Enligt Egen och Andras Erfarenhet. Första Afdelningen.** Stockholm: Joh Beckman, 1849

Hutchinson J: Aneurism of the internal carotid within the skull diagnosed eleven years before the patient's death. Spontaneous cure. **Trans Clin Soc Lond 8**:127-131, 1875

Hutchinson J: Four lectures on compression of the brain. Clinical lectures and reports of the medical and surgical staff of the London hospital. **Lond Hosp Rep 4**:10-55, 1867

Huxham J: **On the malignant, ulcerous sore-throat.** London: J Hinton, 1750

Ibn-al-Nafis: Ibn an Nafis und seine Theorie des Lungenkreislaufs. **Quell Stud Gesch Med 4**:37-88, 1933

Jackson JH: Discussion of paper by Bennett AH, Godlee RS. Case of cerebral tumour. The surgical treatment. **Br Med J 1**:988-989, 1885

Jackson JH: **On the Anatomical and Physiological Localisation of Movement in the Brain.** London, 1875 (Reprinted)

Jackson JH: **Selected Writings of John Hughlings Jackson.** (J Tayler, ed). New York, NY: Basic Books, 1958

Jackson JH: Unilateral epileptiform seizures beginning by a disagreeable smell. **Med Times Gaz 2**:168, 1864

Jackson JH: Unilateral epileptiform seizures, attended by temporary defect of sight. **Med Times Gaz 1**:588-589, 1863

Jaggi OP: **History of Science, Technology, and Medicine in India. Vol 3, Folk Medicine.** Delhi/Lucknow: Atma Ram & Sons, 1982, 228 pp

Jamnagar SG: **The Caraka Samhita.** India: Azurvedic Society, 1949 (reviewed by **J Hist Med 8**:

350-352, 1953) (Expounded by the worshipful Atreya Punarvasu, compiled by the great sage Agnivesa and redacted by Caraka and Drdhabala)

Jansen A: Optische Aphasie bei einer otitischen eitrigen Entzündung der Hirnhäute am linken Schläfenlappen mit Ausgang in Heilung. **Berl Klin Wochenschr 32**:763-765, 1895

Jastrowitz M: Beiträge zur Localisation im Grosshirn und über deren praktischen Verwerthung. **Dtsch Med Wochenschr**, 1888

Jefferson G: The prodromes of cortical localization. **J Neurol Neurosurg Psychiatry 16**:59-72, 1953

Joffroy A: Hospice de la Sâlpetrière clinique nerveuse. Leçons faites en Décembre 1891, 1. **Prog Med (2nd ser) 22**:61-62, 1894

John of Gaddesden, in Lennox WG: John of Gaddesden on epilepsy. **Ann Med Hist (3rd ser) 1**: 283-307, 1939 (1314, orig)

John of Mirfield: **Surgery.** (JB Cotton, trans). 1969

Jones WHS: Ancient Roman folk medicine. **J Hist Med 12**:459-472, 1957

Kadyi H: **Ueber die Blutgefässe des Menschlichen Rückenmarkes.** Lemberg: Gubrynowicz and Schmidt, 1889

Kalmus JA: **Tafel anatomia.** 1647

Karplus JP, Kreidl A: Über Totalextirpation einer und beider Grosshirnhemisphären an Affen (macacus rhesus). **Arch Physiol Leipz**:155-212, 1914

Keen WW: Three successful cases of cerebral surgery including (1) the removal of a large intracranial fibroma, (2) exsection of damaged brain tissue and (3) exsection of the cerebral center for the left hand. With remarks on the general technique of such operations. **Trans Am Surg Assn 6**: 293-347, 1888

Kenyon JH: Endothelioma of the brain three years after operation. **Ann Surg 61**:106-107, 1915

Kernig VM: Ein Krankheitssymptom der acuten Meningitis. **St Petersburg Med Wochenschr 7**:398, 1882

Keswani NH: **Medical Education in India Since Ancient Times.** 1968

Key A, Retzius G: **Studier i Nervsystemets Anatomi.** Stockholm: PA Norstedt & Soneo, 1872, 68 pp

Key A, Retzius MG: **Studien in der Anatomie des Nervensystems und des Bindegewebes.** Stockholm: Samons & Wallin, 1875-1876, 2 Vols

Khairallah AA: Arabic contributions to anatomy and surgery. **Ann Med Hist 4**:409-412, 1942

King JEJ: The treatment of brain abscess by unroofing and temporary herniation of abscess cavity with the avoidance of usual drainage methods, with notes on the management of hernia cerebri in general. **Surg Gynecol Obstet 39**:554-568, 1924

Klebs E: Die Einschmelzungs-Methode, ein Beitrag zur mikroskopischen Technik. **Arch Mikrosc Anat 5**:164-166, 1869

Kleine W: Periodische Schlafsucht. **Mschr Psychiatr Neurol 57**:285-320, 1925

Klippel M, Feil A: Un cas d'absence des vertebres cervicales avec cage thoracique remontant jusqu'a la base du crâne. **Nouv Iconogr Salpetr 25**:223-250, 1912

Klotz O: Abrecht von Haller (1708-77). **Ann Med Hist 8**:10-26, 1916

Klüver H, Bucy PC: "Psychic blindness" and other symptoms following bilateral temporal lobectomy in rhesus monkeys. **Am J Physiol 119**:352-353, 1937

Knoblauch A: **De Neuromate et Gangliis Accessoriis Veris, Adjecto Cujusvis Generis casu novo atque Insigni.** Frankfort-a-Main, 1843, 39 pp

Kölliker RA von: **Mikroskopisches Anatomie.** Leipzig: Englemann, 1850-1854, 3 Vols

Korsakov SS: Etude médico-psychologique sur une forme des maladies de la mémoire. **Rev Philos 28**:501-530, 1889

Krause F: **Chirurgie des Gehirns und Rückenmarkes nach eigenen Erfahrungen.** Berlin: Urban & Schwarzenberg, 1908 (Vol 1), 1911 (Vol 2)

Krause F: Entfernung des Ganglion Gasseri und des zentral davon gelegenen Trigeminus-stammes. **Dtsch Med Wochensch 19**:341-344, 1893

Krause F: **Surgery of the Brain and Spinal Cord Based on Personal Experiences.** (H Haubold and M Thorek, trans). New York, NY: Rebman, 1909-1912, 3 Vols

Krogius A: Du traitement chirurgical des tumeurs de la fossa latérale moyenne. **Rev Chir 16**:434-445, 1896

Kühne W: **Ueber die Peripherischen Endorgane der Motorischen Nerven.** Leipzig: W Engelmann, 1862

Kulmus JA: **Anatomische tabellen.** Angspurg: JJ Lotters, 1740

Kundrat H: **Arhinencephalie als Typische Art von Missbildung.** Graz: Von Leuschner und Lubensky, 1882

Kussmaul A, Maier R: Ueber eine bisher noch nicht beochriebene eigenthü mliche Arteriener-krankung (Periarteritis nodosa), die mit Morbus Brightii und rapid fortschreitender allgmeiner Muskellähmung einhergeht. **Dtsch Arch Klin Med 1:**484-518, 1866

Kussmaul A: **Die Störungen der Sprache.** Leipzig: FCW Vogel, 1877

Lancisi GM: **De subitaneis mortibus. Libri duo.** Rome: JF Buagni, 1707

Landry O: Note sur la paralysie ascendante aiguë. **Gaz Hebd Med (Paris) 6:**472-474, 486-488, 1859

Lanfranc of Milan: **Science of Cirurgie.** Berlin: Asher and Co, 1894, 360 pp

Langhans T: Ueber Hohlenbildung im Rückenmark in Folge Blutstauung. **Arch Pathol Anat Physiol 85:**1-25, 1881

Langier: **Séance de l'Académie des Sciences.** Paris, 1864

Langley JN: On the union of cranial autonomic (visceral) fibers with the nerve cells in the superior cervical ganglion. **J Physiol 23:**240-270, 1898

Langley JN: **The Autonomic Nervous System.** Cambridge: W Heffer, 1921

Lannelongue M: **De l'Ostéomyélite Aiguë Pendant la Croissance.** Paris: Asselin et Cie, 1879

Lanzino G, DiPierro CG, Laws ER Jr: One century after the description of the "sign": Joseph Babinski and his contribution to neurosurgery. **Neurosurgery 40:**822-828, 1997

Larrey DJ: **Surgical Memoirs of the Campaigns of Russia, Germany, and France.** (JC Mercer, trans). Philadelphia, Pa: Carey and Lea, 1832, 293 pp

Laws ER Jr: The contributions of neurosurgeons to medical history. **Acta Neurochir 124:**172-175, 1993

Laws ER Jr: The neurosurgeon and endocrinology. **Clin Neurosurg 27:**3-18, 1980

Lawson R: On the symptomatology of alcoholic brain disorders. **Brain 1:**182-194, 1879

Le Dran HF: **Traité des óperations de chirurgie.** Paris: Charles Osmont, 1742

Lebert H: **Physiologie Pathologique on Recherches Cliniques, Expérimentales et Microscopiques sur l'Inflammation, la Tuberculisation, les Tumeurs, la Formation du Cal, etc.** Paris: JB Baillière, 1845, 2 Vols

Lebert H: Ueber Krebs und die mit Krebs Verwechselten Geschwülste in Gehirn und Seinen Hüllen. **Virchows Arch Pathol Anat 3:**463-569, 1851

Leeuwenhoek A van: **Epistolae physiologicae super compluribus naturae arcanis.** Delft: Beman, 1719

Legallois JJC: **Expériences sur le Principe de la Vie. Notamment sur Celui des Mouvements du Coeur, et sur le Siège de ce Principe.** Paris: D'Hautel, 1812, 364 pp

Lenhossek von: **Der Feiner Bau des Nervensystems in Lichte neuester Forschungen.** Berlin: Fischer, 1895

Leonardo RA: **History of Surgery.** New York, NY: Froben Press, 1943, 504 pp

Leuret F: **Anatomie Comparée du Système Nerveux Considerée dans ses Rapports avec l'Intelligence.** Paris: Baillière, 1839

Levin M: Narcolepsy (Gélineau's syndrome) and other varieties of morbid somnolence. **Arch Neurol Psychiatr 22:**1172-1200, 1929

Leyden E von: **Klinik der Ruckenmarks-Krankheiten.** Berlin: A Hirschwald, 1874-1876

Leydig F: **Lehrbuch der Histologie des Menschen und der Thiere.** Hamm: G Grote, 1875

L'Hermitte J: Un cas de syndrome thalamique á évolution régressive; l'ataxie résiduelle. **Rev Neurol 28:**1256-1259, 1921

Lichtenstern: Progressive pernicious anaemia in tabetic patients. **Dtsch Med Wochenschr,** 1884

Lichtheim L: Pathologie und Therapie der perniciösen Anamie. **Neuralbl Zentralbl 6:**235, 1887

Liepmann HK: Das Krankheitsbild der Apraxie (motorische Asymbolie) auf Grund eines Falles von einseitiger Apraxie. **Monatschr Psychiat Neurol 8:**15-44, 1900

Lissauer H: Ein Fall von Seelenblindheit nebst einem Beitrage zur Theorie derselben. **Arch Psychiatr Nervenkr 1:**222-270, 1890

Lister J: On a new method of treating compound fracture, abcess, etc. with observations on the conditions of suppuration. **Lancet 1:**326-329, 357-359, 387-389, 507-509; **2:**95-96, 1867

Lister J: On the antiseptic principle in the practice of surgery. **Lancet 2:**353-356, 1867

Littré A: **Histoire de l'academie royale des sciences.** Paris, 1705

Liveing E: **On Megrim, Sick-Headache, and Some Allied Disorders. A Contribution to the Pathology of Nerve Storms.** London: J & A Churchill, 1873

Locke J: The celebrated Locke as a physician. **Lancet 2**:367, 1829

Locock C: [Contribution to discussion on paper by EH Sieveking.] **Lancet 1**:528, 1857

Loeb J: Die Sehstörungen nach Verletzungen der Grosshirnrinde. **Pfluegers Arch 34**:67-172, 1884

Loewi O: Ueber humorale Uebertragbarkeit der Herznervenwirkung. **Pfluegers Arch Ges Physiol 189**:239-242, 1921

Long CW: An account of the first use of sulphuric ether by inhalation as an anaesthetic in surgical operations. **South Med J 5**:705-713, 1849

Lopez Pinero JM: **La Trepanacion en España.** Madrid, Spain: Editorial Tecnica Española, SA, 1967, 480 pp

Lopez RV: **La Craniectomia à Través de los Siglos.** Valladolid Editorial, 1949, 148 pp

Lorry AC: Sur les mouvements de cerveau et de la dure-mere. **Mem Acad R Sci 3**:277, 1760 (2nd publ)

Louis: Sur les tumeurs fongueuses de la dure-mere. **Mem Acad R Chir 5**:1-95, 1774

Lowenthal MS, Horsley VAH: On the relations between the cerebellar and other centers (namely cerebral and spinal) with special reference to the action of antagonistic muscles. (Preliminary account.) **Proc R Soc Lond 61**:20-25, 1897

Lower R, King E: An account of the experiment of transfusion practiced upon a man in London. **Phil Trans 2**:557, 1667

Lower R: **De Catarrhis.** (R Hunter and J Malcalpine, trans from Latin). London: Dawsons, 1672

Lower R: **Tractatus de corde item de motu & colore sanguinis, et chyli in cum transitu.** Amsterdam: D Elzevirum, 1669, 232 pp

Lucas K: **The Conduction of the Nervous Impulse.** London: Longmans, Green & Co, 1917

Luciani L, Sepalli L: **Le Localizzazioni Funzionali del Cervello.** Naples: Vallardi, 1885

Luciani L: **Il Cervelletto. Nuovi Studi di Fisiologia Normale e Patologico.** Florence: Successori le Monnier, 1891, 320 pp

Lund JC: "**Chorea Sancti Viti i Saetesdalen.**" Beretning om Sundhetsstilstanden og Medicinalforholdene i. Norge, 1859

Lund JC: **In Beretning om Sundhetsstilstanden og Medicinalforholdene i Norge i 1860.** Christiania: Trykt i Det Steenske Bogtrykkeri, 1863

Luschka H: **Der Hirnanhang und die Steissdrüse des Menschen.** Berlin: G Reimer, 1860, 97 pp

Luschka H: **Die Structur der Serösen Häute des Menschen.** Tübingen: Laupp & Siebeck, 1851, 98 pp

Luys JB: Atrophie musculaire progressive. Lésions histologique de la substance grise de la moëlle épinière. **Gaz Med (Paris) 15**:505, 1860

Luys JB: **Recherches sur le Système Nerveux Cérébro-Spinal: sa Structure, ses Fonctions, et ses Maladies.** Paris: JB Baillière et Fils, 1865, 660 pp

Lyon IW: Chronic hereditary chorea. **Am Med Times 7**:289-290, 1863

Maas H: Zur Casuistik und Therapie der Gehirnabscesse nach eigenen Erfahrungen. **Berl Klin Wochenschr 6**:127-129, 140-143, 1869

Macewen W: Case presentation before the Glasgow Pathological and Clinical Society Dec. 22, 1885 **Glasgow Med J (new ser) 25**:210, 1886

Macewen W: Discussion of paper by Bennett AH, Godlee RS: Case of cerebral tumour. The surgical treatment. **Br Med J 1**:988-989, 1885

Macewen W: Intra-cranial lesions, illustrating some points in connexion with the localisation of cerebral affections and the advantages of antiseptic trephining. **Lancet 2**:541-543, 581-583, 1881

Macewen W: **Pyogenic Infective Diseases of the Brain and Spinal Cord. Meningitis, Abscess of the Brain, Infective Sinus Thrombosis.** Glasgow: J Maclehose & Sons, 1893, 354 pp

Macewen W: Tumour of the dura mater—convulsions—removal of tumour by trephining—recovery. **Glasgow Med J 12**:210-213, 1879

Macht DI: Moses Maimonides, physician and scientist. **Bull Hist Med 3**:585-598, 1935

Magatus (Magati) C: **De rara medicatione vulnereum, sur de volneribus raro tractandis, libri duo.** Venicetiis: A and B Dei, 1616

Magendie F: Expériences sur les fonctiones des racines des nerfs rachidiens. **J Physiol Exp Pathol 2:** 276-279, 1822

Magendie F: **Leçons sur les Fonctions et les Maladies du Système Nerveux.** Paris: Lecaplain, 1841, 2 Vols

Magendie F: Mémoire sur un liquide qui se trouve dans le crâne et le canal vertébral de l'homme et des animaux mammifères. **J Physiol Exp Pathol 5:**27-37, 1825; **7:**1-29,66-82, 1827

Magendie F: **Rechereches Philosophiques et Cliniques sur le Liquide Céphalorachidien ou Cérébro-spinal.** Paris: Méquignon-Marvis, 1842

Maggius B: **De vulnerum sclopetorum et bombardarum . . . curatione tractatus.** Bononiae: B Bonardum, 1552, 114 pp

Magnus R: Welche Teile des Zentralnervensystems müssen für das Zustandekommen der tonischen Hals- und Labyrinthreflexe auf die Körpermuskulatur vorhanden sein. **Pfluegers Arch 159:** 224-249, 1914

Maimonides M: **Hoc in volumine hec continentur aphorismi Rabi Moysi.** Venice: Hammon, 1500

Major RH: **A History of Medicine.** Springfield, Ill: Charles C Thomas, 1954

Malacarne CG, Malacarne VG: **Memorie Storiche Inforno alla vita e alle Opere di Michele Vincenzo Giacinto Malcarne da Saluzzo, Anatomico e Chirurgo.** Padua: Tip del Seminario, 1819

Malpighi M: **De cerebroepistola, in tetras anatomicarum epistolarum de lingua et cerebro.** Bologna: Benati, 1665

Malpighi M: **Opera omnia.** London: Scott, 1686

Marburg O: Die Adipositas cerebralis. Ein Beitrag zur Kenntnis der Pathologie der Zirbeldrüse. **Dtsch Z Nervenheilk 36:**114-121, 1908

Marcé: Mémoire sur quelques observations de physiologie pathologique tendant à démontrer l'existence d'un principe coordinateur de l'écriture et ses rapports avec le principe coordinateur de la parole. **Compt Rend Soc Biol (Paris)** :93-115, 1856

Marchal CJ: **De Calve Recherches sur les Accidents Diabétiques et Essai d'une Théorie Générale de Diabète.** Paris: P Asselin, 1864

Marie P: De l'ostéo-arthropathie hypertrophiante pneumonique. **Rev Med 10:**1-36, 1890

Marie P: De l'engagement des amygdales cérébelleuses a l'enterieur du trou occipital dans les cas ou la pression intracranienne se trouve augmenté. **Rev Neurol 8:**252, 1900

Marie P: La troisième circumconvolution frontale gauche ne joue aucun rôle spécial dans la fonction du langage. **Sem Med (Paris) 26:**241-247, 1906

Marie P: Sur deux cas d'acromégalie; hypertrophie singulière non congénitale des extrémités supérieures, inférieures et céphaliques. **Rev Med 6:**297-333, 1886

Marie P: Sur l'hérédit-ataxia cérébelleuse. **Sem Med (Paris) 13:**444-447, 1893

Marie P: Sur la spondylose rhizoméliqus. **Rev Med 18:**285-315, 1898

Massa N: **Liber introductorius anatomiae, sive dissectionis corporis humani, nunc primum ab ipso auctore in lucem aeditus.** Venice: Bindonus and Pasinus, 1536, 108 pp

Matteucci C, von Humboldt FHA: Sur le courant eletrique des muscles des animaux vivants et récemment tués. **Compt Rend Acad Sci (Paris) 16:**197-200, 1843

Maunsell HW: Subtentorial hydatid tumour removed by trephining recovery. **N Zeal Med J 2:** 151-156, 1888-1889

Mayer E: Clinical experience with Adrenalin. **Phila Med J 7:**819-820, 1901

Mayow J: **Tractus quinque medico-physici quarum primus agit de sal-nitro, et spiritu nitro-ceres.** Oxford, 1674

Medin O: En epidemi af infantil paralysi. **Hygiea 52:**657-658, 1890

Ménière P: Sur une forme particulière de surdité grave dépendant d'une lésion de l'oreille interne. **Gaz Med Paris (3rd ser) 16:**29, 1861

Mercuriale H: **Medicina practica.** Lugduni, 1623

Meschede JF: **Die Paralytische Geistes Krankheit und ihre Arguniske Grundlage.** Berlin: G Reimer, 1865, 102 pp

Mestrezat W: **Le Liquide Céphalo-rachidien Normal et Pathologique.** Paris: A Maloine, 1912, 681 pp

Metschnikoff E, Roux PPE: Études expérimentales sur la syphilis. **Ann Inst Pasteur 17:**809-821, 1903

Meyer L: Die epithels-granulationen der arachnoidea. **Virchows Arch Pathol Anat 17:**209-227, 1859

Meynert T: Vom Gehirne der Saugethiere, in Stricker S (ed): **Handbuch der Lehre von den Geweben des Menschen und der Thiere.** Leipzig: Engelmann, 1872, Vol 2, pp 694-808

Meynert TH: **Psychiatrie Klinik der Erkrankungen der Vorderhirns.** Wien: W Braumüller, 1884

Michel V: Ueber eine Hyperplasie des Chiasma und des rechten Nervus opticus bei Elephantiasis. **Arch Ophthalmol 19:**145-164, 1873

Middeldorpf AT: Ueberblick über die Akidopeirastik eine neue Untersuchungs-Methode mit Hilfe Spitziger Werkzeuge. **Z Klin Med 7:**321-330, 1856

Miller C: Case of hydrocephalus chronicus with some unusual symptoms and appearances on dissection. **Trans Med Chir Soc Edinburgh 2:**243-248, 1826

Millington: Sir Thomas, 1628-1704, in Feindel W (ed): **The Origin and Significance of Cerebri Anatome.** 1965, pp 20-21

Mills CK: Aphasia and other affections of speech, in some of their medico-legal relations, studies largely from the stand-point of localization. **Rev Insan Nerv Dis (Sept/Dec):**10-181, 1891

Mills CK: **The Nervous System and Its Diseases.** Philadelphia, Pa: JB Lippincott, 1898, 1056 pp

Mingazzini G: **Der Balken, eine Anatomische, Physiologische und Klinische Studie. Hft 28 Monogr Gesamtgeb Neurol Psychiat.** Berlin: Springer, 1922

Minkowski M: Zur Physiologie der Sehsphäre. **Arch Ges Physiol 141:**171-372, 1911

Minkowski O: Uber einen Fall von Akromegalie. **Berl Klin Wochenschr 24:**371-374, 1887

Miraillié C: Sur le mécanisme de l'agraphie dans l'aphasie motrice corticale. **Compt Rend Soc Biol:**2250-252, 1895

Mistichelli D: **Trattato dell'apoplessia.** Rome: A de Rossi, 1709

Mitchell SW, Morehouse GR, Keen WW: **Gunshot Wounds and Other Injuries of Nerves.** Philadelphia, Pa: JB Lippincott, 1864, 377 pp

Miyake H: [Removal of a glioma in the motor cortex of the left cerebral hemisphere.] **J Jpn Surg Soc:**243-260, 1907 (Jpn)

Mohr B: Hypertrophie der Hypophysis cerebri und dadurch bedingter Druck auf die Hirngrundfläche, insbesondere auf dei Sehnerven chiasma derselben und den linkseitigen Hirnschenkel. **Wochenschr Ges Heilhldk 6:**565-571, 1840

Monakow C von: Ueber einige durch Extirpation circumscripter Hirnrindanregionen bedingte Entwicklungshemmungen des Kaninchengehirns. **Arch Psychiatr 12:**141-156, 1881

Mondino d'Luzzi: Anathomia overo dissectione del corpo humano, in: **Petrus de Montagnana's fasciculi di medicina.** Venice, 1493

Mondino d'Luzzi: **Anothomia overo dissectione del corpo humano. Fasciculo di Medicina.** (C Singer, trans). Florence: R I Lier and Co, 1925 (orig 1315)

Monro A Secundus: **Observations on the structure and functions of the nervous system.** Edinburgh: W Creech & Johnson, 1783

Moodie RL: **Paleopathology; an Introduction to the Study of Ancient Evidences of Disease.** Urbana, Ill: University of Illinois Press, 1923

Moodie RL: Studies in paleopathology. XVIII. Tumors of the head among pre-Columbian Peruvians. **Ann Hist Med 8:**394-412, 1926

Morand SF: **Opuscles de chirurgie.** Paris: Guillaume Desprez, 1768

Morgagni GB: **Adversaria anatomica omnia.** Pattavii: Excudebat Jesephus cominus, 1719

Morgagni GB: **Adversaria anatomica, Bk 6, Lugdunum Batavorum. Animadversio XIV.** 1740

Morgagni GB: **De sedibus et causis morborum per anatomen indagatis. Libri quinque.** Venice: Remondini, 1762, 2 Vols

Morgagni GB: **Epistolae anatomicae duodeviginti.** 1740

Morgagni GB: **The seats and causes of diseases investigated by anatomy: in five books, containing a variety of dissections, with remarks.** (B Alexander, trans). London: A Millar and T Cadell, Johnson and Payne, 1769, 868 pp

Morton CA: The pathology of tuberculous meningitis, with reference to its treatment by tapping the subarchnoid space of the spinal cord. **Br Med J 2:**840-841, 1891

Morton SG: **Crania Americana; or a Comparative View of the Skulls of Various Aboriginal Nations of North and South America.** Philadelphia, Pa: J Dobson; London: Simpkon, Marshall & Co, 1839, 296 pp

Müller J: Bestätigung des Bell'schen Lehrsatzes, das die doppelten Wurzeln der Rückenmarksnerven verschiedene Fuctionen haben, durch neue und Entscheidende Experimente. **Notiz Gebiete Nat Heilk 30:**113-117, 1831

Munk H: **Ueber die Funktionen der Grosshirnrinde.** Berlin: A Hirschwald, 1881, 133 pp

Nasse CF: **Sammlung zur Kenntnis der Gehirn- und Rückenmarkskrankeiten aus Englishchen und Franzosischen von Andr. Gottsschalk** . . . Stuttgart, 1837-1840

Needham J: **Science and Civilisation in China.** Cambridge, Engl: Cambridge University Press, 1954, Vol 1, 318 pp

Nélaton A: Affection singulière des os du pied. **Gaz Hop Paris 25:**13, 1852

Netter M: Diagnostic de la méningite cérébro-spinale (signe de Kernig, ponction lombaire). **Sem Med 18:**281-284, 1898

Nicolaier A: Ueber infectiösen Tetanus. **Dtsch Med Wochenschr 10:**842-844, 1884

Nissl F: Ueber die Veränderungen der Ganglienzellen am Facialiskern des Kaninchens nach Ausreissung der Nerven. **Allg Z Psychiatr 48:**197-198, 1892

Nothnagel H: Experimentelle Untersuchungen über die Functionen des Gehirns. **Arch Pathol Anat Physiol Klin Med 57:**184-214, 1873

Obersteiner H: On allochiria. A peculiar sensory disorder. **Brain 4:**153-163, 1882

Ogle W: Anosmia; or cases illustrating the physiology and pathology of the sense of smell. **Med Chir Trans 53:**263-290, 1870

Ogle W: Aphasia and agraphia. **St Georges Hosp Rep 2:**83-122, 1867

Ollivier d'Angiers CP: **De la Moëlle Epinière et de ses Maladies.** Paris: Chez Crevot, 1824

Ollivier d'Angiers CP: **De la Moëlle Epinière et de ses Maladies. Ouvrage Couronné par la Société Royale de Médicine de Marseille dans sa Séance Publique du 23 Octobre 1823, revue Corrigée et Augmentee.** 3rd ed. Paris: Méquignon-Marvis & Fils, 1837, 2 Vols

Oppenheim H, Krause F: Ueber Einklemmung bzw. Strangulation der Cauda equina. **Dtsch Med Wochenschr 35:**697-700, 1909 (change from 1906 in text)

Oppenheim H, Vogt C: Nature et localisation de la paralysie pseudobulbaire congenitale et infantile. **J Physiol Neurol Suppl 18:**293-308, 1911

Oppenheim H: Beiträge zur Prognose der Hemikranie. **Charite Ann 15:**201-296, 1888

Oppenheim H: **Die Geschwulste der Gehirns.** Wien: A Holder, 1896, 271 pp

Oppenheim H: **Lehrbuch der Nervenkrankheiten.** Berlin: S Karger, 1894 (2nd ed, 1898)

Oppenheim H: Ueber allgemeine und localisierte Atonie der Musckulatur (Myotonie) im frühen Kindesalter. **Monatschr Psychiat Neurol 8:**232-233, 1900

Oppenheim H: Ueber eine durch klinisch bisher nicht verwerthete Untersuchungsmethode ermittelte Form der Sensibilitätsstörung. **Neurol Centralbl 4:**529-533, 1885

Oppenheim H: Ueber eine eigenartige Krampfkrankheit des kindlichen und jungendlichen Alters (dysbasia lordotica progressiva, dystonia musculorum deformans). **Neurol Centralbl 30:** 1090-1107, 1911

Oppenheim H: Ueber Hirnsymptome bei Carcinomatose ohne nachweisbare Veränderungen im Gehirn. **Charite Ann 13:**335-344, 1888

Oribasius: **Ouevres d'Oribase.** (Bussemaker and CH Daremberg, trans). Paris: JB Baillière & Fils, 1851-1876, 6 Vols

Osler W: **The Evolution of Modern Medicine: A Series of Lectures Delivered at Yale University on the Stillman Foundation in April, 1913.** New Haven, Conn: Yale University Press, 1922, 243 pp

Owen R: **On the Anatomy of Vertebrates.** London: Longmans, Green & Co, 1866-1868, 3 Vols

Pacchioni A: **Dissertationes binae ad spectatissimum virum D. Joannem, Fantomun datae, cum ejusdem responsione illustradis durae meninges, ejusque glandularum structurae, atque usibus concinnatae.** Rome: R Gonzagam, 1713, 140 pp

Packard FR: **From Barber-Surgeon to Surgeon. The Evolution of Surgery. Landmarks in Medicine.** New York, NY: Appleton-Century, 1939, pp 3-35

Papavoine: **Propositione sur les Tubercules.** 1830

Paracelsus: **Four Treatises.** Baltimore, Md: Johns Hopkins Press, 1941, 256 pp

Paracelsus: **Grosse wund artzney von allen wunden, stich, schussz.** . . . Ulm: Hans Varnier, 1536

Paré A: **Des monstres et prodiges. Deux livres de chirurgie. II.** Paris: Andrè Wechel, 1573

Paré A: La methode curative des playes et fractures de la teste humaine. Paris: J le Royer, 1561

Paré A: La methode de curer les combustiones principalement faictes par la pouldre à Canon. Paris: Jean de Brie, 1551

Paré A: La methode de traicter les playes faictes par hacquebutes et aultres bastons à feu. Paris: Chésviuant Gaulterot, 1545

Paré A: Oeuvres Complètes d'Ambroise Paré. Révués et Collationées sur Toutes les Éditions avec les Variantes by J.-F. Malgaigne. Paris: JB Baillière, 1840-1841, 3 Vols

Parkinson J: An Essay on the Shaking Palsy. London: Sherwood, Neely, and Jones, 1817, 66 pp

Parry CH: Collected Works. London, 1825

Pasteur L: Sur la rage. Compt Rend Acad Sci (Paris) 92:1259-1260, 1881

Paul of Aegina: The Seven Books of Paulus Aegineta. (F Adams, trans). London: Sydenham Society, 1844-1877, 3 Vols

Pellizzi GB: La syndrome epifisaria "macrogenitosomia precoce." Riv Ital Neuropatol 3:193-250, 1910

Perthes GC: Ueber die Ursache der Hirnstörüngen nach Karotisunterbindung und über Arterienunterbindung ohne Schädigung der Intima. Arch Klin Chir 114:403-415, 1920

Petit JL: Oeuvres Complètes de J.L. Petit, etc. Paris: Frédéric Prévost, 1844, 882 pp

Petrén K: Ueber die Bahnen der Sensibilität im Rückenmarke, besonders nach den Fällen von Stichverletzung studiert. Arch Psychiat 47:495-557, 1910

Phelps C: Traumatic Injuries of the Brain and Its Membranes. New York, NY: D Appleton & Co, 1897, 582 pp

Phillips T: An account of a tumor situated on the lumbar vertebrae, of a very extraordinary size and singular appearance, which ensued from a fall (with an engraving). N Lond Med J 1:144-148, 1792

Piccolomini A: Anatomicae praelectiones explicantes mirificam corporis humani fabricam. Rome: Bonfadinus, 1586

Pick A: Beiträge zur Lehre von den Sprachstörungen. Arch Psychiat Nervenkr 23:896-918, 1892

Pietro: Clerica practica. 1035

Pitres A: Considérations sur l'agraphie. A propos d'une observation nouvelle d'agraphie motrice pure. Rev Med 4:855-873, 1884

Plato: The Dialogues of Plato, 3rd ed. (B Jowett , trans). Oxford: Clarendon Press, 1924

Platt WB: Fabricius Guilhelmus Hildanus; the father of German surgery. Bull Johns Hopkins Hosp 16:7, 1905

Pliny the Elder: The Natural History of Pliny. (J Bostock and HT Riley, trans.) London: Bohn, 1856-1893

Pölchen: Gehirnerweichung nach Vergiftung mit Kohlendust. Berl Klin Wochenschr 26:1881

Portal A: Cours d'Anatomie Médicale. Paris: Beaudoin, 1803

Pott P: Remarks on that kind of palsy of the lower limbs which is frequently found to accompany a curvature of the spine and is supposed to be caused by it; together with its method of cure; etc. London: J Johnson, 1779, 84 pp

Pott P: The Chirurgical Works of Percivall Pott, F.R.S. (Earle J, ed). Philadelphia, Pa: J Webster, 1819

Pourfour de Petit F: Lettres d'un Médecin des Hôpitaux du Roi, à un Autre médecin de ses Amis. Naumur: Charles G Albert, 1710

Pourfour du Petit F: Mémoire dans lequel il est démonstré que les nerfs intercostaux fournissent des rameaux qui portent des esprits dans les yeux. Hist Acad R Sci Paris:1-19, 1727

Praxagorus: The Fragments of Praxagorus of Bos and His School. (F Steckerl, col, ed, and transl). Leiden: EJ Brill, 1958

Proust, Tillaux: Opening an abscess of the brain. Med Times Hosp Gaz Lond 2:126-127, 1877

Prunières PB: Sur les objets de bronze, ambre, verre, etc. mêles aux silex et sur les races humaines dont on trouve les debris dans les dolmens de la Lozère. Compt Rend Assoc Franc Avanc SC 2: 683-705, 1873

Prunières: Sur les crânes artifiellements perforés à l'époque des dolmens. Bull Mem Soc Anthropol Paris 9 (2nd ser):185-205, 1874

Puchelt FA: Über partielle Empfindungslähmung. Hdlbg Med Annal 10:485-495, 1844

Quesnay F: Histoire de l'Origine et des Progrès de la Chirurgie en France. Paris: Ganeau, 1749, 520 pp

Quincke H: Die Lumbalpunction des Hydrocephalus. Berl Klin Wochenschr 28:929-933, 965-968, 1891

Quincke H: Ueber Lumbalpunction. **Berl Klin Wochenschr 32:**889-891, 1895

Ramon y Cajal S: **Histologie du Systèm Nerveux de l'Homme et des Vertébrés.** Paris: A Maloine, 1909-1911, 2 Vols

Ranke O: Status corticis verrucosus deformis. **Z Ges Neurol Psychiatr 28:**635-750, 1905

Ranvier LA: Contributions á l'histologie et à la physiologie des nerfs periphériques. **Compt Rend Acad Sci (Paris) 73:**1168-1171, 1871

Ray P, Gupta HN, Roy M: **Susruta Samhita (A Scientific Symposium).** New Delhi, India: National Science Academy, 2nd publication, 1980, 459 pp

Ray P, Gupta HN: **Caraka Samhita (A Scientific Symposium).** New Delhi, India: National Science Academy, 1980, 124 pp

Reed CAL: Some typical recoveries in Iowa from chronic convulsive toxemia (epilepsy) following surgical correction of abdominal viscera. **J Iowa Med Soc 10:**204-208, 1920

Reil JC: Mangel des mittleren und freyen Theils des Balken in Menschengehirn. **Arch Physiol 11:** 241-244, 1812

Reil JC: Ueber den Bau des Hirns und der Nerven. **Neues J Phys Leipzig 1:**96-114, 1795

Remak R: **Observationes Anatomicae et Microscopicae de Systematis Nervosi Structura.** Berlin: Reimer, 1838

Remak R: Vorläufige Mittheilung microscopischer Beobachtungen über den innern Bau der Cerebrospinalnerven und über die Entwicklung ihrer Formelemente. **Arch Anat Physiol,** pp 145-161, 1836

Rhazes: **Liber continens.** Lugduni: J de Ferrariis, 1511, 284 pp

Richter WM von: **Geschichte de Medicin in Russland.** 1813-1817

Riddoch G: The reflex functions of the completely divided spinal cord in man, compared with those associated with less severe lesions. **Brain 40:**264-402, 1917

Rio-Hortega P del: **Bol Real Soc Espan Hist Nat 21:**63-93, 1921

Riverius L: **Medicina practica.** Basel: J Wesenfels, 1663, 582 pp

Riverius L: **The compleat practice of physick.** (N Culpeper, A Cole, W Rowland, trans). London: Peter Cole, 1655, 645 pp

Robert A: Mémoire sur la nature de l'écoulement aqueux très abondant qui accompagne certaines fractures du crâne. **Mem Soc Chir Paris 1:**563-615, 1847

Roberts JB: The field of limitation of the operative surgery of the human brain. **Trans Am SA 3:** 1-108, 1885

Roger Frugardi of Salerno, in Sudhoff K (ed): **Studien zur Geschichte der Medicin.** Leipzig: JA Barth, 1918, 685 pp

Rokitansky C von: Ueber einige der Wichtigsten Krankheiten der Arterien. **Dnksch Akad Wiss Wien 4:**1-72, 1852

Rolando L: **Saggio Sopra la Vera Struttura del Cervello dell'Uomo e degl'Animali, e Sopra le Funzioni del Sistema Nervoso.** Sassari: Stamperia Priviligiata, 1809, 98 pp

Rollo J: **An account of two cases of diabetes mellitus, with remarks as they arose during the progress of the cure.** London: C Dilly, 1797, 2 Vols

Romberg MH: **A Manual of the Nervous Diseases of Man.** (EH Sieveking, trans and ed). London: Sydenham Society, 1853, 2 Vols

Romberg MH: **Klinische Ergebnisse.** Berlin: A Förstner, 1846

Romberg MH: **Lehrbuch der Nervenkrankheiten des Menschen.** Berlin: A Duncker, 1840-1846 (2nd ed, 1851)

Rosenbaum S: Beiträge zur Aplasie des Nervus opticus. **Ztschr Augenheikld 7:**200-213, 1902

Ross R: On some peculiar pigmented cells found in two mosquitoes fed on malarial blood. **Br Med J 2:**1786-1788, 1897

Rossolimo GI: **The Brain Tipograph (a Device for Projection of Brain Parts on the Skull Surface).** Ezheg: Ekterin Bolnizi, 1907, pp 63-65

Roth N: Erasistratus. **Medtronic News,** 1983, pp 20-22

Rothman M: Demonstration des grosshirnlosen Hundes. **Berl Klin Wochenschr 48:**1302, 1911

Roux J: Observation sur une opération de trépan au crâne, faite avec succès dans un cas d'epanchement de pus circonscrit dans la cavité de l'arachnoïde lequel existait depuis quatre ans. **Nouv J Med Chir**

Pharm 12:3-20, 1821

Roy CS, Sherrington CS: On the regulation of the blood-supply of the brain. **J Physiol 11**:85, 1890

Rudolphi KA: **Entozoorum, sive Verminum Intestinalium, Historia Naturalis.** Amstelodami, 1808-1810, 2 Vols

Rufus d'Ephesus: **Oeuvres de Rufus d'Ephèse.** (Ch Daremberg, trans). Paris: JB Baillière & Fils, 1879, 290 pp

Russell D, Batten FE, Collier JSR: Subacute combined degeneration of the spinal cord. **Brain 23:** 39-110, 1900

Russell DS, Donald C: Mechanism of internal hydrocephalus in spina bifida. **Brain 58**:203-215, 1935

Sanderson JB: Note on the excitation of the surface of the cerebral hemispheres by induced currents. **Proc R Soc Lond 22**:368-370, 1873-1874

Sano K: **History of Neurosurgery (Japanese). A Monograph.** Chugai-Seiyaki, 1988, pp 30-43

Saucerotte N: **Mémoire sur les contre-coups dans les lésions de la tête.** 1769

Schäfer EA: On the alleged sensory functions of the motor cortex cerebri. **J Physiol 23**:310-314, 1898

Schaudinn FR, Hoffmann E: Vorläufiger Bericht über das Vorkommon von Spirochaetenen in syphilitischen Krankheitsprodukten und bei Papillomea. **Arb Gesundh Amte 22**:527-534, 1905

Schiff M: **Lehrbuch der Physiologie des Menschen. Muskel- und Nervenphysiologie.** Lahr: M von Schauenburg, 1858-1859, 424 pp

Schmidt MB: Ueber die Pacchion'schen Granulationen und ihr Verhältniss zu den Sarcomen und Psammomen der Dura mater. **Virchows Arch Pathol Anat 170**:429-464, 1902

Schupman A: Case of hypertrophy of brain in child. **Lancet 2**:490-491, 1838

Schwalbe E, Gredig M: Über Entwicklungsstörungen des Klienhirns, Hirnstamms und Halsmarks bei Spina bifida (Arnold'sche und Chiari'sche Missbildung). **Beitr Pathol Anat Pathol 40:** 132-194, 1907

Schwalbe MW: **Eine Eigenthümliche Tonische Krampfform mit Hysterischen Symptomen.** Inaugural Dissertation, Berlin, 1907

Schwann T: **Mikroskopische Untersuchungen über die Uebereinstimmung in der Struktur und dem Wachsthum der Thiere und Pflanzen.** Berlin: GE Reimer, 1839

Sekino H: Surgical text in Meiji-Era. First brain surgery in Japan. **No Shinkei Geka 16**:115-116, 1988

Sellier J, Verger H: Recherches expérimentales sur la physiologie de la couche optique. **Arch Physiol Norm Pathol (5th ser) 10**:706-713, 1898

Senn: **La méningité argué des enfants.** 1825

Sherrington CS: **The Integrative Action of the Nervous System.** New Haven, Conn: Yale University Press, 1906

Sigerist HE: **A History of Medicine.** New York, NY: Oxford University Press, 1951-1961, 564 pp

Simon T: Ueber Syringomyelie und Geschwulstibildung in Rückenmark.

Sinclair WW: Abnormal associated movements of the lids. **Ophthalmol Rev 14**:307, 1895

Singer C, Underwood EA: **A Short History of Medicine, 2nd ed.** Oxford: Clarendon, Press, 1962

Singer CJ: A short history of anatomy and physiology from the Greeks to Harvey. **Rev J Hist Med 15**:442, 1960

Singer CJ: Brain dissection before Vesalius. **J Hist Med 11**:261-274, 1956

Slawyk: Ein Fall von Allgmeininfection mit Influenzabacillen. **Z Hyg Infektkr 32**:443-448, 1899

Soemmerring ST von: **De basi encephali et originibus nervorum cranio egredientium.** Gottingen: A Vendenhoeck, 1778, 184 pp

Soemmerring ST von: **Von Hirn und Ruckenmark.** Mainz: Winkopp, 1788

Soranus: On acute and chronic diseases.

Souques A: **Etapes de la Neurologie Dans l'Antiquité Grecque.** Paris: Masson et Cie, 1936, 247 pp

Spencer H: **The Principles of Psychology.** London: Longman, Brown, Green and Longmans, 1855

Spillane JD: **The Doctrine of the Nerves. Chapters in the History of Neurology.** Oxford: Oxford University Press, 1981

Spiller WG, Frazier CH: Cerebral decompression. Palliative operations in the treatment of tumors of the brain, based on the observation of fourteen cases. **Univ Penn Med Bull 19**:146-167, 1907

Spiller WG, Martin E: The treatment of persistent pain of organic origin in the lower part of the body by division of the anterolateral column of the spinal cord. **JAMA 58**:1489-1490, 1912

Spiller WG, Potts P: **Univ Penn Med Bull 16:**362-366, 1903

Spiller WG: The location within the spinal cord of the fibers for temperature and pain sensations. **J Nerv Ment Dis 32:**318-320, 1905

Spiller WG: Two cases of partial internal hydrocephalus from closure of the interventricular passages. **Am J Med Sci (new ser) 124:**44-55, 1902

Spink MS, Lewis GL: Albucasis on surgery and instruments. **J Hist Med 29:**345-350, 1974

Stalpart Van der Weil C: **Observations rares de médicine, d'anatomie et de chirurgie.** (M Planque, trans). Paris: Nyon and LaPorte, 1780, 548 pp

Starr MA: **Brain Surgery.** New York, NY: William Wood & Co, 1893, 295 pp

Stein SAW: **De Thalamo et Origine Nervi Optici in Homine et Animalibus Vertebratis.** Copenhagen: S Trier, 1834, 66 pp

Steno N: **A dissertation on the anatomy of the brain.** Copenhagen: Busck, 1950

Steno N: **Dissertatio de cerebri anatomae. . . .** Gallico examplari Parisiis edito an, 1669

Stephanus C: **De dissectione partium corporis humani.** Paris: Colinaeum, 1545, 375 pp

Stern M: **Acromegaly.** London: New Sydenham Society, 1899

Stilling B: **Neue Untersuchungen über den Bau des Rückenmarks.** Kassel: von Heinrich Hotop, 1859

Stilling J: **Untersuchungen über die Entstehung der Kurzsichtigkeit.** Wiesbaden: Bergmann, 1887

Strümpell A: **Dtsch Z Neurol 12:**115-149, 1898

Sugita G, Royotoku M: **Keitai Shinsho.** 1774

Swan J: **A Dissertation on the Treatment of Morbid Local Affections of Nerves.** London: J Drury, 1820, 196 pp

Swedenborg E: **The Brain, Considered Anatomically, Physiologically, and Philosophically.** (RL Tafel, trans and ed). London: Speirs, 1882-1887, 2 Vols

Sydenham T: **Observationes medicar.** London, 1676

Sydenham T: **The Entire Works of Dr. Thomas Sydenham.** London: E Cave, 1753, 672 pp

Takayasu M: A case with peculiar changes of the central retinal vessels. **Acta Soc Ophthalmol (Jpn) 12:**554, 1908

Taruffi C: **Storia Della Teratologia.** Bologna: Regia Tipographia, 1891-1894, 8 Vols

Tello JC: **Craniectomia Prehistorica Entre los Hauyos.** London: International Congress of America, 1912

Temkin O: **The Falling Sickness. 2nd ed.** Baltimore, Md: Williams and Wilkins, 1971, 467 pp

Theodoric: Incipt Cyrurgia edita et compilata a divino Fratre Theodorico Episcope Cerviensi Ordinis Praedicatorum, in: **Cyrurgia Guidonis de Cauliaco.** Venetiis, 1499, pp 97-134

Theodoric: **The Surgery of Theodoric, ca 1267.** (E Campbell, J Colton, eds). New York, NY: Appleton-Century-Crofts, 1955-1960, 233 pp

Thierry F: **J Med Chir Pharm 2:**337-346, 1755

Thomas A: **Le Cervelet: Etude Anatomique, Clinique et Physiologique.** Paris: G Steinheil, 1897

Thomas JP: Drainage of cerebral abscess. **Med News (Phila) 46:**193-195, 1885

Thudichum JLW: **A Treatise on the Chemical Constitution of the Brain.** London: Baillière, Tindall & Cox, 1884

Tissot SA: **An essay on onanism: or a treatise upon the disorders produced by masturbation or the effects of secret and excessive venery.** (A Hume, trans). Dublin: J Williams, 1722, 149 pp

Todd RB: **Clinical Lectures on Paralysis, Certain Diseases of the Brain, and Other Afflictions of the Nervous System.** Philadelphia, Pa: Lindsay & Blakiston, 1855

Todd RB: **Clinical Lectures on Paralysis, Certain Diseases of the Brain, and Other Afflictions of the Nervous System. 2nd ed.** London: John Churchill, 1856, pp 284-307

Tooth HH: **The Peroneal Type of Progressive Muscular Atrophy.** London: HK Lewis, 1886

Tourette G Gilles de la: Jumping, latah, myriachiat. **Arch Neurol 8:**68-74, 1884

Trotter W: Chronic subdural hemorrhage of traumatic origin and its relation to pachymeningitis hemorrhage interna. **Br J Surg 2:**271-291, 1914

Trousseau A: De l'aphasie, maladie décrite récemment sous le nom impropre d'aphémie. **Gaz Hop 37:** 13-14, 25-26, 37-39, 48-50, 1864

Trousseau A: Mémoire sur un cas de trachéotomie pratiquée dans la période extrême de croup. **J Connaise Med Chir 1:**541, 1833

Türck L: Ueber sekundäre Erkrankung einzelner Rückenmarkstränge und ihrer Fortsetzungen zum Gehirne. **Z Ges Arzte Wien 9**:289-317, 1853

Türk S: Ueber Retractions-bewegungen der Augen. **Dtsch Med Wochenschr 22**:199, 1896

Turner W: **The Convolutions of the Human Cerebrum Topographically Considered.** Edinburgh: Maclachlan & Stewart, 1806

Uematsu S: The dawn of brain surgery in Japan. History prior to World War II. **Neurosurgery 26**: 162-172

Underwood M: Debility of the lower extremities, in: **Treatise on the diseases in children.** London: J Mathews, 1789, Vol 2, pp 53-57

Unterharnscheidt F, Jacknik D, Gött H: **Der Balkenmangel Vol 128, Monogr Gasamtgeb Neurol Psychiat.** Berlin: Springer, 1968

Unverricht H: Experimentalle und Klinische Untersuchungen uber die Epilepsie. **Arch Psychiat 14:** 175-262, 1883

Valentin GC: Uber den Verlauf und die letzten Ende der Nerven. **Nova Acta Phys Med Acad Caes 18:**51-240, 1836

Valsalva AM: **Joannis Baptistae Morgagni epistolarum anatomicarum duodeviginti ad scripta perinentium celeberrimi viri Antonii Marie Valsalvae pars altera.** Venice: F Pitterus, 1741

Vara Lopez R: **La Craniectomía a Través des los Siglos.** Valladolid, Spain: Editorial, Ebanisteria, 1949, 148 pp

Varolio C: **De nervis opticis nonnullisque aliis praeter communem opinionem in humano capite observatis epistolae.** Padua: Meiti, 1573

Velpeau AALM: Observation sur une maladie de la moëlle épinière tendant à démontrer l'isolement des fonctions des racines sensitives et motrices des nerfs. **Arch Gen Med (old ser) (Paris) 7:** 68-82, 1825

Vesalius A: **De humani corporis fabrica. Libri septum.** Basel: Johannes Oporinus, 1543, 663 pp

Vesalius A: **Opera omnia anatomica et chirurgica.** Batavorum: J du Vivie & J and H Verbeek, 1725, 2 Vols

Vesling J: **Syntagma anatomicum.** Padua: Pauli Frambotti, 1647

Veyssière R: **Recherches Clinique et Expérimentales sur l'Hémianesthésie de Cause Cérébrale.** Thèse No 380. Paris: A Delahaye, 1874, 88 pp

Vicq d'Azyr F: Recherches sur la structure du cerveau, du cervelet, de la moelle elongée, de la moelle épinière, et sur l'origine des nerfs de l'homme et des animaux. **Hist Acad R Sci:**495-622, 1781

Vicq d'Azyr F: **Traité d'anatomie et de physiologie avec des planches coloriées réprésentant au natural les divers organes del'home et de animaux.** Paris: FA Didot d'Aine, 1786

Vieussens R de: **Neurographia universalis.** Lyon: J Carte, 1684

Vieusseux G: Mémoire sur la malade qui a régné à Genève au printemps de 1805. **J Med Chirurg Pharm (Paris) 11:**163-182, 1805

Vigo G da: **Practica in arte chirurgica copiosa . . . continens novem libros.** Rome: Guillirett et H Bononiansem, 1514

Vigo J de : Opera, in: **Chyrurgia.** Lugdini: J and F Giuncta, 1525, 279 pp

Virchow R: **Die Cellularpathologie in ihrer Begründung auf Physiologische und Pathologische Gewebelehre.** Berlin: A Hirschwald, 1859, 440 pp

Virchow R: **Die Krankhaften Geschwülste.** Berlin: A Hirschwald, 1863-1867, 3 Vols

Virchow R: Ein Fall von Progressiver Muskelatrophie. **Arch Pathol Anat Physiol 8:**537-540, 1855

Wachsmuth H: Uber progressive Bulbärparalyse und Diplegia facialis. Dorpat, 1864 (Inaugural thesis)

Wagner W: Die temporäre Resektion des Schädeldaches an Stelle der Trepanation. **Zentralbl Chir 16:**833-838, 1889

Waldeyer HWG: Ueber einige neuere Forschungen im Gebiete der Anatomie des Centralnervensystems. **Dtsch Med Wochenschr 17:**1213-1218, 1244-1246, 1267-1269, 1287-1289, 1331-1332, 1352-1356, 1891

Walker A: New antomy and physiology of the brain in particular, and of the nervous system in general. **Arch Univ Sci 3:**172, 1809

Walker AE (ed): **A History of Neurological Surgery.** Baltimore, Md: Williams and Wilkins, 1951, 583 pp

Waller AV: Experiments on the section of the glosso-pharyngeal and hypo-glossal nerves of the frog and observations on the alterations produced thereby in the structure of their primitive fibres. **Phil Trans R Soc Lond (Pt 2) 140:**423-429, 1850

Wallman H: Eine colloid Cyste im dritten Hirnventrikel und eine Lipoma in Plexus Chorioides. **Virchows Arch Pathol Anat 14:**385-388, 1858

Warkany J: **Congenital Malformations.** Chicago, Ill: Year Book Medical, 1971, 1309 pp

Wassermann A, Neisser A, Bruck C: Eine serodiagnostische Reaktion bei Syphilis. **Dtsch Med Wochenschr 32:**745-746, 1906

Wassermann A: Eine serodiagnostische Reaktion bei Syphilis. **Dtsch Med Wochenschr 32:**745-746, 1906

Weed LH: The cerebrospinal fluid. **Physiol Rev 2:**171-203, 1922

Weeds JF: Case of cerebral abscess. **Nashville J Med Sci (new ser) 9:**156-171, 1872

Weichselbaum A: Ueber die Aetiologie der akuten Meningitis cerebro-spinalis. **Fortschr Med 5:** 573-583, 620-626, 1887

Weigert C: Uber eine neue Untersuchungsmethode des Centralnervensystems. **Centralbl Med Wissensch 20:**753-757, 772-774, 1882

Weigert F: Zur Lehre von der Tumoren der Hirnanhaenge. **Virchows Arch Pathol Anat 65:**212-219, 1875

Weir RF, Seguin EC: Contribution to the diagnosis and surgical treatment of tumors of the cerebrum. **Am J Med Sci (new ser) 96:**25-38, 109-138, 219-232, 1888

Weir RF: Four month's operative work at the New York Hospital. **Med News Phila 50:**271-277, 1887

Weisenberg TH: Tumors of the third ventricle, with the establishment of a symptom complex. **Brain 33:**236-260, 1911

Weiss P: **La Cirugia del Craneo Entre los Antiguos Peruanos.** Lima, 1949, 34 pp

Welt L: Über Charakterveränderungen des Menschen infolge der Läsionen des Stirnhirns. **Dtsch Arch Klin Med 42,** 1888

Wepfer JJ: **Observationes anatomicae, ex cadaveribus eorum, quos sustulit apoplexia.** Schaffhausen: JC Suturi, 1658, 304 pp

Werdnig G: Zwei frühinfantile hereditäre Fälle von progressiver Muskelatrophie unter dem Bilde der Dystrophie, aber auf neurotischer Grundlage. **Arch Psychiatr Nervenkr 22:**437-480, 1891

Wernher: Pneumatocele cranii, supramastoidea, chronische Luftgeschwulst von enormer Grösse durch spontane Dehiscenz der Zellen des Processus mastoideus entstranden. **Dtsch Z Chir 3:** 381-401, 1873

Wernicke C, Hahn E: Idiopathischer Abscess des Occipitallappens durch Trepanation entleert. **Virchows Arch Pathol Anat 87:**335-344, 1882

Wernicke C: **Der Aphasische Symptomenkomplex.** Breslau: Cohn & Weigert, 1874, 72 pp

Wernicke C: **Lehrbuch der Gehirnkrankheiten fur Aerzte und Studierende.** Berlin: Fischer, 1881-1883, 3 Vols

West JF: Case of meningocele associated with cervical spina bifida, cured by aspiration. **Lancet 2:** 552-553, 1985

Westphal C: Ueber einen Fall von intracraniellen Echinococcen mit Ausgang in Heilung. **Berl Klin Wochenschr 10:**205-208, 1873

Westphal CFO: Ueber eine dem Bilde der cerebrospinalen grauen Degeneration ähnliche Erkrank ung des centralen Nervensystmes ohne anatomischen Befund, nebst einigen Bemerkungen uber paradoxe Contraction. **Arch Psychiatr Nervenkr 14:**87, 1883

Westphal CFO: Ueber einige durch mechanische Einwirkung auf Sehnen und Muskel hervorge brachte. **Arch Psychiatr Nervenkr 5:**803-834, 1875

White WH: One hundred cases of cerebral tumor with reference to cause, operative treatment, mode of death and general symptoms. **Guys Hosp Rep 43:**117-142, 1886

Whytt R: **An essay on the vital and other involuntary motions of animals.** Edinburgh: Hamilton, Balfour & Neill, 1751

Whytt R: **Observations on the dropsy in the brain.** Edinburgh: J Balfour, 1768

Whytt R: **Observations on the most frequent species of the hydrocephalus internus viz. The dropsy of the ventricles of the brain. The works of Robert Whytt, M.D.** 2nd ed. Edinburgh: J Balfour, 1768, 762 pp

Whytt R: Observations on the nature, causes, and cure of those disorders which have been commonly called nervous, hypochondriac or hysteric; to which are prefixed some remarks on the sympathy of the nerves. 2nd ed. Edinburgh: T Becket, Hondt & Balfour, 1765

Whytt R: The Works of Robert Whytt, M.D. published by his son. Edinburgh: Balfour, Auld and Smellie, 1768

Wickman OI: Studien über Poliomyelitis acuta. Arb Path Inst Univ Helsingfors 1:109-292, 1905

Widal, Sicard, Ravaut: Cytologie du liquide céphalo-rachidien. Au cours de quelques processus méningés chroniques (paralysie générale et tabes). Bull Mem Soc Med Hop (Paris) (3rd ser) 18: 31-33, 1901

William of Saliceto, in Sudhoff K (ed): Studien zur Geschichte der Medizin. Leipzig: JA Barth, 1918, 685 pp

William of Saliceto: Cyrurgia. (F di Pietro, trans). Venice, 1474

Willis T: A description of an epidemical fever . . . 1661, in: Practice of Physick. London: T Dring, 1684, Treatise VIII, pp 46-54

Willis T: Cerebri anatome: cui accessit nervorum descriptio et usus. London: J Flesher, 1664, 456 pp

Willis T: The anatomy of the brain, in: Dr. Willis's Practice of physick, being the whole works of that renowned and famous physician . . . now translated by S. Portage [sic]. London: T Dring, C Harper and J Leigh, 1684

Willis T: The London Practice of Physick Contained in the Works of Dr. Willis, faithfully made English, and printed together for the publick good. London: T Basset and W Crooke, 1685

Willis T: The practice of physick. (S Portage, trans). London, 1684

Wilson SAK: Progressive lenticular degeneration, a familial nervous disease associated with cirrhosis of the liver. Brain 34:295-509, 1912

Winiwarter F von: Ueber eine eigenthümliche Form von Endarteriitis und Endophlebitis mit Gangrän des Fusses. Arch Klin Chir 23:202-206, 1879

Wiseman R: A treatise of wounds. London: R Norton, 1672

Wiseman R: Severall Chirurgical Treatises. London: E Fleisher and J Macock, 1676

Witkowski L: Ueber Gehirnschütterung. Virchows Arch Path Anat 69:498-516, 1877

Witzel O: Die operative Behandlung der phlegmonösen Meningitis. Mitt Grenzgeb Med Chir 8: 388-392, 1901

Wolff E: Luftansammlung im rechten Seitenventrikel des Gehirns (Pneumozephalus). Munch Med Wochenschr 61:899, 1914

Wood W: Observations on neuroma. Trans Med Chir Soc Edinburgh 3:367-434, 1828/1829

Wren C: Life and Works of Sir Christopher Wren. (EJ Enthoven, ed). London: E Arnold. 1903

Wu Ti: in Bouger DC (ed): History of China. London, 1881, Vol 1, p 106

Würtz F: Practica der Wundartzney. Basel, 1563

Wynter WE: Four cases of tubercular meningitis in which paracentesis of the theca vertebralis was performed for the relief of fluid pressure. Lancet 1:981-982, 1891

Yamagiwa K: Beitrag zur Aetiologie der Jackson'schen Epilepsie. Virchows Arch Pathol Anat 119: 447-460, 1890

Yperman J: Cyrurgia. 1825

Zaufal E: Verein deutscher Aerzte in Prag. Ein Vortrag Prag Med Wochenschr 5:517, 1880

Zernov DN: [Encephalometer. A device for estimating parts of the brain in man.] Proc Soc Physicomed (Moscow Univ, Moscow) 2:70-80, 1889 (Russ)

Zinn JG, Haller A: Mémoires sur les parties sensibles et irritables du corps animal. Laussane: C d'Aunay, 1760, 500 pp

APPENDIX A
The Arts in the Evolution of Neuroscience

A. Earl Walker, MD

From ancient times, the arts have played a role in the training and practice of a healer. In primitive tribes, the chants and dances of the medicine-man were as important as his herbal therapies. As knowledge increased in the Middle Ages, art and music were used more commonly by physicians. After examination of the dead became legal, the morphological changes in the brain were depicted in artistic drawings. The pompous physician examining a flask of urine was often ridiculed in the theater and in the art of the 17th century. Whether it be tom-toms to drive away evil spirits or soothing chords to ease jangled nerves, music has been effectively applied to alleviate suffering from time immemorial. Recently, the rational basis for this therapy has been explored.

At the height of Greek culture, education implied a broad knowledge of the humanities—grammar, dialect (logic), and rhetoric (speaking)—as well as the practical arts—geometry, arithmetic, and astronomy. Upon a knowledge of these subjects, a career in law, medicine, and especially religion could be founded. Accordingly, they were considered not subsidiary to, but the essence of, professional training. After such a basic education, the healer-to-be sat at the feet of one or more master physicians for an indefinite period, often at a prestigious medical center. Note that Galen, after completing his education in the arts, traveled to Alexandria, where for five years he listened to lectures but never got near the sick. Yet, he returned to Pergamon a trained surgeon and, within a year, was appointed physician to the gladiators.

Early Medical Art

Although the Egyptians of the 11th and 12th dynasties supplemented their writings with sketches or paintings of the body, they apparently left no illustrations of their ritualistic transnasal removal of the brain after death in order to implant preservatives within the skull. Those peoples of other lands who made holes in the skull for various reasons (social, medical, or tribal prestige) left neither graphic evidence of their techniques nor script to indicate the mode or reason for their cranial violations. Perhaps the earliest representation of an operation on the head is a huaco of a Mohican of 600 AD perforating the skull with a tumi. Another graphic figure from the New World would seem to be an anencephalic monster.

The ancient Greeks and Romans, although describing the structure of the cranium and its surgical mutilation, left no illustrations of their operative procedures. In the latter part of the first Christian millenium, surgeons, unfamiliar with the anatomy of the head, avoided performing cranial procedures which earlier Greek physicians had skillfully carried out (Jones). In the medical writings of the Arabs, few drawings are found. Since dissection was taboo, knowledge of the nervous system had to be gleaned from sullied translations of Greek and Roman manuscripts. Being written by hand, the medical texts of the Middle Ages contained only a few crude sketches and miniature paintings but none of the nervous system. The earliest European drawings and paintings of the head with rough scribblings to indicate its contents were probably those of the Salernitans in the 13th century. Sometime later the body was drawn upon wood and the location of diseased, wounded, or abnormal states was noted by superimposed lettering. Such "disease-men" became common in the 15th century. On a sketch of the head, faculties of the brain were indicated by circular or quadrilateral "cells," identified by superimposed or adjacent lettering. The presumed mental processes were placed in cells, common sense (sensus communis) included the special and general senses and was placed rostrally, fantasy or imagination in the next cell—sometimes associated with judgment and thinking, and posteriorly, memory was consistently located. In early sketches, these faculties were superposed around or on the head; somewhat later, they were assigned within the brain or cerebral ventricles.

Rather crude sketches of trephines and surgical instruments first appeared in the texts of Cordobian surgeons of the 14th century. Even cruder and more fanciful illustrations of the nervous system were to be found in Asiatic manuscripts.

Renaissance Art in Neurology

Choulant states that medical arts were introduced as a schematic aid to memory, to give representation of an individual and to establish anatomical norms. The first anatomy text by Mundinus had no illustrations. Even after printing and woodcuts were introduced, the few figures were quite schematic. Real-life sketches of the brain drawn by Leonardo da Vinci initiated the normal representation of the brain. As Italy was the birthplace of painting it is natural that in Florence, artists should have formed a section of the "Guild of Physicians and Apothecaries" and associated with doctors during autopsies.

The "science of the sepulchre" pursued by Castagno (1390-1457) and Verraschio (1435-1488) was illustrated by artists of that time. Michaelangelo made a number of dissections but left no illustrations of his anatomical works. In the first printed figures, Fries in 1519 drew a striking facial expression but rather crude cephalic sketches to demonstrate the techniques of removing the brain from the skull. A few years later, Berengario da Carpi drew two sections of the cut brain based upon personal dissections which, although somewhat inaccurate, founded anatomical illustrations to replace the earlier schematic and diagrammatic drawings. Depiction of the cortical and subcortical structures was no longer marred by "cells" and modern artistry replaced the disease-men.

The Italian school of anatomists, stimulated by the appealing *Fabricius* of Vesalius, discovered many anatomical secrets of the human body, and in so doing, corrected some of Galen's errors. They popularized the use of artistic illustrations to demonstrate the practice of medicine. Sketches of surgical instruments and procedures, even trephining, were found in medical treatises. Occasionally, a neurological disorder such as acromegaly or facial spasm was depicted on canvas or in stone.

At the same time in Louvain, André Vesalius was dissecting the human body and making such remarkable preparations that Jan Calcar was able to illustrate the corporeal and neurological structures in a few beautiful plates, several of which Vesalius drew himself. A number of Galen's errors were eliminated. Vesalius's anatomical descriptions were far superior to the previous accounts and stimulated explorations by later anatomists.

The baroque artists, while satisfying their patrons with grandiose and flattering court portraits, also painted subjects as they looked. Thus, Velasquez showed the toothy idiot, the deformed achondroplastic, and the cretin. Pieter Brueghel, the elder, and Hieronymous Bosch depicted cripples and others with neurological infirmities. Rubens painted a microcephalic dwarf. The foibles of the medical profession were characterized. Urine-casting was a favorite subject of the 16th century Dutch painters, whose canvases showed a pale, chlorotic maiden gazing wide-eyed upon a handsome, fur-capped physician in colorful robes surveying a urine flask. The charlatan surgeon is shown removing stones from the head of a feeble-minded lad.

Although the artists were stimulated by the stirring spirit of the Renaissance, the healing arts were slower to advance. The basic sciences had to develop a foundation for the clinical sciences. Not until the 17th century was attention given to precise anatomical depiction of cerebral structures. Thus, Caspar Bartholin described the large groove in the lateral surface of the brain and named it the fissure of Sylvius. In its depths, Johann Christian Reil noted the insular convolutions in 1795. Rolando numbered the gyri and called attention to the prominent central fissure to which his name was given. In 1806, Turner in Edinburgh defined the more constant sulci which were precisely outlined by Gratiolet and Ecker with the aid of a camera lucida.

Modern Neurological Art

Physicians were slow to use the available art in their clinical writings. In the 18th century, a few authors inserted sketches, often of instruments, to complement their clinical descriptions. Whytt in 1768 wrote on the motion of animals without using illustrations. In the same year, Percivall Pott in a text on injuries of the head had only three plates of surgical instruments used in cranial operations. In the next century, both John and Charles Bell drew beautiful illustrations for their textbooks. Richard Bright was an accomplished landscape and medical artist. Henle not only prepared the drawings for his manuscripts, he drew artistic sketches on a blackboard with chalk to illustrate his lectures. In 1852, Chouland prepared a history of anatomical illustrations which contained neurological art of interest. Although in the latter part of the 19th century, manuscripts had more and better figures, some writers still relied upon lengthy descriptions and few illustrations. Consider that Oppenheim in his 270-page book on brain tumors, published in the 1890s, used only 14 figures, most of which were line drawings. Cushing, early in the 20th century, after completing an operation would make several sketches to illustrate his procedure with such talent that his professional artist felt envious of his work.

Photography by that time was gaining such popularity that artistic and faithful reproductions of both gross and microscopic preparations were possible. Foerster on his ward rounds had an assistant carry a camera so that he could snap a photograph of interesting cases. As a result, his lengthy papers in the *Handbuch für Neurologie* were amply illustrated with photographs of his subjects. At about the same time, Brödel and his school of medical illustrators at Johns Hopkins Hospital, after spending hours in the dissecting and operating rooms, produced artistic and detailed drawings of surgical procedures showing minutiae that even the assistants at surgery had not seen. Thus, modern art enhanced medical instruction.

The Neurosciences in the Theater

From time immemorial, the doctor has been treated both kindly and, again, rudely in drama. Aristophanes in *Clouds* wrote that physicians were lazy, long-haired fops. In Roman times, the medical profession was, at first not very highly regarded. Later it became specialized and was, according to Celsus, highly respected. However, as Roman life degenerated, the practice of medicine declined and was kept alive only in the monasteries. Drama was neglected as the populace entertained themselves by story-telling, dancing, singing, or chanting. In some countries of the world, religious plays were performed. The physician was, however, not involved. It was not until the Renaissance that the theater showed an interest in the medical profession. Shakespeare, in his numerous plays, occasionally refers to physicians, but rarely to surgeons. Shakespeare does make infrequent references to the nervous system when medical subjects are at issue. In *Hamlet*, he has Falstaff decry—"this apoplexy, as I take it, is a kind of lethargy, an't please your lordship, a whoreson tingling .... It hath its origin from much grief, from study, and from perturbation of the brain. I have read the cause of his effects in Galen."

Later, however, French writers found the medical profession a ready target for their satire. Molière in the 17th century railed at the pedantic physicians who paraded across the stage of five of his comedies extolling the merits of the clyster, lancet and purge. Consider Le Sage's Dr. Sangrado in *Gil Blas*—"the tall, withered, wan executioner of the sisters three" who bled "the old canon to death's door in less than two days by drawing off 18 good porringers of blood" (a porringer is a small soup bowl).

Occassionally, members of the medical profession ventured to enter the theater. Claude Bernard in his early days produced a play, which after a few performances flopped; he was advised to try some other profession. So medicine gained a brilliant physiologist.

In modern times, as the stage became a popular source of entertainment, drama (which played an increasing role in the lives of the populace) rarely involved the physician. An occasional playwright, such as George Bernard Shaw, did discuss medical problems, as in *The Doctor's Dilemma*, but the serious side of life was in general avoided.

The Place of Music in Neurology

Music of various types—the beat of the drums or the chants of the medicine-man—was used to dispell sickness by peoples of all parts of the world, centuries before Christ. Pythagorus, who delved into the physical basis of sound, recognized the soothing effect of music on the troubled mind and prescribed "musical medicine." For psoitis and sciatica, Pythagorus advocated playing pipes over the painful area until it throbbed and pulsed, thereupon the pain would be relieved. Theophrastus (c. 370-280 BC) wrote that wild, passionate music played near a paining member would alleviate a person's suffering. Although later Romans such as Soranus doubted the efficacy of such therapy, Aesclepiades in the first century after Christ wrote that sorrows could be dispelled by music, cymbals, and noise. In a treatise on acute and chronic disease 600 years later, Aurelianus stated that earlier writers thought that music might relieve mania; however, he questioned this for he had noted that priests as they chanted seemed to become possessed of a mania. A few centuries later, the Arabs used music in their mental hospitals to tame their patient's passions. In the Middle Ages, war and disease so occupied the nations of the world that music was confined to the religious songs and chants of the monasteries. Early in the 14th century, Henri de Mondeville admonished his students to "keep up your patients' spirits by music of viols and ten stringed psaltery."

As the plague swept through Europe decimating the population, the arts were neglected. Not until the Renaissance was music resurrected and passed from the home and church to the professional stage, where it was supported by the ruling classes. In Italy, the religious music of the monasteries gave way to secular madrigals which people sang in the streets. Physicians, as well as all educated persons, played musical instruments. In this age, church music, elaborated by the organ and the violin, blossomed into the opera. To this art, the doctor's most notable contribution was Giovanna Baptista della Porto's invention of the opera glasses in 1590. Opera, at least grand opera, did not exploit physicians whose role on the stage was purely professional, such as in *Traviata* when the physician pronounced the death of Violetta.

Until the Middle Ages, music was believed to be appreciated in the ear. Willis, noting that people with musical talents had soft cerebella and that those lacking musical talents had hard cerebella, placed the center for music in the cerebellum. Gall and Spurzheim, who assigned many functions to the brain, located the appreciation of music to the cerebral cortex. However, Gall's theory, although unfounded, had just sufficient appeal to stimulate more investigation. Later studies of the speech disorders occasionally referred to musical disabilities. Head reported that the aphasic usually could produce a melody and sing it in time and tune, but if the score was needed, was unable to read or sing to it.

The neuroanatomical basis of music has been explored recently. In brief, the appreciation of music, like speech, may be differentially affected by hemispheric lesions. For example, when right-handed individuals are injected with amytal in the right internal carotid artery while counting, they lose control of tonality and pitch, although still conscious and talking normally; however, when the left hemisphere is injected with Amytal, speech, comprehension, vocalization, and singing cease, and then return to normal in a few minutes. In general, the greater the musical sophistication of a person, the greater the role of the left hemisphere. Melodies, as well as single notes, are represented in the right hemisphere of the naive subject; however, in trained individuals, such functions are represented in both hemispheres. Musical integration, intimately related to vocalization and pragmatic meaning, Pribram affirmed was processed in the left frontolimbic cortices, by different topographical and structural mechanisms than natural language. However, subcortical circuits play a role, for Head reported that "music is liable to make different reactions" on the two sides of the body in patients with thalamic lesions. He maintained that musical capacity (by which he meant the ability to recall a melody and hum it in time and in tune), was not necessarily impaired in speech defects. He noted that singing words might fail but still the melody might be whistled.

Although music, neither punitive not threatening, has been a therapeutic agent in psychiatry and pediatrics and, more recently, in anesthesiology, little basic investigation has been carried out to determine its effects upon brain activity. An interesting study of the influence on the electroencephalogram of "passionate" and "soothing" musical compositions has been reported to show more beta activity in the records of persons listening to calm rather than exciting lyrics (Bruys).

Conclusions

Throughout the ages, the medicine-man (in whatever garb) has played a significant part in human life. During the evolution of art, drama, and music, the physician used graphic arts to instruct followers, drama to appeal to the populace, and music to dissipate the mechancholies of patients. In his ministrations to the sick, the physician's ostentatious and flamboyant dress has heartened his patients even if he had little therapy to offer. In the early part of the 16th century, the bearded physicians donned plumed hats and long cloaks; later, they wore ornately decorated costumes, covered their heads with large wigs, and prominently displayed a gold-headed cane in their hands. No wonder the physician was considered the flower of civilization!

Music, from as early as the tom-toms of the savage to the recent modern rap and rock'n'roll of the screeching pop singers, has stimulated the brain of man. That such cacophonies may have a place in the armamentarium of physicians treating the diseased brain is now being examined scientifically in the clinic and the neurosurgical operating room. At some unsure time, is it possible that appropriate soothing musical tones could so dull the algetic centers of the brain that the current pain-killers will no longer be necessary?

References

Aurelianus C: **On Acute Diseases and Chronic Diseases.** (IE Drabkin, trans). Chicago, Ill: University of Chicago Press, 1950, 1019 pp

Bartholin C: **Institutiones anatomicae.** Leiden: Hack, 1641, 496 pp

Berengario da Carpi: **Commentaria cum amplissimis additionibus super anatomia Mundini una cum texta ejusdem in prietinum et verum nitorem redacto.** Bologna: H de Benedictis, 1521, 528 pp

Borchgrevink HM: Prosody and musical rhythm are controlled by the speech hemisphere, in Critchley M, Hanson (eds): **Music, Mind and Brain.** New York, NY: Plenum Press, 1982

Bruys MA, Swertsen B: Evaluating the effect of music on electroencephalogram patterns of normal subjects. **J Neurosurg Nurs 16:**96-100, 1984

Ecker A: **Die Hirnwindung des Menschen nach eigenen Untersuchungen insbesondere über die Entwicklung derselben beim Fötus.** Braunschweig Vieweg Sohn, 1869, 56 pp

Foerster O: Motorische Felder und Bahnenin, in Bumke O, Foerster O (eds): **Handbuch der Neurologie.** Berlin: Springer-Verlag, 1936, Vol 6

Fries L: **Spiegel der Arztny.** Strassburg: J Grieninge, 1519

Gall FJ, Spurzheim JC: **Anatomie et Physiologie du Système Nerveux en Général, et du Cerveau en Particulier.** Paris: F Schoell et al, 1810-1819, 4 Vols

Gratiolet LP: **Mémoires sur les Plis Cérébraux de l'Homme et des Primates.** Paris: Bertrand, 1854

Head H: **Aphasia and Kindred Disorders of Speech.** Cambridge, Engl: University Press, 1926, 549 pp

Jones WHS: Ancient Roman folk medicine. **J Med Hist 3:**525-546, 1948, **12:**459-472, 1957

Oppenheim H: **Die Geschwulste der Gehirns.** Wien: A Holder, 1896, 271 pp

Pribram K: Brain mechanisms in music. Prolegomena for a theory of the meaning of meaning, in Critchley M, Hanson (eds): **Music, Mind and Brain.** New York, NY: Plenum Press, 1982, Vol 2, pp 21-35

Reil JC: Uber den Bau des Hirns und der Nerven. **Neues J Phys Leipzig 1:**96-114, 1795

Rolando L: **Saggio Sopra la Vera Struttura del Cervello dell'Uomo e degl'Animalii, e Sopra le Funzioni del Sistema Nervoso.** Sassari: Stamperia Privilegiata, 1809, 98 pp

Turner W: **The Convolutions of the Human Cerebrum Tomographically Considered.** Edinburgh: Maclachlan & Stewart, 1806

Vesalius A: **De humani corporis fabrica. Libri septum.** Basel: Johannes Oporinus, 1543, 663 pp

Willis T: **Cerebri anatome: cui accessit nervorum descriptio et usus.** London: J Flesher, 1664, 456 pp

APPENDIX B

Medical Fees
Throughout the Ages

A. Earl Walker, MD

As long as the healing art was in the hands of the clergy, any compensation was considered voluntary contribution to the religious order. But when medical practice separated from priestly duties and left the temples, it became a trade governed by the rules of commerce. In the earliest known code of law, that of Hammurabi of Babylon about 2250 BC, medical practice was regulated. It was recognized that all persons were not equal and so it was determined that services to a gentleman, freeman, or slave should be recompensed on different bases depending upon the social status of the individual and the result of treatment.

Ancient royalty either maintained one or more physicians at court for personal services or had a well-known physician in the community available to treat a member of the royal family. Herodotus related how Darius of Persia, suffering from a sprained ankle, could not obtain any relief from the treatment of his Egyptian court physicians. Finally, he learned of a Greek captive, Democedes of Cretona, who was reputed to be an excellent physician for the care of such injuries. He ordered this bedraggled person to be brought from prison to examine him. Democedes applied fomentations and soothing medications which gave immediate relief. Darius was so grateful that he took the physician into his household, but desirous of retaining his services, refused to grant his freedom.

The fees of Persian physicians were regulated according to the severity of the case and the status of the patient. Nobility, assumed to be wealthy, often paid their bills with livestock or chattel. In Greece, when the sick visited the temples of Asklepios, they were expected to leave an offering of some kind, such as gold, coins, rings, and ornaments of all types. Poets, philosophers, and artists left their works in gratitude for their services. These emoluments often included gold or other casts of the diseased organ—ovaries, uterus, abdominal viscera—which might be of any size or composition.

The Greek physicians were, at times, independent of the sovereigns. Thus Hippocrates is said to have refused to go to Persia at the request of the King when that country was in the midst of a plague.

From the time of Constantine the Great, monarchs attached to their court one or more physicians called archiaters. Other public archiaters, in charge of medical practices in the cities or towns, regulated the licensing of medical practitioners. The latter, paid by the state, cared for the poor gratuitously but collected a fee for services from other persons.

In Roman times, Cato and Pliny wrote caustically of their doctors who were suspected of poisoning their patients. The annual fee at that time ranged from the equivalent of $156,000 for treating royalty to approximately $10,000 for a private practitioner. The higher fees for attending emperors and kings were understandable when the dangers and inconvenience of such services are considered. Later, notable Romans, such as Galen, might charge the equivalent of $2,000 for attending an illness.

With the decline of the Roman Empire, the practice of medicine, except for the Greek physicians attending the Roman legions and the upper classes, fell into the hands of poorly educated and inadequately trained laity. The presence of these unlicensed practitioners prompted the introduction of a code to govern the practice of medicine: "If, he [the physician] happens to harm a gentleman, he must pay a forfeit of a hundred sous. If the patient dies as the effects of this operations, the physician should be handed over to the relatives of the deceased, who may do with him whatever they please. If, in any way, he cripples a serf or cause his death, he is held accountable for the restoration of another to the lord."

After the Roman era, the physician was often considered to be "money hungry." Consider Rhazes, who dabbled in alchemy and injured his eye, necessitating the services of a doctor who charged him 500 dinars. Rhazes commented that he had found the true alchemy and the way to make gold; thereupon, he took up the practice of medicine. Chaucer describes a similar money-seeking physician in his Canterbury tales. Of course, not all doctors were so money conscious. Some had grateful and generous patients. Yet, there must have been some foundation for the feeling, for it is stated in a Salernitan treatise written about 1200 AD that "patients who show themselves ungrateful to the physician after being cured, may be made to suffer again." At that school, the candidate upon receiving his master's degree to practice medicine, took an oath to give gratuitous care to the poor and not to share in the apothecaries' charges. Most royal patients were generous but some neglected to pay their physician's fee, according to Henri de Mondeville. For that reason, the latter recommended that a clear understanding regarding the fee should be made before starting treatment. Moreover, the stipulated fee should be twice the amount that the physician expected to receive.

Since, in medieval times, surgery was looked down upon and the surgeons often received neither recompense nor honor, it is understandable that they often depended upon payment in kind for their services. Ambroise Paré began his career as a follower of the armies of Henry II without rank or source of pay. His recompenses consisted of casks of wine, horses, jewels and, from his army patients, small coins. True, when royal persons were involved. Paré's rewards were quite generous—300 crowns and a promise of future favors. But not all physicians were so well treated by their lords or kings. King Charles II of England when seized with an apoplectic attack was immediately bled by his physician, Sir Edmund King. However, court regulations at that time required that another physician be consulted before such indignities were performed upon a royal person. Although the king recovered, it required an act of the Privy Council to pardon the transgression of Sir Edmund and to approve a fee of one thousand pounds, which incidentally was never paid. On another occasion, the physician to Queen Anne, Peter Chamberlen, complained that for years of service to their Majesties, he had never received any stipend. But royal individuals were not always so parsimonious. Louis XIV of France was generous to his physicians and for an operation on a fistula gave the equivalent of $200,000 to his surgeons and assistants.

At times, payment for a successful operation was made by a life-time annuity (e.g., thirty pounds per annum); occasionally, in the case of royalty, for large amounts. Quarin received an annuity of 10,000 pounds per annum and was made a baron for a consultation on Joseph II of Germany. Dimsdale of London, at the request of Empress Catherine of Russia, introduced inoculation against smallpox, for which he received a fee of 10,000 pounds, miscellaneous expenses, and an annuity of 500 pounds a year. Thomas Willis in 1792, summoned to Lisbon to attend the mentally deranged Queen of Portugal, requested a stipend of 1000 pounds a month and expenses; should his treatment be successful, he was promised an additional 20,000 pounds.

In the 19th and 20th centuries, consultation fees for attending wealthy internationally known persons varied greatly. A few noted physicians refused large checks and accepted only a modest fee commensurate with the time and personal expenses involved; some have given their services gratis to famous persons.

Guy de Chauliac in the 14th century wrote regarding a physician's fee "let his reward be according to his work, to the means of the patient, to the quality of the issue, and to his own dignity."

The Language of Medical Writings

The standing of the physician in the community was to some extent related to his image in society, which in turn hinged upon his learning a language. By the Middle Ages, Latin was the tool of physics and jealously guarded by the physician. In England, however, after the Norman Conquest in 1066, French became the language of society and politics although Latin was used in medicine and the universities. However, the regional vernacular continued to be heard in the home and on the street. As a result, the public demanded that medical texts be written in medieval English, a request which was accentuated when printing became common. Thus, in England, not only did the Latin and English medical manuscripts differ, but the language in professional and social circles diverged, for Chaucer created a language of poetry and nuance quite distinct from the language of science and medicine. The schism between the classicists and the laity, at times, led to serious consequences. A plaque on the wall of a street in Birmingham attests to the fact that Thomas Brown was burned at the stake for writing in English.

Medical books in the pre-Renaissance era were too expensive for the ordinary citizen, so a number of authors wrote lesser treatises for poor scholars, physicians, or lay persons. Many of these texts were composed by clergy who may also have been physicians. Accordingly they were gentlemen uninterested in material gains and careful in their deportment, especially with the fair sex. There were, of course, some money-conscious writers of vernacular medical texts which were full of empty words, fables, and lies.

APPENDIX C

Historical Glossary of Neurological Syndromes

A. Earl Walker, MD

A syndrome represents a group of symptoms and/or signs indicative of a lesion or disorder. It differs from a disease in that the cause or etiology of the latter is specified. A syndrome may be due to any of a number of agents (e.g., vascular or neoplastic).

Aberrant sympathetic regeneration syndrome. In 1757, Duphénix noted that a person with a penetrating injury of the parotid gland would sweat on the ipsilateral cheek when eating. More than a hundred years later, Frederick Parkes Weber reported the occurrence of a rash and sweating in the preauricular and temporal regions, with a feeling of warmth, within minutes of tasting certain foods, particularly acid or sweet aliments, after an injury in the parotid region. In such cases, the sweating occurred in the distribution of the auriculotemporal branch of the trigeminal nerve or, less commonly, of the greater auricular nerve. As a result of injury, these nerves received regenerating nerve fibers, normally innervating the parotid gland, which had made misdirected connections with sweat glands. Other sympathetic responses have been noted to occur after parotid surgery or facial palsy as the result of aberrant connections. The precise path of these fibers is not established. (See Crocodile tears and Marcus Gunn phenomenon.)

Argyll Robertson pupil. The Argyll Robertson syndrome (Douglas M.C.L. Argyll Robertson, 1837-1909) is characterized by constricted pupils reactive to accommodation but not to light or the application of atropine, physostigmine, and methacholine. The site of the lesion is uncertain but probably is in the midbrain.

Bell's facial palsy. Sir Charles Bell (1774-1842), in 1836, described an acute paresis of one side of the face unassociated with other neurological impairments. The palsy was usually preceded by a slight malaise and earache, or pain on the affected side of the face. The facial droop usually cleared in a few weeks in children, but might persist longer or never completely resolve in adults. Closure of the affected eye was the earliest sign of returning function, and the lower facial muscles were the last to recover.

Benedikt's syndrome. This classical syndrome, which Moritz Benedikt (1835-1920) described in 1889, is the result of a lesion of the red nucleus, particularly its posterosuperior part through which the oculomotor nerve passes to reach the interpeduncular fossa. Contralateral choreiform, tremulous, athetotic, or ballistic hyperkinesias, and ipsilateral third nerve paralysis are the constant findings; however, hemiparesis, hemianesthesia, and other evidence of neighboring involvement may occur. (See Claude's syndrome.)

Bertolotti-Garcin's syndrome (hemibase syndrome). The Bertolotti-Garcin's syndrome is a paralysis of all twelve cranial nerves due to a lesion on one side along the base of the skull, although one or more nerves may commonly be spared. In spite of the extensive involvement, there is no evidence of intracranial or intraspinal extension. Bertolotti-Garcin's syndrome is due to a neoplasm at the base of the skull, either primary or secondary, usually a metastatic carcinoma of the breast.

Brachial plexus syndrome. In 1779, Smellie described a baby delivered by forceps with such compression of the head that "rendered the arms paralytic for several days." In another case, Smellie stated that a baby girl was delivered by the feet. That the baby was not able to move one of her arms, he attributed to a dislocation of the shoulder at the time of delivery; however, it may have been a brachial plexus injury.

Lesions of the upper brachial plexus were better described by Guillaume B.A. Duchenne in 1872 and Wilhelm H. Erb a few years later. In 1885, Augusta Dejerine-Klumpke reported injury to the lower part of the brachial trunk causing a Horner's syndrome, weakness and atrophy of the intrinsic hand muscles, and sensory impairment of the ulnar aspect of the forearm and of the fourth and fifth fingers. Complete lesions of the brachial plexus with a paralyzed, flail, and insensitive arm have been reported.

Bremer's syndrome (status dysraphicus or Bremer's status dysraphicus). A forme fruste of syringomyelia, Bremer's syndrome is characterized clinically by Horner's syndrome, heterochromia of the iris, and paralysis of the fifth, sixth, and seventh cranial nerves. It is assumed to be due to cavitation or softening within the pons, which may extend rostrally.

Cerebellopontine angle syndrome. This term was introduced by Henneberg and Koch in 1902 to describe the recess between the tentorium, the brainstem, the posterior wall of the petrous bone, the middle cerebellar peduncle, the cerebellum, and the occipital bone with the associated cranial nerves. Lesions of the cerebellopontine angle usually arise from the acoustic nerve, from the meninges, and, less commonly, from vascular structures.

Cervical rib syndrome. Cervical ribs were said to have been noted by both Galen and Vesalius, but the first detailed report was made by Hunauld in 1744. The condition was treated medically by Cooper in 1818; in 1861, Coote operated to relieve such a condition. Bramwell in 1903 noted that a normal first rib might compress the lower components of the brachial plexus, and Murphy seven years later excised a rib in a patient with this condition. A comparable syndrome involving the lumbosacral plexus may result from obstetrical maneuvers or compression by the fetal head in the pelvis.

Citelli's syndrome. Citelli's syndrome is a lesion of the foramen lacerum causing Gradenigo-Lennois syndrome.

Claude's syndrome. Claude's syndrome (Henri C.J. Claude, 1869-1945) results from the involvement of the red nucleus and brachium conjunctivum producing an ipsilateral third nerve paralysis and contralateral asynergia, ataxia, dysmetria, and dysdiadochokinesia. Claude's syndrome is the result of thrombosis of a perforating branch of the posterior cerebral artery. (See Benedikt's syndrome.)

Crocodile tears. After partial recovery from a facial palsy, a copious flow of tears may be initiated by eating. An uncommon sequela of Bell's palsy, crocodile tears (Chorobski) may occur following other causes of facial paralysis such as herpes zoster and is said to be due to misdirected regenerated fibers. (See Aberrant sympathetic regeneration syndrome.)

Eye retraction syndrome (Stilling-Türk-Duane syndrome). Alexander Duane in 1905 described a patient who had restriction of adduction, with upshooting on attempted adduction, retraction of the eyeball, and impaired abduction. This is probably due to paradoxical innervation of the adductors.

Foville's inferior pontine syndrome. The tegmentum of the caudal pons is involved in Foville's syndrome (Achille L.F. Foville, 1799-1878) so that the fibers of the sixth cranial nerve, the nuclei of the sixth and seventh cranial nerves, the spinothalamic tract, the medial lemniscus, the spinal trigeminal root, and the inferior cerebellar peduncle are all implicated. A minor variant is characterized by paralysis of ipsilateral conjugate gaze and paralysis of the sixth and seventh cranial nerves; in some cases there is also involvement of the pyramidal and spinothalamic tracts.

Fuchs' sign. Fuchs' sign (Ernst Fuchs, 1851-1930) is indicated by a peculiar, uncoordinated movement of the drooping upper lid in third nerve regeneration.

Gradenigo-Lennois syndrome. In 1904, Giuseppe Gradenigo (1859-1926) described a syndrome consisting of pain in the ipsilateral eye and side of the head, and ipsilateral sixth cranial nerve paralysis due to an acute or chronic otitis media; however, the syndrome may also be secondary to a neoplastic lesion at the petrous apex. (See Citelli's syndrome.)

Grenet syndrome (crossed sensory paralysis). The lesion in Grenet's syndrome is in the middle third of the pons, damaging the sensory nucleus of the trigeminal nerve, the spinothalamic tract, the medial lemniscus, the motor nucleus of the trigeminal nerve, and the superior cerebellar peduncle. It is characterized clinically by homolateral facial anesthesia for pain and temperature, and patchy loss of pain and temperature on the contralateral trunk. There may be homo-lateral paralysis of muscles of mastication and other pontine signs.

Holmes-Adie pupil (tonic or myotonic pupil). In 1906, Markus described a pupillary abnormality which later was termed the Holmes-Adie pupil (Sir Gordon M. Holmes, 1876-1965; William J. Adie, 1886-1935). It is believed to occur mainly in women in the third decade of life. One pupil is usually slightly larger than the other and reacts slowly through a normal range to accommodation and very slowly, if at all, to light. If the person is kept in a dark room for some time, the affected pupil may slowly dilate and when brought into the light constrict feebly. The pupil usually constricts slowly to metha-choline instilled in the conjunctival sac, indicating a hypersensitivity to acetyl-choline.

Horner's syndrome. In 1869, Johann F. Horner (1831-1886) described a syn-drome consisting of an ipsilateral miotic pupil, ptosis, anhidrosis of the ipsilat-eral face, and enophthalmos. Claude Bernard noted a similar syndrome in experimental animals in which the cervical sympathetic chain was excised.

Internuclear palsies or internuclear ophthalmoplegia. This syndrome may pre-sent anteriorly or posteriorly and is presumed to be due to abnormalities of the medial longitudinal fasciculus. It is characterized by paralysis of the medial rectus muscle for lateral gaze but not for convergence. Dissociated nystagmus (in the abducted eye) is present so that the optic axes are parallel in the pri-mary position.

Magendie-Hertwig squint position. A result of posterior fossa injuries, the Magendie-Hertwig squint condition (François Magendie, 1783-1855; Richard Hertwig, 1850-1937) is characterized by the eye on the affected side looking down and "in" and the other eye looking up and "out." The lesion, being supranuclear, causes no diplopia.

Marchiafava-Bignami syndrome. Toward the end of the 19th century, a chronic dementia was reported in Italians who drank a local wine (Carducci). In 1903, Ettore Marchiafava (1847-1935) and Amico Bignami (1862-1929) noted that the corpus callosum in these patients was necrotic. In sporadic cases of Italians and natives of other nations who developed the condition, a rapid dementia and, at times, dysarthria and rigidity of the limbs occurred. In these cases, the corpus callosum and the third layer of the cerebral cortex were necrotic.

Marcus Gunn phenomenon (jaw-winking). The Marcus Gunn phenomenon (Robert Marcus Gunn, 1850-1909) is characterized by an associated move-ment of one eyelid when the patient eats, chews, or moves the jaw toward the normal eye. An inverted Marcus Gunn phenomenon may occur during chew-ing with the palpebral fissure narrowing. It is usually congenital, but may occur after facial palsy as a result of misdirection of regenerating fibers.

Marie-Foix syndrome (cerebellar hemiparesis). The Marie-Foix syndrome

(Pierre Marie, 1853-1940; Charles Foix, 1882-1927) is usually due to thrombosis involving the lateral pons and the middle cerebellar peduncle, the trigeminal root and, at times, adjacent tracts. Clinically, there are ipsilateral cerebellar signs (i.e., dysdiadochokinesis, dysmetria, and incoordination).

Medulla oblongata syndromes. A number of syndromes of the medulla oblongata were reported in the earlier literature but many had no pathological verification. A few had multiple lesions. On critical analysis, only two syndromes were established—the lateral medullary and the medial medullary syndromes.

When critically analyzed, other medullary syndromes—described by Avellis, Babinski-Nageotte, Bonnier, and Cestan—are found to have been based on inadequate evidence or to have been misinterpreted. Cases reported by Schmidt, Tapia, Jackson, and Barré are probably due not to medullary but to extramedullary lesions.

Lateral medullary syndrome. This syndrome, described by Wallenberg in 1895, was the result of thrombosis of the posterior inferior cerebellar artery or, rarely, of a branch of the vertebral artery. It commonly begins with acute vertigo, nausea, vomiting, dysphagia, dysarthria, unsteadiness, hiccoughs, occasionally diplopia, facial weakness, and numbness of the ipsilateral side. Within a few days, only the unsteadiness, dysphagia, dysarthria, and sensory disturbances such as numbness of the ipsilateral face and contralateral half of the body persist.

Medial medullary syndrome. Dejerine described a disturbance due to an infarct in the distribution of a rostral perforating branch of the anterior spinal artery. The clinical findings are weakness of the tongue secondary to hypoglossal nerve or nucleus involvement, contralateral hemiplegia, and impaired posterior column sensation. Dejerine described a second type in which the lateral and medial medullary syndromes are combined. The third type described by Dejerine was the result of bilateral medial lesions.

Mesencephalic syndrome. This syndrome is usually the result of vascular occlusion of the branches of the basilar artery—the medial perforating vessels supplying the paramedian structures, oculomotor nuclei and fibers, and midline nuclei; the paramedian branches supplying the red nucleus and lateral aspects of the cerebral peduncle; the lateral circumflex arteries supplying the cerebral peduncle and posterior red nucleus; and the tectal branches arising from the superior cerebellar or posterior cerebral artery. The clinical syndrome described as the result of a mesencephalic lesion does not always correlate with the presumed vascular insult, probably because of the numerous and variable collateral vessels. Although several syndromes have been described, they are often partially combined with evidence of involvement of other tracts or nuclei of the mesencephalon. Experimental lesions in monkeys have confirmed, in general, the basis of the clinical syndromes.

Melkersson's syndrome. Melkersson's syndrome (Ernst Melkersson, 1898-

1932) is characterized by infranuclear facial palsy, at times bilateral, and is an affliction of young persons, especially girls. It tends to recur after months or years and may be associated with a painless edema of the face, most noticeable in the lower lip. Various other cephalic disturbances may be present.

Millard-Gubler syndrome (ventral pons syndrome). The Millard-Gubler syndrome (Auguste L.J. Millard, 1830-1915; Adolphe M. Gubler, 1821-1879) is usually due to a thrombotic lesion and is characterized by ipsilateral peripheral facial paresis and external rectus paralysis causing impaired abduction of the ipsilateral eye. If the lesion is hemorrhagic or neoplastic, other pontine structures are often involved.

Nothnagel's syndrome. This varied syndrome described by Carl W.H. Nothnagel (1841-1905) is characterized by uncoordinated gait (e.g., reeling or rolling gait) and oculomotor palsies and is often associated with nystagmus. It is considered to be due to a tectal or neighborhood tumor pressing upon the cerebellar vermis or quadrigeminal plate. It is rarely seen.

Oculofacial palsies (Moebius syndrome). This infantile nuclear syndrome described by Paul Moebius (1853-1907) in 1889 consists of unilateral or bilateral ocular palsies and paralysis of other cranial nerves, usually the facial nerve. The nature and site of the lesion are not clear but it probably occurs early in embryonic life (within the first four weeks).

Oculogyric crises. These tonic eye movements consist of an upward or, less commonly, a lateral spasmodic deviation of the eyes which may last more than half an hour. The episode may be initiated by an emotional outburst and may be associated with loss of consciousness or head posturing.

Opsoclonus. Myoclonic movements of the eyes, designated "opsoclonus" by Orzechowski, have also been called ocular myoclonus and lightning eye movements, ataxic conjugate movements, saccadomania, and dancing eyes. The eye movements are characterized by arrhythmic, irregular, "chaotic" saccades occurring with the eyes open or closed, in sleep or awake, and are often accompanied by myoclonus of other muscles, such as the platysma, sternocleidomastoid, or palate. They are associated with a number of neurological conditions including encephalitis, neuroblastomas, and remote carcinomas. Similar jerking movements which may occur with poor vision are not considered true opsoclonus. The movements, usually conjugate and accompanied by blinking of the eyelids, differ from nystagmus in their irregularity.

Superior orbital fissure syndrome. This syndrome is characterized by slight exophthalmos, partial or total ophthalmoplegia, severe pain, and sensory loss in upper divisions of the trigeminal nerve and a constricted pupil not dilated by cocaine.

Palatal nystagmus or myoclonus. Palatal nystagmus, or myoclonus, consists of bilateral palatal, pharyngeal, and laryngeal rhythmic myoclonia at 30 to 200/min while awake or asleep; it may be due to a lesion of the pons, cerebellar nuclei, or inferior olive.

Parinaud's syndrome. Parinaud's syndrome (Henri Parinaud, 1844-1905) consists of paralysis of conjugate upward gaze due to a lesion of or pressure upon the superior colliculi muscle. When associated with pubertas praecox, paralysis of conjugate deviation, weakness of convergence, and pupils unresponsive to light, it is usually due to a pineal tumor.

Paroxysmal transitory psychic disorder. A number of transitory disordered states occur with the subject seemingly normal at all times. Such phenomena including some manifestations of epilepsy, disturbed perception in migraine, transitory episodes of amnesia, and impaired consciousness in narcolepsy are striking but transient abnormalities of conduct, which leave the individual in a normal physical and mental state when they have passed.

Amnesia is a prime example of the temporary disturbances of function. For centuries, it has been known that blows to the head (which may or may not produce a loss of consciousness) can impair memory for a short period before and after the insult. Boxers have been known to continue a bout after receiving a sharp blow to the head and yet later have no recollection of their ostensibly normal conduct after the injury—a state that may last for several hours. As the result of an intense emotional event, such as a homicide, a person may be unable to recall what happened. During depressed conditions of the brain caused by anesthesia, blood loss, or a state of shock, a patient while seemingly unconscious may experience vivid memories of floating about or hearing the conversations of attending physicians and associates. Somewhat similar trance states may be induced by hypnosis. Such isolated amnestic events, sometimes emotionally tinged, have been recognized for years. Weir Mitchell wrote of a military officer who, after sustaining a right median nerve paralysis as the result of a bullet wound of the arm which bled little, talked incoherently about extraneous matters and "had not the least remembrance of having been shot or of any event which followed within an hour afterwards."

During seizures, memory is generally considered to be lost, but many patients are able to recall the beginning or aura of their attacks. Long periods of amnesia may occur in such attacks, during which patients may perform quite complicated behavior of which they have no recall.

Pes cavus (familial). Pes cavus has been defined as an abnormally high longitudinal arch of the foot associated with clawing of the toes; this condition has been variously termed claw foot, cave foot, high arched foot, and pes arcuatus. Familial pes cavus is commonly seen in certain heredofamilial neurological disorders such as Friedreich's ataxia, peroneal muscular atrophy, hereditary spastic paraplegia, myelodysplasia accompanying spina bifida, heredopathia atactica polyneuritiformis, or formes frustes of the above disorders. The condition may occur independently or be associated with another developmental abnormality such as lymphedema.

Phantom limb syndrome. Although amputations were common in the days of hand-to-hand combat, it is surprising that phantom sequelae were not mentioned before the 15th century. The earliest descriptions of phantom limbs are credited to Ambroise Paré, Rene Descartes, and Albrecht von Haller; however, more detailed accounts have been given by Gueniot (who described telescoping of amputated limbs), Weir Mitchell, and later French authors. Even Paré, who must have performed many amputations, makes only passing reference that the amputee may still feel the limb which may be quite painful and subject to spasms.

The first detailed account of phantom limbs was given by Weir Mitchell in 1871. He stated that most amputees have a sensory ghost or phantom of the excised member, which may become apparent either immediately following the amputation or up to three weeks later. The phantom limb may be abruptly recalled if the stump is struck or is stimulated by a faradic current, or if additional amputation is performed. It may be so real that the person attempts to use it only to become rudely aware of its absence. As time passes, usually the phantom limb is foreshortened so that an arm consists only of the forearm and hand attached to the shoulder. The retained distal parts may assume grotesque and/or painful positions which are variously described. Weir Mitchell emphasized that the stump is hypersensitive to movement, temperature changes, pin-prick (especially if repeated), and to phantom movements of the stump. The missing limb assumes various postures, often related to the position at the time of injury, and can be moved at will with or without pain. The small digits (e.g., fingers and toes) are the most commonly moved, but in many phantom limbs these parts are fixed in a painful or cramped attitude. Occasionally, the stump contracts spasmodically or remains in a tetanic painful or painless position. Weir Mitchell recognized that reoperation was "by no means encouraging."

Because the phantom limb was described mainly in war victims of adult age, young amputees were thought not to have such sensations. However, more recent studies have indicated that the body schema is a fundamental process and that phantom limbs may be appreciated in both congenital aplastic limbs and limbs amputated in childhood.

Pontine syndrome. Prior to the 17th century, the pons was included with the cerebellum as the caudal part of the brain. The earliest known reported abnormality of the pons was a patient reported by Kingston, a shoemaker in his early teens who died suddenly and at postmortem examination was found to have a walnut-sized aneurysmal dilatation of the right internal carotid artery and the basilar artery, which had compressed and softened the pons. The pontine cases described by Huyem contained few details of the clinical disturbances. Subsequent isolated cases added some features, but it was Marburg's detailed report that described the syndromes secondary to lesions at various levels of the basilar artery.

Pontine infarctions were usually due to thrombosis of branches of the basilar artery causing an ischemic infarct. These softenings, infrequently multiple, involved the basilar system, which irrigates many pontine nuclei and fiber tracts through small feeding vessels which produce complex symptomatology.

Pontine hemorrhage must have occurred many times before Cheyne first described the condition. Oppenheim gave a good clinical description of the hemorrhagic lesions of the pons, which are quite extensive and more deadly than those produced by ischemia. The various pontine syndromes have been named after the neurologists who described them—Millard-Gubler ventral pons syndrome, Foville pontine tegmental syndrome, Grenet midpontine syndrome, Raymond-Cestán syndrome of the rostral pons, Marie-Foix lateral pontine syndrome, and Gasperini syndrome of the caudal tegmentum.

Progressive external ophthalmoplegia. Apparently the term was used by Beaumont, but the first case was reported in 1856 by Albrecht von Graefe (1828-1870), after whom the disorder was named. Hutchinson, in 1879, described a case, but without autopsy findings. Fuchs in 1896 regarded the condition as a neuronal degeneration or a muscular dystrophy. Subsequent autopsied cases, however, have not clarified the atrophic or dystrophic nature of the disorder, which may occur in association with myotonic dystrophy, hereditary oculopharyngeal dystrophy, Bassen-Kornzweig syndrome, Refsum's syndrome, familial ataxia, Moebius syndrome, progressive supranuclear palsy, and symptomatic ophthalmoplegia.

Raymond-Cestán syndrome (superior Foville's syndrome). In the Raymond-Cestán syndrome (Fulgence Raymond, 1844-1910; Raymond Cestán, 1872-1934), the rostral third of the pons is involved, damaging the medial lemniscus, the spinothalamic tract, the superior cerebellar peduncle, and the supranuclear oculomotor tract. Clinically, ipsilateral hemiasynergy, contralateral hemiplegia, and hemianesthesia (with paralysis of gaze toward the lesion) are present.

Restless legs syndrome. Although Thomas Willis may have refered to "restless legs" as Critchley avers, it was more than a century and a half before the complaint was again mentioned. In 1849, Magnus Huss wrote of three alcoholics who complained when lying down of creeping sensations and an irrepressible desire to move the legs. At night, to get relief, the victims had to get up and walk about. In 1861, Wittmar referred to "anxietas tibiarum" by which he was probably referring to restless legs. Although later writers mentioned the condition, K.A. Ekbom gave the first detailed description. He noted that the principal complaint was a peculiar creeping sensation beneath the skin in the muscles, even in the bones of both legs, although not necessarily occurring simultaneously. Rarely, it was present in the arms. The annoying creeping sensation might be associated with a weak or heavy feeling of the involved members. It only occurred when the individual was at rest, usually in the evening when tired or in bed. The feeling might persist for hours, keeping the patient awake. Walking about or massaging the legs might afford some relief; cold applications, even cold air, helped. The affliction might affect patients of either sex for years. In rare cases, an iron deficiency was responsible, but usually no cause could be found. Various conditions aggravated the complaints, which did not respond well to the many drugs prescribed.

Rochon-Duvigneaud syndrome. This orbital apex syndrome, called the Rochon-Duvigneaud syndrome, is characterized by severe supraorbital pain, absent corneal reflex, ptosis, and diplopia.

Sicard-Collet syndrome. The Sicard-Collet syndrome (Jean A. Sicard, 1872-1929; Frédéric J. Collet) occurs as the result of a lesion involving all of the structures passing through the jugular foramen and anterior condylar canal. Clinically, there is loss of sense of taste in the posterior part of the ipsilateral tongue, dysphagia, dysphonia, and palate, the vocal cord, trapezius and sternocleidomastoid paralysis, and atrophy. The condition may be associated with tumor, trauma, or vascular and inflammatory lesions which implicate other nerves at the base of the skull.

Superior cerebellar artery syndrome. This rare syndrome is the result of thrombosis of the superior cerebellar artery damaging the upper pons and midbrain (mainly the superior cerebellar peduncle and in some cases the adjacent spinothalamic tract and sympathetic tract), causing a Horner's syndrome.

Superior orbital fissure syndrome. This syndrome, described by Rochon-Duvigneaud in 1896, is characterized by the following: paralysis of the third, fourth, and sixth cranial nerves causing a complete ophthalmoplegia including ptosis; sensory loss in the first division of the trigeminal nerve; sympathetic paresis in some cases; and exophthalmos secondary to obstruction of the ophthalmic vein. There may be visual impairment or loss giving an orbital apex syndrome. It is caused by trauma, infection, tumor, or aneurysm.

Vestibular syndrome. Probably the earliest vestibular syndrome recognized as such was reported in 1861 by Prosper Ménière, a Parisian superintendent of a deaf and dumb hostel who wrote of a patient having paroxysmal attacks of vertigo with vomiting. These attacks were associated with tinnitus and deafness in an ear and recurred at intervals, with normal intervening periods. Although Ménière reasoned that the cause of the attack was a disturbance of the labyrinth, neither he nor later writers of that time knew its nature. That was not resolved until centuries later when the temporal bones of afflicted persons were examined; at that time, it was discovered that the saccule was distended, the perilymph space obliterated, Reisner's membrane was absent from the cochlea due to distention of the scala media displacing the membrane against the bony wall of the scala vestibuli, and Corti's organ was compressed and the tunnel occupied by a vague coagulum.

Villaret's syndrome. In Villaret's condition (Maurice Villaret, 1877-1946), the lower four cranial nerves as well as the cervical sympathetic nerves are damaged, producing the Sicard-Collet syndrome as well as Bernard-Horner's syndrome. It is usually the result of trauma, neoplasm, or inflammatory lesions.

Weber's syndrome. Hermann D. Weber (1823-1918) described a patient who had a contralateral hemiplegia and oculomotor palsy on the side of a lesion in the ventromedial part of the cerebral peduncle. This syndrome came to be called Weber's syndrome.

A number of other conditions—postural nystagmus, vestibular neuronitis, ear infections, vascular accidents involving the labyrinth, otosclerosis, and drug intoxications—may give rise to such vertiginous attacks. Localized cerebral lesions, usually involving the angular and supramarginal gyri, produce opto-kinetic nystagmus in which the directional preponderance is most often toward the side of the lesion. Positional paroxysmal benign nystagmus was first described by Bárány in 1921. When the head is placed in a certain position, after a latent period of a few seconds, a horizontal and rotatory nystagmus appears toward the lower ear and rapidly adapts. It was believed to be due to vascular occlusion, trauma, or a low-grade infection of the otolith.

Other syndromes. Syndromes such as facial hemispasm and crossed hemiplegia, described in 1908 by Edouard Brissaud and Jean A. Sicard, and crossed paralysis of the eighth cranial nerves, described by Marie-Ernst Gelle, are rare and the result of multiple lesions.

As the emotions were considered to reside in the somatic organs and not the brain, a hearty laugh suggests the origin of the emotion. Although Hippocrates placed the joys and sorrows in the brain, subsequent philosophers and physicians made little effort to localize such feelings. The phrenologists placed such emotions in the cerebral cortex. Vladimir M. von Bechterew in 1887 postulated that facial expressions were a thalamic function. Alfons Jakob explored the brains of patients exhibiting pathological laughter and crying and found lesions in the basal ganglia in more than half of the cases. The locus and ganglia involved in emotional expression, however, remained unresolved at the beginning of the 20th century.

References

Argyll Robertson D: On an interesting series of eye symptoms in a case of spinal disease, with remarks on the action of Belladonna on the iris, etc. **Edinb Med J** 14:646-708, 1869

Avellis G: Klinische Beiträge zur halbseitigen Kehlkopflähmung. **Berl Klin** 40:1-26, 1891

Babinksi J, Nageotte J: Hémiasynergie, latéropulsion et myosis bulbaires avec hémianesthésie et hémiplégie croisées. **Rev Neurol** 10:358-365, 1902

Benedikt M: Tremblement avec paralysie croisée du moteur oculaire common. **Bull Med (Paris)** 3:547-548, 1889

Bernard C: Des phénomènes oculopupillaires products par la section du nerf sympathique cervical; ils son indépendents des phenomenes vasculaires caloriques da la tête. **Compt Rend Acad Sci** 55: 381-382, 1869

Bonnier P: Un nouveau syndrome bulbaire. **Presse Med** 11:174-177, 1903

Bramwell E: A case of meralgia paresthetica (Bernhardtsche Sensibilitätsstörung) with a short account of condition. **Edinb Med J** 14:26-33, 1903

Bremer FW: Klinische Untersuchung zur Aetiologie der Syringomyelia. **Dtsch Z Nervenheilk** 95, 1926

Brissaud EA, Sicard JA: Type special de syndrome alterne. **Rev Neurol** 16:86, 1908

Cestan R: Le syndrome protubérantiel superieur. **Rev Neurol** 11:1053-1054, 1903

Chorobski J: The syndrome of crocodile tears. **Arch Neurol Psychiatry** 65:299-318, 1951

Citelli S: Vegetazioni adenoidi e sord omutis mo. **Boll Med Orecchio Gola Naso** 22:141-150, 1904

Claude HCJ: Syndrome pédonculaire de la région du noyau rouge. **Rev Neurol** 23:311, 1912

Collet FJ: Sur un nouveau syndrome paratytique pharyngolaryngé par blessure de guerre. **Lyon Med** 124:121-129, 1916

Coote H: Pressure on the axillary vessels and nerve by an exostosis from a cervical rib—Interference with the circulation of the arm—Removal of the rib and exostosis—Recovery. **Med Times Gaz** 2: 108, 1861

Duane A: Congenital deficiency of adduction associated with impairment of abduction, retardation movements, contractions of the palpebral fissure and oblique movements of the eye. **Arch Ophthalmol** 34:133, 1905

Duphénix M: Observations sur les fistules du canale salivaire de Stenon. I. Sur une plaque compliquée à la joue où le canal salivaire fut déchiré. **Mem Acad R Chir** 3:431, 1757

Ekbom K: Akroparestesier och restless legs under graviditet. **Lakartidningen** 57:2597-2603, 1960

Ekbom KA: Asthenia crurum paraesthetica ("irritable legs"): a new syndrome consisting weakness, sensation to cold and nocturnal paresthesia in legs, to certain extent to treatment with priscol and doryl. **Acta Med Scand** 118:197-209, 1944

Erb W: Ueber eine eigenthümliche Localisation von Lähmungen im Plexus brachialis. **Verh Naturh Med** 1:130-136, 1874-1876

Foville ALF: Note sur une paralysie peu connue de certains muscles de l'oeil, et sa liasion avec quelques points de l'anatomie et da physiologie de la protubérance annulaire. **Bull Soc Anat (Paris) (2nd ser)** 33:393-414, 1858

Fuchs E: Ueber Blepharochalasis (Erschlaffung der Lidhaut). **Wein Klin Wochenschr** 9:109, 1896

Gradenigo G: Sulla leptomeninge circonscritta e sulla paralisi dell' abducente di origine otitica. **Gior R Accad Med Torino** 10:59-84, 1904

Gubler AM: De l'hémiplégie alterne envisagée comme sign de lésion de la protubérance annulaire et comme preuve de la décussation des nerfs faciaux. **Gaz Hebd Med** 3:749-789, 811, 1856

Gueniot M: D'une hallucination du toucher (ou héterotopie subjective des extremités) particulière à certains amputés. **J Physiol (Paris)** 4:725-730, 1861

Henneberg and Koch: Über 'Central'-Neurofibromatose und die Geschwülste des Kleinhirnbrücken-winkels. (Acusticus-Neurom). **Arch Psychiatry Nervenkr** 36:251-304, 1902

Hertwig H: Expierimenta que dam de effectibus laesionum in partibus encephali singularibus et de verdsimili harum partium functione, Bertolini, formis Feisteridnis et Eiserdorffianis (1926). **Int Cat Surg Gen (1st ser)** 6:185, 1885

Horner JF: Ueber eine Form von Ptosis. **Klin Monatsbl Augenheilk** 7:193-198, 1869

Hunauld FJ: **Communication to the Royal Academy of Sciences, 1740.** Amsterdam, 1744

Kingston PN: Case of fatal encephalitis with hemiplegia immediately excited by cantharides, in consequence of intense predisposition from basilar and internal carotid aneurysm. **Edinburgh Med J** 57:69-77, 1842

Klumpke A: Contribution à l'etude des paralysies radiculaires du plexus brachial; paralysies radiculaires totales; radiculaires inférieures; de la participation des filets sympathiques oculopupillaires dans ces paralysies. **Rev Med** 5:591-616, 739-790, 1885

Marburg O: Zur pathologie der Spinalganglien. **Arb Neurol Instit Univ** 8:103-139, 1902

Marchiafava E, Bignami A: Sopra un alterazione del corpo calloso osservata in soggeti alcoolisti. **Riv Patol Nerv Ment** 8:544-549, 1903

Marcus Gunn R: Congenital ptosis with peculiar associated movements of the affected lid. **Trans Ophthalmol Soc UK** 3:283-286, 1883

Markus C: Notes on a peculiar pupil phenomenon in cases of partial iridoplegia. **Trans Opthalmol Soc UK** 26:50-56, 1906

Melkersson E: Ett fall av recidiverande facialispares i samband med angioneurotiskt odom. **Hygiea 90**:737-741, 1928

Mitchell SW: Phantom limbs. **Lippincotts Mag 8**:563-569, 1871

Moebius PJ: Ueber engeborene doppelseitige Abducens-Facialis-Laehmung. **Munch Med Wocherschr 35**:91-94, 108-111, 1888

Murphy T: Brachial neuritis caused by pressure of the first rib. **Aust Med J 15**:582-585, 1910

Nothnagel H: **Topische Diagnostik der Gehirnkrankheiten: eine Klinische studie.** Berlin: A Hirschwald, 1879

Paré A: **La Manière de Traicter les playes faictes tat par hacquebutes que par fléche** . . . Paris: Ieau de Brie, on Arnoul l'Angelier, 1552

Parinaud H: Paralysie des mouvements associés des yeux. **Arch Neurol (Paris) 5**:145-172, 1883

Raymond F, Cestan R: Le syndrome protubé rantiel supérieur. **Gaz Hop 76**:829-834, 1903

Raymond F, Cestán R: Trois observations de paralysie des mouvements associés des globes oculaires. **Rev Neurol 9**:70-77, 1901

Rochon-Duvigneaud A: Quelques cas de paralysie de tous lef nerfs orbitaires (ophtalmoplégie totale avec amaurose et anesthésie dans le domaine del'ophtalmique), d'origine syphitique. **Arch Optalmol (Paris) 16**:746-760, 1896

Sicard JA: Syndrome du carrefour condylo-déchiré postérieur (type par de paralysie des quatre nerfs craniens). **Mars Med 53**:385-397, 1916/1917

Smellie W: A collection of preternatural cases and observations in midwifery, new edition, in: **Treatise on theory and pract of midwifery.** London: W Strahan, T Cadell, and G Nicol Strand, 1779

Villaret M: Le syndrome nerveux de l'espace rétro-parotidien postérieur. **Rev Neurol (Pt 1) 23**: 188-190, 1916

von Bechterew V: Die Bedeutung der Sehhügel auf Grund von experimentellen und pathologischen Daten. **Virchows Arch Pathol Anat 110**:102 and 322, 1887

Wallenberg A: Acute bulbaraffection (Embolie der Art. cerebellar. post. inf. sinistr.) **Arch Psychiat Nervenkr 27**:505-540, 1895

Weber HD: A contribution to the pathology of the crura cerebri. **Med Chir Trans 46**:121-139, 1863

Wittmar T: **Pathologie und Therapie der Sensibititat. Neurosen.** Leipzig: Schafer, 1861, p 45

APPENDIX D

Bibliography of Writings by A. Earl Walker

University of Alberta, 1926 (A.B.), 1930 (M.D.), 1952 (LL.D.(Hon.))
The Johns Hopkins University, 1985 (D.H.L.)
University of Chicago, 1931-34 (Resident training)

Instructor to Professor of Neurological Surgery, University of Chicago, 1937-47
Professor of Neurological Surgery, The Johns Hopkins University, and
Neurological Surgeon-in-Charge, The Johns Hopkins Hospital, 1947-72
Visiting Professor, University of New Mexico, 1972-83

Member:

American Academy of Neurological Surgery, Secretary, 1942-45, President, 1946
American Association of Neurological Surgeons, President, 1970
American Association of Neuropathologists, President, 1950
American Board of Neurological Surgery, Chairman 1956-59
American College of Surgeons
American Electroencephalographic Society, President, 1955
American Neurological Association, Vice President, 1952, President, 1966
Congress of Neurological Surgeons, Honored Guest, 1958
Eastern Association of Electroencephalographers, President 1950-51
International League Against Epilepsy, Vice President, 1954, President, 1956
Society of Neurological Surgeons, Historian 1952, President, 1966-67
World Federation of Neurosurgical Societies, President, 1966-69

Books:

The Primate Thalamus. Chicago, Ill: University of Chicago Press, 1938, 321 pp (with HC Johnson)

Penicillin in Neurology. Springfield, Ill: Charles C Thomas, 1946, 201 pp

Post-Traumatic Epilepsy. Springfield, Ill: Charles C Thomas, 1949, 86 pp

A History of Neurological Surgery. Baltimore, Md: Williams and Wilkins, 1951, 583 pp (editor)

A Follow-Up Study of Head Wounds in World War II. Washington, DC: US Government Printing Office (VA Medical Monograph), 1961, 179 pp

Transtentorial Herniation. Springfield, Ill: Charles C Thomas, 1961, 162 pp

Head Injury Conference Proceedings. Philadelphia, Pa: JB Lippincott, 1966, 589 pp (AE Walker and WF Caveness, editors)

The Late Effects of Head Injury. Springfield, Ill: Charles C Thomas, 1969, 560 pp (AE Walker, WF Caveness, and McD Critchley, editors)

Head Injured Men Fifteen Years Later. Springfield, Ill: Charles C Thomas, 1969, 118 pp (with F Erculei)

Manual of Echoencephalography. Baltimore, Md: Williams and Wilkins, 1971, 149 pp (with S Uematsu)

Stereotaxy of the Human Brain, 2nd edition. Stuttgart: Georg Thieme Verlag, 1982 (G Schaltenbrand and AE Walker, editors)

Cerebral Death, 3rd edition. Baltimore/Munich: Urban and Schwarzenberg, 1985, 206 pp

The History of the World Federation of Neurological Societies. Albuquerque, NM: University of New Mexico Press, 1985, 141 pp (AE Walker, historian)

Functional and Stereotactic Surgery. EI Kandel. New York/London: Plenum Medical Books, 1989, 695 pp (translation editor)

Stedman's Medical Dictionary, 25th edition. Baltimore, Md: Williams and Wilkins, 1990, 1784 pp (consultant for neurology, neuropathology, and neurosurgery)

Publications

Attachments of the dura mater over base of the skull. **Anat Rec 55:**291-295, 1933

The pathology of spasmodic torticollis with a note on respiratory failure from anesthesia in chronic encephalitis. **J Nerv Ment Dis 78:** 630-637, 1933 (with Grinker)

Congenital dermal sinuses: a source of spinal meningeal infection and subdural abscesses. **Brain 57:**401-421, 1934 (with Bucy)

Encephalography in children. **Am J Roentgenol Radium Ther 32:**437-456, 1934

The thalamic projection to the central gyri in macacus rhesus. **J Comp Neurol 60:** 161-184, 1934

Estudio estadístico de una serie de 230 casos consecutivos de tumor intracraneal. **Rev Cirurg Barcelona 10:**197-213, 1935 (with Ley)

Statistical review of two hundred and thirty consecutive cases of intracranial tumor. **Acta Neuropathol Eston 60:**52-67, 1935 (in honorem Ludovici Puusepp) (with Ley)

The retrograde cell degeneration in the thalamus of macacus rhesus following hemidecortication. **J Comp Neurol 62:**407-419, 1935

The thalamic projection to the cortex cerebri in macacus rhesus. **Trans Am Neurol Assoc 61:** 45-48, 1935 (with Bailey and Poljak)

An experimental study of the thalamo-cortical projection of the macaque monkey. **J Comp Neurol 64:**1-39, 1936

Convulsive seizures in adult life. **Arch Int Med 88:**250-268, 1936

Cysticercosis cellulosae in the monkey. **J Comp Pathol Ther 49:**141, 1936

Hypertension and brain tumor: case report. **J Iowa Med Soc 26:**303-307, 1936 (with Abbott, Anderson, and Van Epps)

The external configuration of the cerebral hemispheres of the chimpanzee. **J Anat 71:** 105-116, 1936 (with Fulton)

A note on the thalamic nuclei of macaca mulatta. **J Comp Neurol 66:**145-155, 1937

A study of the cerebello-cerebral relationships by the oscillographic method. **J Physiol 90:** 39-40, 1937

Experimental anatomical studies of the topical localization within the thalamus of the chimpanzee. **Proc Kon Akad Wetensch Amsterdam 40:**1937

The projection of the medial geniculate body to the cerebral cortex in the macaque monkey. **J Anat 71:**319- 331, 1937

The syndrome of the superior cerebellar peduncle in the monkey. **Brain 60:**329-353, 1937 (with Botterell)

The thalamus in relation to the cerebral cortex in Macaque monkey. **J Nerv Ment Dis 85:** 249-261, 1937

Tumors of the posterior cranial fossa. **J Iowa Med Soc 27:**55-61, 1937

An oscillographic study of the cerebello-cerebral relationships. **J Neurophysiol 1:**16-23, 1938

Electrical excitability of the motor face area: a comparative study in primates. **J Neurophysiol 1:**152-165, 1938 (with Green)

Hemidecortication in chimpanzee, baboon, macaque, potto, cat and coati: a study in encephalization. **J Nerv Ment Dis 87:** 676-700, 1938 (with Fulton)

The anatomical basis of the thalamic syndromes. **J Belge Neurol Psychiatr 2:**89-95, 1938

The effects of ablation of the cortical motor face area in monkeys. **J Neurophysiol 1:**252-280, 1938 (with Green)

The thalamus of the chimpanzee. I. Terminations of the somatic afferent systems. **Confin Neurol 1 (Fasc 2):**99-126, 1938

The thalamus of the chimpanzee. II. Its nuclear structure, normal and following hemidecortication. **J Comp Neurol 69:**487-507, 1938

The thalamus of the chimpanzee. III. Metathalamus, normal structure and cortical connections. **Brain 61:**250-268, 1938 (with Fulton)

The thalamus of the chimpanzee. IV. Thalamic projections to the cerebral cortex. **J Anat 73:** 37-93, 1938

Anatomy, physiology and surgical considerations of the spinal tract of the trigeminal nerve. **J Neurophysiol 2:**234-248, 1939

Astrocytosis arachnoideae cerebelli. **Arch Neurol Psychiatr 45:**520-532, 1941

Early diagnosis of brain tumors. **Ill Med J 80:** 1941

Lipoblastic meningioma. **Arch Surg 48:**371-378, 1941 (with Haverfield)

The immediate and late effects of the intrathecal injection of iodized oil. **JAMA 116:**2247-2254, 1941 (with Marcovich and Jessico)

The myelographic diagnosis of intramedullary spinal cord tumors. **Am J Roentgenol Radium Ther 45:**321-331, 1941 (with Jessico and Marcovich)

Topical arrangement within the spinothalamic tract of the monkey. **Arch Neurol Pyschiatr 46:**877-883, 1941 (with Weaver)

Vascular anomalies of the spinal cord in children. **Am J Dis Child** 61:928-932, 1941 (with Buchanan)

Central representation of pain. **Res Publ Assoc Res Nerv Ment Dis** 23:63-85, 1942

Congenital atresia of the foramens of Luschka and Magendie. **Arch Neurol Psychiatr 48:** 583-611, 1942 (with Taggart)

Congenital atresia of the foramina of Luschka and Magendie. **Trans Am Neurol Assoc 58:** 146-151, 1942 (with Taggart)

Effects of intensity and wave length on driving cortical activity in monkeys. **J Neurophysiol** 5:483-486, 1942 (with Halstead, Knox, and Woolf)

Lissencephaly. **Arch Neurol Psychiatr 48:** 13-29, 1942

Mesencephalic tractotomy. **Arch Surg 44:** 953-962, 1942

Modification of cortical activity by means of intermittent photic stimulation in the monkey. **J Neurophysiol** 5:349-356, 1942 (with Knox and Halstead)

Pathogenesis of chorea. **J Pediatr** 20:555-575, 1942 (with Buchanan and Case)

Relief of pain by mesencephalic tractotomy. **Arch Neurol Psychiatr** 48:865-883, 1942

Somatotopic localization of spinothalamic and secondary trigeminal tracts in the mesencephalon. **Arch Neurol Psychiatr 48:** 884-889, 1942

The topical organization and termination of the fibers of the posterior columns in macaca mulatta. **J Comp Neurol** 76:145-158, 1942 (with Weaver)

Treatment of penetrating wounds of the head. **War Med** 2:454-464, 1942

El valor clinico de la electroencefalografia. **Rev Argentino-Norteamericana Ciencias Medicas** 1:472-479, 1943 (with Lambros and Case)

Localization of taste in the thalamus of macaca mulatta. **Yale J Biol Med** 16:175-191, 1943 (with Blue and Ruch)

Mechanism of temporal fusion effect of photic stimulation on electrical activity of visual structures. **J Neurophysiol** 6:213-220, 1943 (with Woolf, Halstead, and Case)

Neurogenic polycythemia. **Ann Int Med** 19: 470-481, 1943 (with Carpenter and Schwartz)

Sciatica. **Bull Winnebago Med Soc** 4:5-14, 1943

The clinical value of electroencephalography. **Dis Nerv Sys** 7:202-206, 1943 (with Case and Lambros)

A case of congenital atresia of the foramina of Luschka and Magendie. **J Neuropathol Exp Neurol** 3:368- 373, 1944

Afferent connections, in Bucy PC (ed): **The Precentral Motor Cortex.** Urbana, Ill: University of Illinois Press, 1944, pp 111-132

Dilatation of the vertebral canal associated with congenital anomalies of the spinal cord. **Am J Roentgenol Radium Ther** 52:571-582, 1944

Electroencephalographic alterations following cerebral concussion. **Trans Am Neurol Assoc** 60:1944

Experimental hypogeusia from Horsley-Clarke lesions of the thalamus in macaca mulatta. **J Neurophysiol** 7:171-184, 1944 (with Patton and Ruch)

Neurogenic polycythemia. **J Neuropathol Exp Neurol** 3:425-426, 1944

Neurological and psychological effects of cerebral injuries in: **Medicine and the War.** Chicago: University of Chicago Press, 1944 (with Halstead)

Photic driving. **Arch Neurol Psychiatr** 52: 117-125, 1944 (with Woolf, Halstead, and Case)

Physiology of concussion. **Soc Trans Arch Neurol Psychiatr** 52:78-79, 1944 (with Kollros and Case)

Psychosurgery. **Surg Gynecol Obstet** 78:1-11, 1944

The physiological basis of concussion. **J Neurosurg** 1:103-116, 1944 (with Case and Kollros)

Convulsive factor in commercial penicillin. **Arch Surg** 50:69-73, 1945 (with Johnson)

Cranioplasty; collective review. **Int Abstr Surg** 81:1-23, 1945 (with Woolf)

Penicillin convulsions. The convulsive effects of penicillin applied to the cerebral cortex of monkey and man. **Surg Gynecol Obstet** 81: 692-701, 1945 (with Johnson and Kollros)

Principles and practice of penicillin therapy in diseases of the nervous system. **Ann Surg** 122:1125-1135, 1945 (with Johnson)

The effects of lesions of the visual system on photic driving. **J Neuropathol Exp Neurol** 4: 59-67, 1945 (with Woolf, Knox, and Halstead)

The relief of facial pain. **Med Clin North Am** 29:73-97, 1945

The syndrome of cerebral conclusion. **Clinics** 4: 361-395, 1945

Convulsive effects of antibiotic agents on the cerebral cortex. **Science** 103:116, 1946 (with Johnson, Case, and Kollros)

Hemilaminectomy. **Surg Clin North Am** 26: 70-77, 1946

Problems of posttraumatic epilepsy in an army general hospital. **Assoc Res Nerv Ment Dis Proc 26:**461-515, 1946 (with Quadfasel)

The effect of antibiotic substances on the central nervous system. **Prog Neurol Psychiatr 1:** 205-210, 1946 (with Johnson)

The physiological basis of cerebral concussion. **Assoc Res Nerv Ment Dis Proc 26:**437-466, 1946

The treatment of motor sensory disturbances. **Prog Neurol Psychiatr 1:**540-545, 1946

Activated electroencephalography. **Arch Neurol Psychiatr 58:**533-549, 1947 (with Kaufman and Marshall)

Extraspinal lumbar meningocele. **J Neurosurg 4:** 80-86, 1947 (with Pendergrass and Bond)

Histopathology of thermocoagulation of the cerebral cortex. **J Neuropathol Exp Neurol 6:** 311-322, 1947 (with Silver)

Normal and pathological after-discharge from frontal cortex. **Assoc Res Nerv Ment Dis Proc 27:**460-475, 1947 (with Johnson)

The treatment of the epileptic veteran. **TB 10-28, Veterans Administration.** Washington, DC, 1947 (with Lennox)

Toxic effects of intrathecal administration of penicillin. **Arch Neurol Psychiatr 58:**39-45, 1947

Follow-up report on a series of posttraumatic epileptics. **Am J Psychiatr 104:**781-782, 1948 (with Quadfasel)

Review of *The Neocortex of Macaca Mulatta.* **J Neurophysiol 11:**149-150, 1948

Surgical treatment of epilepsy. **Am J Surg 75:** 200-218, 1948 (with Johnson)

The epileptic veteran. National Veterans Epilepsy Center, Cushing Veterans Administration Hospital, Framingham, Mass, 1948 (with Lennox)

The new look in epilepsy. **Johns Hopkins Nurses Alumnae Mag 47:**43-44, 1948

Vascular system. **Prog Neurol Psychiatr 3:** 397-408, 1948 (with Johnson)

Afferent connections, in Bucy PC (ed): **The Precentral Motor Cortex. 2nd edition.** Urbana, Ill: University of Illinois Press, 1949, pp 112-132

Brain tumors in children. **J Pediatr 35:**617-637, 1949 (with Hopple)

Cerebral pedunculotomy for the relief of involuntary movements. I. Hemiballismus. **Acta Psychiatr Neurol 24:**723-729, 1949

Electrocorticography. **Bull Johns Hopkins Hosp 85:**344-359, 1949 (with Marshall)

Ménière's syndrome. **J Omaha Mid-West Clin Soc 10:**46-51, 1949

Review of *Atlas of Peripheral Nerve Injuries.* **Bull Johns Hopkins Hosp 85:**405, 1949

Spontaneous ventricular rhinorrhea and otorrhea. **J Neuropathol Exp Neurol 8:**171-182, 1949

Thalamocortical relationships—concluding remarks. **EEG Clin Neurophysiol 1:** 451-454, 1949

Thalamocortical relationships—introductory remarks. **EEG Clin Neurophysiol 1:** 389-390, 1949

The electroencephalogram after head injury. **J Nerv Ment Dis 109:**383-395, 1949 (with Kaufman)

The surgical treatment of pain and motor disorders. **Prog Neurol Psychiatr 4:**1949 (with Culbreth)

Water, nitrogen and electrolyte content of brain following cerebral concussion. **Am J Physiol 156:**129-136, 1949 (with Eichelberger and Kollros)

Behavioral alterations following lesions of the medial surface of the temporal lobe. **Fol Psychiatr Neurol Neuro-chir Nederland 53:** 444-452, 1950 (with Thomson)

Angiographic diagnosis of spontaneous thrombosis of the internal and common carotid arteies. **J Neurosurg 8:**631, 1951 (with Johnson)

Cerebral angiography in "brain tumor suspects." **J Neurosurg 7:**127-138, 1950 (with Culbreth and Curry)

Convulsive activity. **Q J Phila Beta Pi 47:** 108-115, 1950

Convulsive patterns in cerebellum and brainstem. **Assoc Res Nerv Ment Dis Proc 30:** 282-298, 1950 (with Markham, Browne, and Johnson)

Diseases of the nervous system. Neurology. **Annu Rev Med 1:**231-250, 1950

Effect of strychnine on the cat's electrocerebellogram. **Proc Soc Exp Biol Med 73:**97-99, 1950 (with Johnson, Browne and Markham)

Epilepsia post-traumatica. **Arch Neurocir 6:** 137-159, 1950

Herniated lumbar nucleus pulposus, its diagnosis and surgical management. **Philippine J Surg 5:**99-110, 1950 (with Gustilo)

Post-traumatic epilepsy. **Surg Gynecol Obstet 91:**110-112, 1950

Recent advances in the treatment of craniocerebral injuries, in: **Advances in Surgery II.** New York, NY: Interscience Publishers, 1950, pp 221-230 (with Fisher)

Review of *Clinical Electroencephalography.* **Bull Johns Hopkins Hosp 86:**183, 1950

Review of *Diagnosis and Treatment of Brain Tumors and Care of the Neurosurgical Patient.* **Bull Johns Hopkins Hosp 86**:77, 1950

Review of *Skull Fractures and Brain Injuries,* by HE Mock. **Surg Gynecol Obstet 95**:1950

Section of U fibers of motor cortex in cases of paralysis agitans (Parkinson's disease). **Arch Neurol Psychiatr 64**:57-59, 1950 (with Cobb, Pool, Scarff, Schwab, and White)

The electroencephalogram in thalamic hemorrhage. **EEG Clin Neurophysiol 2**:99-102, 1950 Marshall)

The electroencephalographic changes after hemispherectomy in man. **EEG Clin Neurophysiol 2**:147-156, 1950 (with Marshall)

The neurosurgical treatment of intractable pain. **J Lancet 70**:279-282, 1950

Vascular system. **Prog Neurol Psychiatr 5**:1950 (with Silver)

El sindrome de Ménière. **Arch Neurocir 8**:9-16, 1951

Intracranial abscesses, in Cecil RL and Loeb RF (eds): **Textbook of Medicin. 8th edition.** Philadelphia, Pa: WB Saunders, 1951, pp 1479-1482

Intracranial tumors, in Cecil RL and Loeb RF (eds): **Textbook of Medicin. 8th edition.** Philadelphia, Pa: WB Saunders, 1951, pp 1470-1478

Practical considerations in the treatment of head injuries. **Neurology 1**:75-84, 1951

Review of *Acute Head Injuries,* by JP Evans. **J Neuropathol Exp Neurol 10**:1951

Review of *Electroencephalography in Clinical Practice,* by RS Schwab. **Bull Johns Hopkins Hosp 87**:1951

Rhombencephalic convulsive activity. **Bull Johns Hopkins Hosp 89**:442-467, 1951 (with Markham, Browne, and Johnson)

The surgical treatment of pain and motor disorders. **Prog Neurol Psychiatr 6**:337-350, 1951 (with Harrison)

The treatment of epilepsy by cortical excision. **J Pediatr 1**:75-84, 1951

Cerebral arterial shunt. **Arch Neurol Psychiatr 68**:58-65, 1952 (with Browne and Stern)

Cerebral pedunculotomy for the relief of involuntary movements. II. Parkinsonian tremor. **J Nerv Ment Dis 116**:766-775, 1952

Experimental cerebellar seizures. **Arch Neurol Psychiatr 67**:473-482, 1952 (with Johnson, Browne, and Markham)

General summary of the report of the Committee on Research in Epilepsy. **Epilepsia (3rd ser) 1**:108-110, 1952

Head injuries. **Modern Med 20**:91, 1952

Hemangiomas of the fourth ventricle. **J Neuropathol Exp Neurol 11**:103-115, 1952 (with Johnson and Browne)

Introductory remarks. American League Against Epilepsy Symposium. **Epilepsia (3rd ser) 1**: 50, 1952

Introductory remarks. Symposium on photometrazol activation of the electroencephalogram. **EEG Clin Neurophysiol 4**:263-264, 1952

Neuralgia, trigeminal and glossopharyngeal (tic douloureux). **Curr Ther**:643, 1952

Response of experimental epileptic foci to intravenous and topical metrazol. **EEG Clin Neurophysiol 4**:131-139, 1952 (with Johnson)

Surgical aspects of spinal cord disorders. **Cyclopedia Med Surg Specialties 12**:903-915, 1952 (with Johnson)

Surgical clinic on hydrocephalus. **Surg Clin North Am 32**:1347-1361, 1952 (with Bachs)

The diagnosis of brain tumors by angiography. **Brain Nerve 4**:17-19, 1952 (with Amador, Harrison, and Sugar)

The surgical treatment of involuntary movements. **Texas Rep Biol Med 10**:105-109, 1952

The surgical treatment of postural (intermittent) exophthalmos. **Brain Nerve 4**:3-8, 1952

The vascular system. **Prog Neurol Psychiatr 7**: 361-373, 1952 (with McQueen)

Tratamiento quirurgico de las hidrocefalias no neoplasicas. **Arq Neuro-Psiquiatr 10**: 287-304, 1952 (with Bachs)

Behavior and the temporal rhinencephalon in the monkey. **Bull Johns Hopkins Hosp 93**: 65-93, 1953 (with Thomson and McQueen)

Experimental hydrocephalus. **J Neuropathol Exp Neurol 12**:283-292, 1953 (with Bachs)

Histopathologie et pathogénie des anévrysmes arteriels cérébraux. **Rev Neurol 89**:477-490, 1953 (with Allègre)

Keeping up with advances in medicine. **Md State Med J 2**:55, 1953

Photogenic epilepsy: parameters of activation. Report of case. **Arch Neurol Psychiatr 69**: 760-765, 1953 (with Marshall and Livingston)

Review of *Neurosurgery: an Historical Sketch,* by Horrax. **Bull Hist Med 27**:84-85, 1953

Review of *Stereoencephalotomy: Thalamotomy and Related Procedures. Part I. Methods and Stereotaxic Atlas of the Human Brain,* by EA Spiegel and HT Wycis. **Bull Johns Hopkins Hosp 89**:1953

Simian psychomotor epilepsy. **EEG Clin Neu-**

rophysiol Suppl 3:53, 1953 (with Warner)

Surgical treatment of epilepsy. Acta Med Philippina 9:101-115, 1953

The surgical treatment of pain and motor disorders. Prog Neurol Psychiatr 8:363-373, 1953 (with Warner)

Changing role of neurological surgery in medicine. JAMA 156:833-835, 1954

Complications of cerebral angiography. Neurology 4:643-656, 1954 (with Kaplan)

Effect of hypothalamic lesions on canine neurogenic arterial hypertension. Proc Soc Exp Biol Med 85:474-477, 1954 (with Browne and McQueen)

La conducta y el rinencefalo temporal en el mono. Rev Latino-Am Psiquiatr 3:1954 (with Thomson and McQueen)

Role of the brainstem in blood pressure regulation in the dog. Neurology 4:2 13, 1954 (with McQueen and Browne)

The pathology and pathogenesis of cerebral aneurysms. J Neuropathol Exp Neurol 13: 248-259, 1954 (with Allègre)

The propagation of cortical and subcortical epileptic discharge. Epilepsia (3rd ser) 3: 37-48, 1954 (with Faeth)

Vascular system. Prog Neurol Psychiatr 9: 367-381, 1954 (with Faeth)

Cerebral arterial shunt in the monkey. J Neurosurg 12:634-642, 1955 (with Browne and Warner)

Cerebral pedunculotomy for involuntary movements. Surg Gynecol Obstet 100:716-720, 1955

Curso avanzado de epilepsia. Neurocirugia 12: 1-39, 1955

Die nordamerikanische Neurochirurgie der Gegenwart. Dtsch Med Wochenschr 80: 441-443, 1955

El significado del tálamo. Rev Neuro Psiquiatr 18:131-150, 1955

Intracranial tumors (brain tumors), in Cecil RL and Loeb RF (eds.): Textbook of Medicine, 9th edition. Philadelphia/London: WB Saunders, 1955, pp 1600-1608

Intracranial abscesses (brain abscesses), in Cecil RL and Loeb RF (eds.): Textbook of Medicine, 9th edition. Philadelphia/London: WB Saunders, 1955, pp 1608-1612

Les fistules carotico-caverneuses. Ann Ocul 188: 834-848, 1955 (with Allègre)

Pain—the neurosurgeon's viewpoint. J Chron Dis 2:91-95, 1955

Review of The Founders of Neurology, edited by W Haymaker. Bull Hist Med 29:96-97, 1955

The meaning of the thalamus. Proc 6th Latin-Am Neurosurg Cong:926-946, 1955

The surgical treatment of pain and motor disorders. Prog Neurol Psychiatr 10:387-399, 1955 (with Poggio)

Threshold studies on production of experimental epilepsy with alumina cream. Proc Soc Exp Biol Med 88:329-331, 1955 (with Faeth, Kaplan, and Warner)

Tumors of the nervous system. Brain tumors. Curr Ther:533-538, 1955

Observations upon cerebellar convulsive activity induced by strychnine. Yale J Biol Med 28: 419-427, 1955/1956 (with Poggio)

The electroencephalographic concomitants of subcortical epilepsy. Acta Neurol Latino-Am 1:239-255, 1995

A man is as old as his legs. Md Med J 5:73-74, 1956

Carotid-cavernous fistulas. Surgery 39:411-422, 1956 (with Allègre)

Cerebrospinal fluid rhinorrhoea following removal of an acoustic neuroma. A case report. J Neurosurg 13:199-204, 1956

Clinical localization of intracranial aneurysms and vascular anomalies. Neurology 6:79-90, 1956

Experimental subcortical epilepsy. Arch Neurol Psychiatr 75:548-562, 1956 (with Faeth and Warner)

La fisiologia de la epilepsia. Med Cirurg Farmacia (Janeiro) 237:1-15, 1956

Neuralgia, trigeminal and glossopharyngeal (tic douloureux). Curr Ther:521, 1956

The vascular system. Prog Neurol Psychiatr 11: 230-245, 1956

Impairment of memory as a symptom of a focal neurological lesion. Southern Med J 50: 1272-1275, 1957

Motor disorders and pain. Prog Neurol Psychiatr 12:373-386, 1957 (with Lichtenstein)

Physiological principles and results of neurosurgical interventions in extrapyramidal diseases. Premier Congres International des Sciences Neurologiques. Bruxelles. Juillet 21-28, 1957. pp 118-137

Prognosis in post-traumatic epilepsy. A ten-year follow-up of craniocerebral injuries of World War II. JAMA 164:1637-1641, 1957

Recent memory impairment in unilateral temporal lesions. Arch Neurol Psychiatr 78: 543-552, 1957

Sequelae of head injuries. Curr Med Digest 24: 61-67, 1957

Stimulation and ablation. Their role in the history of cerebral physiology. J Neurophysiol

20:435-449, 1957

Studies on effect of the injection of alumina (alum oxide) cream into the basal ganglia. **Arch Neurol Psychiatr 78:**562-567, 1957 (with Faeth)

Subarachnoid hemorrhage and intracranial aneurysms: medical or surgical. **Surgery 41:** 509-511, 1957

The development of the concept of localization in the 19th century. **Bull Hist Med 31:** 99-121, 1957

The vascular system. **Prog Neurol Psychiatr 13:** 239-253, 1957 (with Aronson)

Medicolegal aspects of head injuries. **Postgrad Med 24:**A34-A46, 1958

Post-traumatic epilepsy, administrative considerations, in Medical Department, US Army: **Surgery in World War II. Neurosurgery.** 1958, Vol 1, pp 279-317

Primitive trepanation: the beginning of medical history. **Trans Stud Coll Phys Phila (4th ser)** 26:99-102, 1958

Review of *Congenital Arteriovenous Aneurysms of the Carotid and Vertebral Arterial Systems,* edited by H Olivecrona and J Ladenheim. **J Neuropathol Exp Neurol 17:**538-539, 1958

Review of *The Brain and Human Behavior. Research Publication of the Association for Research in Nervous and Mental Disease,* edited by HC Solomon, S Cobb, and W Penfield. **Bull Johns Hopkins Hosp:**220, 1958

A follow-up of head injured men of World War II. **J Neurosurg 16:**600-601, 1959 (with Jablon)

A simplified approach to pallidotomy. **Southern Med J 52:**136-142, 1959 (with Aronson and McGovern)

Intracranial abscesses, in Cecil RL and Loeb RF (ed): **Textbook of Medicine, 10th edition.** Philadelphia/London: WB Saunders, 1959, pp 1560-1562

Intracranial tumors, in Cecil RL and Loeb RF (ed): **Textbook of Medicine, 10th edition.** Philadelphia/London: WB Saunders, 1959, pp 1551-1560

Propagation of after-discharge between temporal lobes. **J Neurophysiol 22:**538-553, 1959 (with Poblete and Ruben)

Review of *Ciba Foundation Symposium on the Cerebrospinal Fluid. Production. Circulation and Absorption,* by GE Wolsteinholme and CM O'Connor. **Bull Johns Hopkins Hosp (March):**1959

Review of *Epilepsy,* by M Sakel. **Bull Johns Hopkins Hosp (March):**1959

Review of *Speech and Brain-Mechanisms,* by W Penfield and L Roberts. **Bull Johns Hopkins Hosp (Dec):**1959

Subcortical recording in temporal lobe epilepsy. **Arch Neurol 1:**288-302, 1959 (with Lichtenstein and Marshall)

Surgical treatment of epilepsy. **Curr Med Digest 26:**59-68, 1959

The heroic treatment of acute head injuries: a critical analysis of the results. **Am Surg 26:** 184-188, 1959 (with Black)

A critical analysis of electrocorticography in temporal lobe epilepsy. **Arch Neurol 2:**172-182, 1960 (with Lichtenstein and Marshall)

Ménière's syndrome or aural vertigo: Surgical therapy. **J Nerv Ment Dis 130:**567-577, 1960

Obituary. John F. Fulton, 1899-1960. **J Neurophysiol 25:**346-349, 1960

Review of *A History of Neurology (M.D. Monographs on Medical History, No. 2),* by W Riese. **Bull Hist Med 34:**93-94, 1960

Review of *Sir Geoffrey Jefferson: Selected Papers.* **EEG Clin Neurophysiol 3:**326-327, 1960

Review of *The Cerebral Cortex in English. Some Papers on the Cerebral Cortex,* by G von Bonin. **Contemp Psychol:**5, 1960 (trans)

Solitary spinal cord tumors occurring in multiple members of a family. **J Neurosurg 17:** 783-787, 1960 (with Myers, Austin, and Gallagher)

The march of focal motor convulsions. **Trans Am Neurol Assoc,** 1960 (with Udvarhelyi)

The state of consciousness in focal motor convulsions. **Epilepsia 1:**592-599, 1960

Anterolateral chordotomy for relief of pain. **Postgrad Med 29:**485-495, 1961 (with Diemath and Hoppnen)

Histochemical study of tumors of the central nervous system. **Proc Int Cong Neuropathol 1:**95-102, 1961 (with Udvarhelyi, O'Connor, Laws, and Krainin)

Murder or epilepsy. **J Nerv Ment Dis 133:** 430-437, 1961

Review of *Electrical Studies on the Unanesthetized Brain,* edited by ER Ramey and DS O'Doherty. **Bull Johns Hopkins Hosp:**1961

Review of *Essentials of Neurosurgery for Students and Practitioners,* by S Mullan. **J Nerv Ment Dis 133:**453-454, 1961

Review of *Klinik und Behandlung der Raumbeengenden Intrakraniellen Prozesse. Handbuch der Neurochirurgie,* edited by H Olivecrona and W Tonnis. **J Neuropathol Exp Neurol 20:**456-457, 1961

Review of *La trepanacion del crneo en el Antiguo Per,* by J Lastres and F Cabieses. **Bull Hist**

Med 35:575-576, 1961

Stimulation and depth recording in man, in Sheer DE (ed): **Electrical Stimulation of the Brain.** Austin, Tex: University of Texas Press, 1961, pp 498-518 (with Marshall)

Summary, from *Extrapyramidal System and Neuroleptics.* 1961, pp 295-297

Cerebral depth recording in man. **Extrait du Livre Jubilaire du Dr. Ludo von Bogaert:** 844-865, 1962 (with Marshall and Weitz)

Editorial. Observer error, statistical and biological significance. **Curr Med Digest 29:**42-44, 1962

General considerations, in **Pediatric Surgery. Part VII. Nervous System.** Chicago, Ill: Year Book Medical Publishers, 1962, pp 1221-1232

Incidence of post-traumatic epilepsy in Korean veterans as compared with those from World War I and World War II. **J Neurosurg 19:** 122-129, 1962 (with Caveness and Ascroft)

Infections of the nervous system, in **Pediatric Surgery. Part VII. Nervous System.** Chicago, Ill: Year Book Medical Publishers, 1962, pp pp 1265-1268

Miscellaneous conditions, in **Pediatric Surgery. Part VII. Nervous System.** Chicago, Ill: Year Book Medical Publishers, 1962, 1285-1289

Perspectives in neurosurgery. **J Indian Med Profession 9:**4360-4362, 4364-4369, 4347-4374, 1962

Post-traumatic epilepsy. **World Neurol 3:** 185-194, 1962

Review of *The Spinal Cord, Basic Aspects and Surgical Considerations,* by G Austin. **J Neurol 21:**663-664, 1962

Stereotaxic methods for the study of the subcortical activity in epilepsy. **Confin Neurol 22:** 217-222, 1962

The neurosurgical evaluation of the chiasmal syndrome. **Am J Ophthalmol 54:**564-581, 1962

The results of anterior interbody fusion of the cervical spine. **J Bone Joint Surg 44A:** 1569-1587, 1962 (with Robinson, Ferlic, and Wiecking)

The value of electroencephalography in the prognostication and prognosis of post-traumatic epilepsy. **Epilepsia 2:**138-143, 1962 (with Marshall)

Trauma to the nervous system, in: **Pediatric Surgery. Part VII. Nervous System.** Chicago, Ill: Year Book Medical Publishers, 1962, pp 1255-1264

Brainstem reticular formation influence on convulsions in monkey. **Arch Neurol 8:**248-256, 1963 (with Rodriguez-Serrano)

Cerebral peduncle in propagation of convulsions. **Arch Neurol 8:**581-590, 1963 (with Richter)

High frequency thermal induction lesions of the brain. **J Nerv Ment Dis 136:**298-301, 1963

Intracranial abscesses, in Cecil RL and Loeb RF (eds): **Textbook of Medicine, 11th edition.** Philadelphia: WB Saunders, 1963, pp 1663-1666

Intracranial tumors, in Cecil RL and Loeb RF (eds): **Textbook of Medicine, 11th edition.** Philadelphia: WB Saunders, 1963, pp 1675-1683

Posttraumatic epilepsy and early cranioplasty. **J Neurosurg 20:**1085, 1963 (with Erculei)

Review of *Clinical Orthopaedics and Related Research, No. 27,* by DePalma. **Bull Johns Hopkins Hosp 113:**179, 1963

Review of *Operative Neurosurgery,* by ES Gurdjian. **JAMA 188:**764-765, 1963

Review of *Principles of Neurological Surgery,* by L Davis and RA Davis. **JAMA 187:**138-139, 1963

Review of *The Microscopic Anatomy of Tumors of the Central and Peripheral Nervous System,* by P Del Rio-Hortega. **J Nerv Ment Dis 137:** 306, 1963

The late results of cranioplasty. **Arch Neurol 9:** 105-110, 1963 (with Erculei)

The syndrome of the tentorial notch. **J Nerv Ment Dis 136:**118-129, 1963

The use of adhesive tapes of closure of scalp and skin. **J Neurosurg 20:**812-813, 1963 (with Otenasek)

Autotransplantation of gliomas. **J Neuropathol Exp Neurol 23:**324-333, 1964

Post-traumatic epilepsy, in Rowbotham: **Acute Injuries of the Head, Their Diagnosis, Treatment, Complications and Sequela, 4th edition.** Edinburgh: E and S Livingstone, 1964, Vol 15, pp 486-509

Pseudomotor cerebri associated with prolonged corticosteroid therapy. **JAMA 188:**779-784, 1964 (with Adamkiewicz)

Review of *Volume VIII. The Cortex of the Four Year Old Child.* **Nerv Ment Dis 138:**304, 1964

Subcortical recording in experimental focal chronic epilepsy. **Trans Am Neurol Assoc 89:** 37-39, 1964 (with Rivera)

Surgical treatment of epilepsy. **Mod Treat 1:** 1104-1116, 1964

The contribution of depth recording to clinical medicine. **EEG Clin Neurophysiol 16:** 88-99, 1964 (with Marshall)

The neurosurgeon's viewpoint. **J Bone Joint Surg 46(Am):**1806-1810, 1964

The pattern of propogation of epileptic discharges in Schaltenbrand G, Woolsey (eds): **Cerebral Localization and Organization.** Madison, Wisc: The University of Wisconsin Press, 1964, Vol 7, pp 95-111

The VIIIth nerve action potential in Meniere's disease. **Laryngoscope 73:**1456-1464, 1963

Autoimmune response to malignant glial tumors. Preliminary observations. **Neurology 15:**474-476, 1965 (with Mitts)

Chronic post-traumatic headache. **Headache 5:** 67-72, 1965

Cortical projections and paralysis. **Trans Am Neurol Assoc 90:**128-131, 1965 (with Richter)

Dissemination of acute focal seizures in monkey—(II). From subcortical foci. **Arch Neurol 12:**357-380, 1965 (with Udvarhelyi)

Echoencephalography for head trauma. Proceedings of the IIIrd International Congress of Neurological Surgery. **Excerpta Medica Int Cong Series 110:**194-199, 1965 (with Uematsu and Sugar)

Frontal lobe epilepsy. **Psychiatrr Neurol 150:** 321-333, 1965

Review of *Brain Function. Cortical Excitability and Steady Potentials. Relations of Basic Research to Space Biology. UCLA Forum in Medical Sciences, No. 1*, edited by MAB Brazier. **Bull Johns Hopkins Hosp:**1965

Review of *Epilepsia und ihre Randgelbiete in Klinik und Praxis,* edited by W Schultse. **Bull Johns Hopkins Hosp:**1965

The art of selecting technical aids for neurological diagnosis of brain lesions. **Clin Neurosurg 13:**277-290, 1965

The generalization of a seizure. **J Nerv Ment Dis 140:**252-270, 1965 (with Udvarhelyi)

The production of focal brain lesions by induction heating. **Excerpta Medica Int Cong Series 110:**556-560, 1965

The training of a neurosurgeon. A review of an international problem. **J Neurosurg 23:** 54-62, 1965

Critical evaluation of brain scan. **Neurology 16:** 746-748, 1966 (with Abbassioun, Udvarhelyi, and Fueger)

Dural echoencephalography. **J Neurosurg 25:** 634-637, 1966 (with Uematsu)

Grantsmanship. **Clin Neurosurg 13:**55-62, 1966

Induction thermocoagulation of the brain: a new neurosurgical tool. **IEEE Trans Biomed Eng BME 13:**114-120, 1966 (with Burton, Mozley, and Braitman)

Internal structure and afferent relations of the thalamus, in Purpura D, Yahr MD (eds): **The Thalamus.** New York: Columbia University Press, 1966, pp 1-12

Introduction, in Caveness W, Walker AE (eds): **Head Injury Conference Proceedings.** Philadelphia, Pa: JB Lippincott, 1966, pp 1-12

Neurological crossroads of the world. **Trans Am Neurol Assoc 91:** 1-9, 1966 (Presidential Address)

Post-traumatic epilepsy. **Proc Aust Assoc Neurol 4:**1-8, 1966

Pre-frontal lobe epilepsy. **Int J Neurol 5:** 422-429, 1966

Radiofrequency telethermocoagulation. **JAMA 197:**700-704, 1966 (with Burton)

Report of Ad Hoc Committee to study head injury nomenclature. **Clin Neurosurg 12:** 386-394, 1966

Section of the cerebral peduncle in the monkey. **Arch Neurol 14:**231-240, 1966 (with Richter)

Summation of the Symposium on Parkinson's disease. **J Neurosurg 24:**475-477, 1966

Depth EEG studies in a patient with fourteen and six per second positive spikes. **EEG Clin Neurophysiol 22:**86-89, 1967 (with Niedermeyer and Ray)

EEG and behavioral findings in temporal lobe epileptics (before and after temporal lobectomy). **EEG Clin Neurophysiol 23:**493, 1967 (with Niedermeyer et al)

Effects of orbito-frontal ablation on thalamocortical potentials and behavior in the cat. **EEG Clin Neurophysiol 23:**90, 1967 (with Velasco et al)

Experimental petit mal. **Trans Am Neurol Assoc 92:**57-61, 1967 (with Morello)

Introduction and conclusion, in: Recent Advances in Clinical Neurophysiology. **EEG Clin Neurophysiol Suppl 25:**1967

Modern trends in the neurophysiological investigation of brain diseases. Introduction. **EEG Clin Neurophysiol Suppl 25:**101, 1967

Modern trends in the neurophysiological investigation of brain diseases. Conclusion. **EEG Clin Neurophysiol Suppl 25:**205-206, 1967

Review of *The Use of Diagnostic Ultrasound in Brain Disorders,* by CC Grossman. **J Nerv Ment Dis 144:**231-232, 1967

Review of *Thomas Willis. The Anatomy of the*

Brain and Nerves, edited by W Feindel. **Bull Hist Med 1941:**187-188, 1967

Sexual behavior in temporal lobe epilepsy. **Arch Neurol 16:**37-43, 1967

Summation of the symposium on the vertiginous patient. **Arch Otolaryngol 85:**558-560, 1967

Temporal lobectomy. **J Neurosurg 26:**642-649, 1967

The acute head injury: a multidisciplinary problem. **Neurol Med Chir (Tokyo) 9:**7-20, 1967

The propagation of focal cortical seizures in the monkey. **J Nerv Ment Dis 144:**358-373, 1967 (with Ip and Rivera)

The relationship of head trauma to neurological disease. **Bull School Med Univ Md 52:** 64-68, 1967

The significance of post-traumatic epilepsy. **Conn Med 31:**109-114, 1967

Ultrasonic determination of the size of cerebral ventricular system. **Neurology 17:**81-84, 1967 (with Uematsu)

Acute head injury—a multidisciplinary problem. **No To Shinkei 20:**1217-1223, 1968

The anatomy of amnesia. **Neuro-ophthalmology 4:**201, 1968

The neurological manifestations of von Recklinghausen's disease, in: **Brain and Mind Problems.** Il Pensiero Scientifico, 1968, pp 359-380 (with Adamkiewicz)

The pathology of intracranial aneurysms. **Prog Brain Res 30:**283-288, 1968 (with Govaert et al)

The study of potentials in chronic experimental epilepsy. **EEG Clin Neurophysiol 24:**290, 1968 (with Morello et al)

Visual disturbances in temporal lobectomized patients. **Neuro-ophthalmology 4:**230, 1968 (with Walsh)

A prospectus, in Jasper HH, Ward AA, Pope A (eds): **Basic Mechanisms of the Epilepsies.** Boston, Mass: Little, Brown, and Co, 1969, pp 807-814

Brain herniations, in Vinken PJ, Bruyn GW (eds): **Handbook of Clinical Neurology, Vol 1.** Amsterdam: North Holland Publishing, 1969, p 550

Current concepts of pathogenesis of tremor in Parkinson's disease, in: **Third Symposium on Parkinson's Disease.** Edinburgh: E and S Livingstone, 1969, pp 100-105

Depth EEG findings in epileptics with generalized spike-wave complexes. **Arch Neurol 21:** 51-58, 1969 (with Niedermeyer and Laws)

Diagnostic significance of scalp and depth EEG findings in patients with temporal and

frontal lobe epilepsy. **Johns Hopkins Med J 126:**146-153, 1969 (with Laws and Niedermeyer)

Electroencephalography in neurosurgery. **EEG Clin Neurophysiol 27:**643, 1969

Neurosurgical instruction in the medical school. **Neurocirugia 27:**17-20, 1969

Significance of the electroencephalogram in comatose respirator cases. **Curr Med Digest 36:**189-200, 1969

Single unit studies on acute and chronic epileptic foci. Their surrounds and their mirror foci in cats and monkeys. **Trans Am Neurol Assoc 94:**183-184, 1969 (abstract with Ishijima)

The contribution of scalp and depth EEG findings to the surgical treatment of temporal lobe epilepsy. **EEG Clin Neurophysiol 26:** 110, 1969 (with Niedermeyer et al)

The death of a brain. **Johns Hopkins Med J 124:** 190-201, 1969

The results of anterior interbody fusion of the cervical spine. Review of 93 consecutive cases. **J Neurosurg 30:**127-133, 1969 (with Riley, Robinson, and Johnson)

Unit studies on transcallosal spread of epileptic activities in the cat's brain. **EEG Clin Neurophysiol 26:**631, 1969 (with Ishijima et al)

Differential diagnosis of trigeminal neuralgia, in Hassler R, Walker AE (eds): **Trigeminal Neuralgia.** Stuttgart: Georg Thieme Verlag, 1970, pp 30-34

Post-traumatic epilepsy 15 years later. **Epilepsia 11:**17-26, 1970 (with Erculei)

R. Glen Spurling 1894-1968. **Trans Am Neurol Assoc 95:**337-338, 1970

The propagation of epileptic discharge. **Epilepsy Mod Probl Pharmacopsychiatr 4:**13-28, 1970

The role of the cerebral peduncle in movements. **Neurosci Res 3:**175-207, 1970

The slow spike-wave complex as a correlate of frontal and fronto-temporal post-traumatic epilepsy. **Eur Neurol 3:**330-346, 1970 (with Niedermeyer et al)

The unresting specialty. The 1970 AANS Presidential Address. **J Neurosurg 33:** 613-624, 1970

Trauma workshop report: neural trauma. **J Trauma 10:**1069-1071, 1970 (with Ommaya et al)

Carotid-cavernous fistula: a technique for occlusion of fistula with preservation of carotid blood flow. **Trans Am Neurol Assoc 96:** 205-208, 1971 (with Black, Uematsu, and Perovic)

Cerebral blood flow and oxygen consumption. An on-line technique. **Johns Hopkins Med J** **128**:134-140, 1971 (with Pevsner, Bhushan, and Ottesen)

Life expectancy of head injured men with and without epilepsy. **Arch Neurol 24**:95-100, 1971 (with Leuchs, Lechtape-Gruter, Caveness, and Kretschman)

The cerebrospinal fluid from ancient times to the atomic age. **Acta Neurol Latino-Am 1 (Suppl 1)**:1-9, 1971

The cerebrospinal fluid in health and disease. Summary of a symposium. **P Neuro-Psiquiatr 29**:323-336, 1971

The law and the neurosurgical nurse. **J Neurosurg Nurs 3**:83-92, 1971

The life expectancy of head injured men with and without epilepsy. **Zentralbl Neurochir 32**:3-9, 1971 (with Leuchs, Lechtape-Gruter, Caveness, and Kretschman)

The pathological findings in fatal craniospinal injuries. **J Neurosurg 34**:603-613, 1971 (with Davis, Bohlman, Fisher, and Robinson)

The value of electroencephalography for the neurosurgeon. **EEG Clin Neurophysiol** IC-15-27, 1971

A prospective study of post-traumatic seizures in children. **Trans Am Neurol Assoc 97**:4, 1972 (with Black and Shepard)

Cerebral circulation and metabolism at deep hypothermia. **Neurology 22**:1065-1070, 1972 (with Tabaddor and Gardner)

Long term evaluation of the social and family adjustment to head injuries. **Scand J Rehabil Med 4**:5-8, 1972

Neurologic surgery today. **CMD**:799-805, 1972 (with Laws)

Prognostic value of cerebral blood flow (CBF) and cerebral metabolic rate of oxygen. (CMRO$_2$) in acute head trauma. **J Trauma 13**:1953-1955, 1972 (with Tabaddor, Bhushan, and Pevsner)

Summary for the International Symposium on Rehabilitation in Head Injury. **Scand J Rehabil Med 4**:154-156, 1972

The current status of epilepsy in some developing countries. **Epilepsia 13**:99-106, 1972

The libidinous temporal lobe. **Schweiz Arch Neurol Neurochir Psychiatr 111**:473-484, 1972

The technique of temporal lobectomy in psychomotor epilepsy and postoperative sexual changes. **J Neurosurg 5**:9-16, 1972 (Russ)

Carotid-cavernous fistula: a controlled embolus technique for occlusion of fistula with preservation of carotid blood flow. Technical note.

J Neurosurg 38:113-118, 1973 (with Black, Uematsu, and Perovic)

Central phosphenes in man: a report of three cases. **Neuropsychologia 11**:1-19, 1973 (with Chapanis, Uematsu, and Konigsmark)

Echoencephalography, a non-invasive diagnostic procedure of increasing value. **CMD**: 913-927, 1973 (with Uematsu)

Man and his temporal lobe. John Hughlings Jackson lecture. **Surg Neurol 1**:69-79, 1973

Optimal criteria for care of patients with stroke. **JAMA 226**:164-168, 1973 (Stroke Advisory Committee)

A method for the recording of the pulsations of the midline echo in cerebral death. **Johns Hopkins Med J 135**:383-390, 1974 (with Uematsu)

Book review of *The Victim is Always the Same*, by IS Cooper. **J Nerv Ment Dis**:71-72, 1974

Editorial: Guidelines for stroke. **Surg Neurol 2**: 108, 1974

Electrical stimulation of the cerebral visual system in man. **Confin Neurol**:113-124, 1974 (with Uematsu, Chapanis, and Gucer)

Experimental temporal lobe epilepsy. **Brain 97**: 423-446, 1974 (with Velasco and Velasco)

Letter: Guidelines for stroke care. **J Neurosurg 40**:413-414, 1974

Obituary. Percival Bailey, 1892-1973. **Surg Neurol 2**:85-86, 1974

Surgery for epilepsy. *Handbook of Clinical Neurology*, edited by PJ Vinken and GW Bruyn. **Epilepsies 15**:739-758, 1974

Thalamotomy for alleviation of intractable pain. **Confin Neurol 36**:88-96, 1974 (with Uematsu and Konigamark)

The brain team. **J Neurosurg Nurs 6**:49-57, 1974

Cerebral blood flow and brain metabolism as determinants of death, a review. **Johns Hopkins Med J**:107-115, 1975 (with Smith)

Cerebral death, in Tower DB (ed): **The Nervous System**. New York: Raven Press, 1975, Vol II, pp 75-87

Criteria of cerebral death. **Trans Am Neurol Assoc 100**:29-35, 1975 (with Molinari)

Current concepts of epilepsy. **Proc Natl Semin Epilepsy—Bangalore, India 6.7**:9, 1975

D.C. potentials of temporal lobe seizures in the monkey. **J Neurol 209**:199-215, 1975 (with Mayanagi)

Echoencephalography. **Med Trial Tech 21**: 445-465, 1975 (with Uematsu)

Epilepsy: a Canadian viewpoint, in Wada JA (ed): **Modern Perspectives in Epilepsy**. Montreal: Eden Press, 1975, pp 8-23

Long-term effects of temporal lobe lesions on

sexual behavior and aggressivity, in Fields W (ed): **Neural Bases of Violence and Aggression.** St Louis, Mo: WH Green, 1975, pp 392-400 (with Blumer)

Neurosurgical management of the epilepsies. Critique and perspectives. **Adv Neurol 8:** 333-350, 1975

Outcome of head trauma: age and post-traumatic seizures. **Ciba Foundation Symp 34:** 215-226, 1975 (with Black and Shepard)

Past, present and future of epilepsy. **Proc Natl Semin Epilepsy—Bangalore, India 10.1:5,** 1975

Surgical intervention in epilepsy. **Proc Natl Semin Epilepsy—Bangalore, India 8.1:3,** 1975

The localization of sex in the brain, in Zulch KJ, Creutzfeldt O, Galbraith GC (eds): **Cerebral Localization.** Berlin: Springer-Verlag, 1975, pp 184-199 (with Blumer)

The national seminar on epilepsy—a critique. **Proc Natl Semin Epilepsy—Bangalore, India 11.1:261-274, 1975**

The neural basis of sexual behaviour, in Benson F, Blumer D (eds): **Psychiatric Aspects of Neurological Disease.** New York: Grune and Stratton, 1975, Vol 11, pp 199-217

The neurological basis of sex. **Ann Indian Acad Med Sci 9:**152-167, 1975

The neurological basis of sex. Lakshmipathi Oration delivered at W.H.O. Seminar on Epilepsy—Bangalore, India, 1975

The neuropathological findings in irreversible coma. A critique of the "respirator." **J Neuropathol Exp Neurol 34:**295-323, 1975 (with Diamond and Moseley)

Experimental studies on temporal lobe epilepsy in the monkey. **Neurol Med Chir (Tokyo) 16:**255-263, 1976 (with Mayanagi)

Neurosurgical aspects of head pain, in Appenzeller O (ed): **Pathogenesis and Treatment of Headache.** New York,: Spectrum Publications, 1976, pp 146-158

Respirator brain. Report of a survey and review of current concepts. **Arch Pathol Lab Med 100:**61-64, 1976 (with Molinari and Moseley)

The neurological basis of sex. **Neurol India 24:** 1-13,1976

The neurosurgeon's responsibility for organ procurement. **J Neurosurg 44:**1-2, 1976

Intracranial pressure monitoring in neurosurgery, in Fleming DG, Ko WH (eds): **Indwelling and Implantable Pressure Transducers.**

Histological reactions to various conductive and dielectric films chronically implanted in the subdural space. **Med Biol Eng Comput 11:** 195-210, 1977 (with Loeb and Uematsu)

Long-term behavorial effects of temporal lobectomy for temporal lobe epilepsy. **McLean Hosp Bull:**85-103, 1977 (with Blumer)

Sedative drug surveys in coma. How reliable are they? **Postgrad Med 61:**105-109, 1977 (with Molinari)

The middle age of epilepsy, in Penry J (ed): **Epilepsy; Eighth International Symposium.** New York: Raven Press, 1977, pp 81-85

Ancillary studies in the diagnosis of brain death. **Ann NY Acad Sci 315:**228-240, 1978

Pathology of brain death. **Ann NY Acad Sci 315:**272-280, 1978

Pulsatile cerebral echo in diagnosis of brain death. **J Neurosurg 48:**866-875, 1978 (with Uematsu and Smith)

Absence of pulsatile midline-echo as determination of cerebral death. **Ultrasound Med Biol:** 251-256, 1979 (with Uematsu and Smith)

Advances in the determination of cerebral death. **Adv Neurol 22:**167-177, 1979

Clinical evaluation of long-term epidural monitoring of intracranial pressure. **Surg Neurol 12:**373-377, 1979 (with Gucer, Viernstein, and Chubbuck)

The nervous system. General considerations. **Pediatr Surg 3:**1549-1557, 1979 (with Long)

The prediction of post-traumatic epilepsy—a mathematical approach. **Arch Neurol 36:** 8-12, 1979 (with Feeney)

Book review of *Neurological Classics in Modern Translations,* edited by DA Rottenberg and FH Hochberg. **Bull Hist Med 54:**292-293, 1980

Continuous intracranial pressure recording in adult hydrocephalus. **Surg Neurol 13:** 323-328, 1980 (with Gucer and Vierstein)

The national survey of stroke. Clinical findings. **Stroke (Suppl 1) 12:**113-144, 1981 (with Robins et al)

Book review of *Metastatic Tumors of the Central Nervous System,* by K Takakura, K Sano, S Hojo, and A Hirano. **J Nerv Ment Dis 170:** 700-701, 1982

Classification of movement disorders, in Schaltenbrand G, Walker AE (eds): **Stereotaxy of the Human Brain.** Stuttgart: Georg Thieme Verlag, 1982, pp 503-509

Comments on "Chronic pain as a variant of depressive disease: the pain-prone disorder." **J Nerv Ment Dis 170:**424, 1982

Depth recording, in Schaltenbrand G, Walker AE (eds): **Stereotaxy of the Human Brain**. Stuttgart: Georg Thieme Verlag, 1982, pp 661-668 (with Uematsu, Niedermeyer, and MacDonald)

General principles of stereotaxic surgery for epilepsy, in Schaltenbrand G, Walker AE (eds): **Stereotaxy of the Human Brain**. Stuttgart: Georg Thieme Verlag, 1982, pp 645-652

Normal and pathological physiology of the thalamus, in Schaltenbrand G, Walker AE (eds): **Stereotaxy of the Human Brain**. Stuttgart: Georg Thieme Verlag, 1982, pp 181-217

Stereotaxic surgery for tremor, in Schaltenbrand G, Walker AE (eds): **Stereotaxy of the Human Brain**. Stuttgart: Georg Thieme Verlag, 1982, pp 515-521

Book review of *Neurobehavioral Consequences of Closed Head Injury*, by H Levin, A Benton, and R Grossman. **J Nerv Ment Dis 171:** 50-51, 1983

Book review of *The Thalamus and Midbrain of Man*, by RR Tasker et al. **J Nerv Ment Dis 171:**50-51, 1983

Current concepts of brain death. **J Neurosurg Nurs 15:**261-264, 1983

The past four decades—experimental epilepsy. **Res Publ Assoc Res Nerv Ment Dis 61:**1-17, 1983

Book review of *A Textbook of Epilepsy, 2nd edition*, edited by J Laidlaw and R Alan. **J Nerv Ment Dis 172:**114-115, 1984

Book review of *Brain Damage and Recovery*, by S Finger and DG Stein. **J Nerv Ment Dis 172:**117, 1984

Book review of *Hughlings Jackson on Psychiatry*, by K Dewhurst. **J Nerv Ment Dis 172:** 113-114, 1984

Book review of *Management of Pituitary Adenomas*, by ER Laws et al. **J Nerv Ment Dis 172:**114-115, 1984

Dead or alive. **J Nerv Ment Dis 172:**639-641, 1984 (editorial)

The electroencephalographic characteristics of the rhombencephalectomized cat. **EEG Clin Neurophysiol 57:**156-165, 1984 (with Hovda and Feeney)

Book review of *Dandy of Johns Hopkins*, by WL Fox. **Bull Hist Med 59:**559-560, 1985

Epidemiology of brain tumors: the national survey of intracranial neoplasms. **Neurology 35:** 219-226, 1985 (with Robins and Weinfeld)

George B. Udvarhelyi. **Surg Neurol 24:**361-363, 1985 (with Macksey)

Post-traumatic epilepsy. **Prog Clin Neurosci 2:** 91-99, 1985

Book review of *Epilepsy and the Corpus Callosum*, edited by AG Reeves. **J Nerv Ment Dis 174:** 636-638, 1986

Book review of *Surgery of the Mind*, by EA Turner. **J Nerv Ment Dis 174:**55-56, 1986

The neurological basis of amnesia. **Seara Med Neurocir 15:**89-97, 1986 (with Feeney)

The evolution of the World Federation of Neurosurgical Societies. **Acta Neurochir 94:** 99-102, 1988

As I saw it. **Appl Neurophysiol 51:**7-9, 1988

Brain death—an American viewpoint. **Neurosurg Rev (Suppl 1)12:**259-264, 1989

Post-traumatic epilepsy in World War II veterans. **Surg Neurol 32:**235-236, 1989

The fate of World War II veterans with post-traumatic seizures. **Arch Neurol 46:**23-26, 1989 (with Blumer)

Understanding of language, in Carbojal JR, Escobar A (eds): **Homenaje al Doctor y Profesor Manuel M. Velasco Suarez**. SA, Mexico: Editorial Progreso, 1989, pp 671-685 (with Feeney)

Long-term effects of severe penetrating head injury on psychosocial adjustment. **J Consult Clin Psychol 58:**531-537, 1990 (with Tellieer et al)

Congenital anomalies of the cerebellar vermis—the Dandy-Walker syndrome. **Adv Clin Neurosci 1:**1-11, 1991

The death of a brain. First Medico-Legal Argentinian Congress, 1991

Brain death—1992. First International Symposium on Brain Death, Havana, Cuba, 1992

Lapses of Memory. Memory Symposium, The Johns Hopkins University, 1992

Book review of *Neurosurgical Classics*, edited by RH Wilkins. **Bull Hist Med 67:**378-379, 1993

Book review of *Neurobehavioral Problems in Epilepsy*, by DB Smith et al. **Adv Neurol 55:** 496, 1991; **EEG Clin Neurophysiol:**1993

The falling sickness arises. **Surg Neurol 45:** 71-83, 1996

Index

Illustrations are indicated by an *f*, tables by a *t*.

Falret, 97
Fat emboli, 247
Fazio, 143
Fazio-Londe disease, 143
Feil, 210
Feré, 178
Fernel, 71, 171, 212
Fernsides, 187
Ferrara, 151
Ferrier, 92, *92f,* 93, 94, 97, 120, 161, 163, 250, 257, 272
Ferrier, 97
Fetishes, cranial, 8
Finkelnburg, 102
Fischer, 184
Fistula, cerebrospinal fluid, 170
Flechsig, 110, 127
Fleischer, 117
Flourens, 90–91, *90f,* 94, 119, 163, 235
Foerster, 107, 320
Foix, 111, 333
Fontana, 148, 149
Foramen, congenital atresia, 208–209, *209f*
Fourth cranial nerve, 196
Foville's inferior pontine syndrome, 331
France, 234–236, 276–279
Frapolli, 154, 242
Frazier, 269, *270f,* 272
Freud, 102
Friedreich, 141, 142, 282
Friedreich's ataxia, 143
Fries, 319
Fritsch, 91–92, 96, 182, 250, 278
Fröhlich, 259, 279
Frontal lobes, function, 95
Frothingham, 229
Fuchs, 337
Fuchs' sign, 331
Funk, 153
Fürbringer, 169
Fuster, 98

G

Galen, 48–57, 98, 108, 113, 117, 118, 125, 131, 134, 150, 160, 161, 163, 185, 203, 227, 326
  anatomy and physiology, knowledge of, 50–51, 53–55
  cerebellum, description of, 117

  cranial nerves, description of, 159
  epilepsy, description of, 52–53
  gladiators' wounds, treatment of, 48–49
  peripheral nerves, description of, 145
  spinal cord, description of, 51–52, 128
Gall, 89–90, 99–100, 105, 106, 109, 119, 322
Galvani, 148–149, 242
Gamper, 106
Gardner, 189, 213
Gaseous material, abnormal intracranial, 170
Gasperini, 337
Gaubius, 113
Gaupp, 136
Gay, 216
Gélineau, 184
Gelle, 339
Gengou, 225
Gerlach, von, 88
Germany, 239–241, 280–282
Gersdorff, 239
Gibbs, 98
Glazier, 229
Glisson, 146–147
Glossopharyngeal nerve, 163
Godlee, 257, 258, 272
Golgi, 88, 173, *173f,* 252, 256, 271
Goltz, 93–94
Gorman, 114
Gowers, 111, *111f,* 116, 133, 136, 140, 159, 160, 162, 164, 165, 178, 179, 183, 188, 213, 220, 225, 251, 261, 275, 280, 288
  cerebral aneurysm, incidence, report of, 187–188, *188t*
  sleep disorders, description of, 185
Gradenigo-Lennois syndrome, 331
Graefe, von, 140, 196, 249, 337
Graham, 180
Graña, 7, 9–10
Gratiolet, 95
Greek medicine, 21–49
  Alexandrian school, 37–41
    nervous system, concept of, 39–40, *39f*
    physiology, knowledge of, 39–40
    clinics, 23–24
  Hippocratic school, 24–37
    epilepsy, concept of, 27–33
    head wounds, treatment of, 33–34
    nervous system, concept of, 24–26
    neurological disorders
      concept of, 27–32
      description of, 26